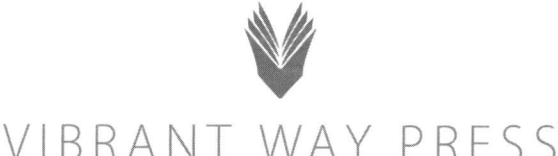

THE THYROID CURE

The Functional Mind-Body Approach to Reversing Your Autoimmune Condition and Reclaiming Your Health!

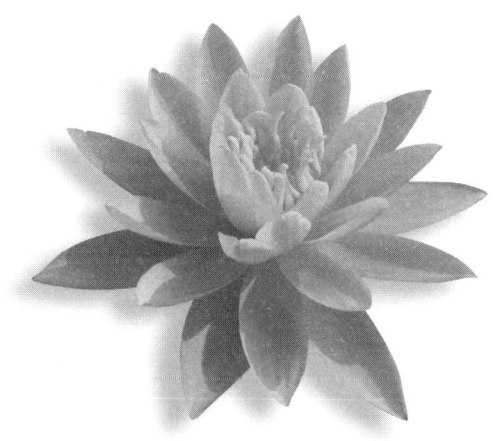

Michelle Corey

VIBRANT WAY PRESS

The Thyroid Cure Copyright © 2014

All rights reserved. No part of this book may be used or reproduced in any manner whatsoever without written permission except in the case of brief quotations embedded in critical articles and reviews.

Printed in the United States of America
Published by
Vibrant Way Press, Inc.
P.O. Box 3413
Taos, NM 87571
ISBN 978-1-939376-00-8
Library of Congress Control Number: 2014936145

Cover art designed by Herb Bigalow
Illustrations by Caroline DeVita • www.carolinedevita.com

*This book is dedicated to Andrew.
Thank you for believing in me and for being
my greatest supporter.*

*This book is also dedicated to the millions
of autoimmune sufferers on the planet. May you
find this information and heal your life.*

Table of Contents

Disclaimer 1
To the Reader 2
Who is This Book For? 3
Prologue: My Story 5
Introduction 31

PART ONE: AWARENESS
The Autoimmune Condition

Chapter 1: Take Charge of Your Health
Become Empowered: The Five Stages of Empowerment in Health 37
Stage One: Get Passionate About Getting Better 40
Stage Two: Step Out of the Victim Role and Take Responsibility 42
Stage Three: Take Action by Challenging the System 44
Stage Four: Become Your Own Health Advocate 50
Stage Five: Make the Necessary Lifestyle Adjustments to Heal! 55

Chapter 2: Consider the Real Cost of Wellness
The Limitations of Health Insurance 57
Fee-for-Service Providers 60
Working Within Your Health Plan 61
Make Your Health a Top Priority 63

Chapter 3: Explore Different Medical Approaches
Western / Conventional / Orthodox / Medicine 65
Alternative Medicine 68
Complementary and Alternative Medicine (CAM) 68
Traditional Medicine 70
Integrative/Holistic and Functional Medicine 71
The Ingredients of a Successful Model of Healing 74
Finding a Practitioner 75

Chapter 4: Discover Your Thyroid
How a Healthy Thyroid Functions 79
Why We Need Optimal Thyroid Hormone Levels..................................... 81

Chapter 5: Understand Your Immune System
Immune System Basics 85
Immunity... 86
The Barriers 86
The GI Tract Illustrated 88
The Liver 90
The Cells of the Immune System.. 91
The Organs 95
The Immune Response Illustrated 96

Chapter 6: Reframe the Autoimmune Process
Is the Autoimmune Process a Condition or a Disease?.............................. 99
Stress and the Autoimmune Process.. 100
The Th1 Versus Th2 Dominance Debate 102
Your Genes Are Not Your Destiny!... 105

Chapter 7: Autoimmune Thyroid Conditions
Graves' (Thyrotoxicosis): Hyperthyroidism... 107
How is Graves' Diagnosed? 108
What is the Conventional Treatment of Graves'? 111
Hashimoto's Thyroiditis 113
How is Hashimoto's Thyroiditis Diagnosed?... 113
What is the Conventional Treatment of Hashimoto's Thyroiditis? 117

Chapter 8: Become Conscious of Stress and Body Burden
The Cause of Autoimmune Conditions:
Chronic Stress in All Its Forms! 119
Our Cup Runneth Over…But Not in a Good Way!............................... 119
Understanding the Physiology of Stress 121

Chapter 9: Uncover the "Splinters" in Your Autoimmunity
The Many Forms of Stress 126

Splinter #1: Chronic Emotional Stress 127
Splinter #2: Unhealthy Coping Patterns 131
Splinter #3: Poor Nutrition 133
Splinter #4: Gastrointestinal (GI) Stress 147
Splinter #5: Adrenal Burnout 155
Splinter #6: Hormonal Stress... 158
Splinter #7: Inflammatory and Infectious Stress 164
Splinter #8: Toxic Stress... 173

Chapter 10: Perform Your Personal Assessments
Emotional Stress Assessment 190
GI Stress Assessment 192
Adrenal Stress Assessment... 194
Infectious Stress Assessment 195
Inflammatory Stress Assessment 197
Toxic Stress Assessment 198
Hormonal Stress Assessment 201

PART TWO: TRANSFORMATION
The Thyroid Cure Repair Program

Chapter 11: Take the Splinters Out!
Identify and Heal the Underlying Causes of Autoimmunity 207

Chapter 12: Test—Don't Guess!
Thyroid Tests.. 209
The Importance of Testing for Antibodies...................................... 210
Other Important Tests for Autoimmunity 211

Chapter 13: The First Steps Toward Reversing your Autoimmune Thyroid Condition
What to Do First If You Are Hypothyroid Due to Hashimoto's............. 215
Choosing a Thyroid Medication 217
Why You May Need Thyroid Replacement Hormones to Get Better...... 219
If You Have Symptoms of Adrenal Fatigue 221

Should You Take High Potency Iodine? 222
Will You Need Thyroid Hormones for Life? 225
What to Do First If You Are Hyperthyroid Due to
Graves' or Hashimoto's 227
Graves' and the Stress Connection 228
Things You Can Do to Start Feeling Better Fast! 228
Thyroid Repair Program at a Glance 229

Chapter 14: Optimize Your Nutrition
The Thyroid Cure Mind-Body Nutrition Program 233
Discover Your Unique Mind-Body Type:
Sensitivity Discovery Program 238
Phase I: *Eating for Your Good Genes* 242
Phase I: *Eating for Your Good Genes* Shopping List 252
Phase II: Sensitivity Discovery 261
Phase III: Vibrant for Life! 269
When You May Need a Health Practitioner 271

Chapter 15: Reduce Stress
Support Your Adrenals 273
Just Breathe! 279
Restorative Sleep 280
Honoring Your Unique Mind-Body Type 285
Mindfulness; Being Present in the Moment 287
Exercise 289
Reconnect with Nature 291
Manage Your Life 291
Cultivate Joy 292
When nothing seems to help 293

Chapter 16: Heal Your Gut
The Gut is Your Immune System's Neighborhood 295
What You can Do on Your Own to Heal Your GI 298
Remove Your GI Splinters! 298
Replace What's Missing! 299

Reinoculate with "Good Bugs" 300
Repair Your Inner Tube! 301
Supplement Suggestions to Heal Your Gut 302
Heartburn Acid Reflux and GERD 304
Self-Healing Program for GERD... 305
When You Need a Practitioner – *Test, Don't Guess!*................................ 309
Functional Testing for GI Splinters... 311

Chapter 17: Restore Your Liver
Your Liver's Key Functions 314
Detoxification and Your Unique Mind-Body Type 317
Methylation 317
Methylation and Glutathione... 320
What You Can Do on Your Own 321
Restore Your Liver 321
Improve Your Methylation 326
Boost Your Glutathione.. 327
When You May Need a Practitioner –*Test, Don't Guess!*........................ 330
Functional Testing for Toxic Splinters 333

Chapter 18: Clear Infections
Infections and Autoimmunity 335
What You Can Do on Your Own 339
Supplements to Fight Infections and Boost Immunity........................... 346
When You Need a Health Practitioner, *Test, Don't Guess!*...................... 347
Functional Testing for Infections 348

Chapter 19: Detox Your Life
Clean Body—Revamp Your Personal Care Products 351
Clean Home.. 352
Drink Clean Water!... 354
Breathe Fresh Air—Not Chemicals!.. 355
Clean Green! 356
Clean Up Electromagnetic Fields in Your Home!................................... 357
Become a Mold Warrior! 359
Living with Pets.. 360

Clean Garden and Garage 362
Clean Office 364
Safe Detox Treatments 365
Conclusion 369

Chapter 20: Putting It All Together 370

PART THREE:
The Mind-Body Connection

Connecting Emotions and Your Health 375
Toxic Shame: The Cycle of Self Loathing 385
Transforming Shame 391
Anger and Hostility 392
Forgiveness 396
Blame vs. Responsibility 397
Is the Imbalance in Your Body or Your Mind? 399
Take Back Your Power and Express Yourself 406
Conclusion 406

PART FOUR:
Interviews with Doctors Who are Curing
Autoimmune Conditions

C. E. Gant, M.D. 411
Susan Blum, M.D. 423
Alexander Haskell, N.D. 435
Conclusion 446
Gratitude 449
Appendix I: Recommended Supplements 452
Appendix II: Recommended Reading and Resources 456
Appendix III: Finding Your ACE Score 466
Endnotes 468
Index 490

Disclaimer

The information in this book is not intended to diagnose, treat, or cure any disease. This book does not offer a cure from the outside. Instead, it arms you with the knowledge to bring the core systems of your body back into balance so that you can cure yourself. This book is not a substitute for quality health care provided by a licensed and knowledgeable health care practitioner. In fact, the author encourages you to review the material in this book with your physician. The author and publisher are not engaged in rendering medical, psychological or any other kind of personal professional services in this book. The author and publisher specifically disclaim all responsibility for any injury, damage or loss that the reader may incur as a consequence of following the guidelines detailed in this book. Before making any decisions based upon the information and recommendations found in this book, you should first check with your own physician.

This book is designed to educate the reader in a "new way of thinking" about autoimmune conditions, and the underlying triggers of autoimmunity. Research about this subject is ongoing and subject to conflicting interpretations. While every effort has been made to provide accurate information, the author and publisher cannot be held responsible for any errors or omissions.

To protect the identities of the people whose stories appear in this book, we have changed names and in some cases created composites.

To the Reader

I touch on many topics in this book, and each section could be a book of its own. I have chosen to include both the physical and emotional aspects of my journey because I believe both are crucial to the healing process.

I firmly believe that if someone with an autoimmune condition, having uncovered the physiological causes of her (or his) condition, were to follow all the physical healing protocols but fail to address the underlying emotional issues, the old emotional patterns would eventually drag her (or him) back to an autoimmune state. Conversely, if someone were to address only the emotional aspects without healing the physical body, the likelihood of a complete recovery would be slim.

Some readers with a medical or scientific background may feel that I have included too much "New Age fluff." Some general readers may feel I've included too much science. It is my hope that by embracing both science and spirit within the context of healing, we can put an end to the epidemic of "incurable" disease and enjoy vibrant health.

Who is This Book For?

"To know the road ahead, ask those coming back."
– Chinese Proverb

The focus of this book is to address thyroid dysfunction caused by the autoimmune conditions known as Graves' disease and Hashimoto's thyroiditis. In Western countries the most common cause of hypothyroidism is Hashimoto's thyroiditis.[1]

Many people diagnosed with hypothyroidism are never told why their thyroid is underactive and can suffer for years with a progressive condition that will eventually destroy their thyroid gland. This book will help you to determine whether your thyroid condition is autoimmune in nature and then help you reverse the autoimmune process.

When I say, "reverse the autoimmune process," what I mean is "cure" your autoimmune thyroid condition. I have done this with myself and I have witnessed hundreds of other people do the same. I believe, with help, you can cure yourself. This book will give you the guidance to begin your journey to health.

While this book addresses autoimmune thyroid conditions, the practical healing protocols will greatly benefit anyone with any autoimmune condition. Current medical research shows that all autoimmune conditions are essentially the same process occurring in the body: the inflamed immune system, under the strain of continual triggers, mistakes healthy tissue as foreign and begins to destroy it. The only difference between various autoimmune conditions is which organ is being attacked. With lupus, it can be the skin, the liver, the joints, etc. With type I diabetes, it's the pancreas; with multiple sclerosis it is the brain and spinal cord; and with ulcerative colitis it is the large intestine and rectum.

In the case of Hashimoto's and Graves', the thyroid is the obvious target, but it's important to note that it's rarely just the thyroid being affected, and that there are typically many conditions happening at the same time.

In this book, you will find a series of steps anyone can take to find the underlying cause of their autoimmune disorder, as well as ways to treat the causes and begin to heal. I believe that the guidelines outlined in this book will help you to find your own path to reversing all of your autoimmune thyroid symptoms and bring your body back into balance.

For those of you who are like me and need to hear it from a medical doctor, I've included a section entitled, "Interviews with Doctors Who Are Curing Autoimmune Conditions." Hopefully their interviews will inspire you and give you even more hope that you can heal. Hope is, after all, one of the most important aspects of healing!

It is my desire that this book will offer a new way of thinking about all autoimmune disease, its causes, and the steps you can take to reverse it.

If you have been sick for a long time…

For those of you who have suffered with an autoimmune condition for years and have experienced significant tissue damage, this book may help you to stop the progression of your condition, but it makes no promises for regenerating what may have been lost during the course of your illness. But there is always hope, so please don't give up, because you can still optimize what you have and feel better!

Prologue

"Love is what we were born with. Fear is what we learned here."
— MARIANNE WILLIAMSON

If you opened this book, chances are that you or someone you love has been diagnosed with an autoimmune thyroid condition and are not getting satisfactory answers from conventional medicine. I understand your pain and confusion because I've been there myself.

As you read my story you may feel overwhelmed by the information and what I went through to get better. I want to ease your mind and let you know that your path will be much easier. I have done the research and spent the time creating a program that essentially streamlines the road to recovery. I have done the work so that you don't have to. I share my journey so that you can get a picture of how I arrived at my conclusions and to illustrate that I know how challenging it is to be an autoimmune sufferer.

In March of 2004, just a few weeks after my 36th birthday, I was diagnosed with Hashimoto's thyroiditis. I didn't know it at the time, but I also had positive autoantibodies indicating early signs of lupus. I was 35 pounds overweight despite rigorous daily cardio workouts, hot yoga and a strict 1500-calorie-per-day organic, vegetarian diet. My face looked like someone had blown it up with a bicycle pump, and I had an unsightly freckle mustache due to a condition called melasma. It wasn't pretty. Other symptoms included chronic sinusitis; foggy thinking; mood swings; carbohydrate and alcohol cravings; relentless hay fever all year long; skin rashes all over my body and on the palms of my hands and feet; swollen, aching joints and insomnia. I was living in Santa Cruz and buckling under the pressure of running my own marketing firm and enduring an unhappy, codependent marriage.

The diagnosis was quite accidental. At the time, my husband had been having strange gastrointestinal (GI) symptoms that left our small beach town doctors stumped. I had been poring over alternative healing books for years, partly out of curiosity and partly to find an answer to my own chronic symptoms. I had just read a book by a well-known alternative physician in the Bay Area. I was convinced that this doctor would be able to figure out what was happening with my husband's digestive system.

I barely even thought of making an appointment for myself. After years of ignoring my own needs and intuition and putting others first, I was so stuck in a victim/martyr role that I all but ignored my own symptoms—even though they were more severe than my husband's. I was used to putting the needs of others before my own and then silently (and sometimes, not so silently) resenting them. Like many people with chronic illness, I frequently neglected my body's many cries for help. I had yet to learn the art of self-love, and was not prepared to take full responsibility for my physical or emotional health.

So, instead of addressing what was happening in my body, I convinced my husband to see an integrative medical doctor, who I'll call Dr. Wake Up, about his GI symptoms. We made an appointment and drove north.

As we sat in Dr. Wake Up's office discussing my husband's travels around Southeast Asia, he turned to me and said,

"How are you feeling?"

Surprised that the focus was now on me, I blurted out, "Lousy, but my doctor thinks I'm just depressed."

"What do YOU think is wrong?" he asked in a genuinely inquisitive tone.

I was taken back by the question—I couldn't believe he was asking me for my opinion. I said, "I think I have a chronic Candida infection and it's ruining my health, but all the doctors I've seen say that's impossible."

"Okay, let's run some tests for that and check your thyroid, too."

I felt a combination of surprise and relief, because this doctor was actually listening to me. I had been to so many doctors over the years, both alternative and conventional, who completely ignored my intuition about my own health. I felt hopeful, but I didn't have any expectations. My attitude toward my health tended to be defeatist and self-pitying: Woe is me—nobody will ever figure out what's wrong with me!

A few weeks later, on the day of my diagnosis, I sat in my doctor's private office waiting for the results of the blood work I had taken. As he looked over my labs, he raised one eyebrow and said,

"Well, it looks like you do have a Candida infection—and you have Hashimoto's thyroiditis, which is a form of autoimmune disease. Unfortunately, there is no cure for Hashimoto's, and your thyroid gland will eventually be destroyed by your immune system. The only treatment we can offer you is thyroid replacement hormones, which you will have to take indefinitely."

I was shocked, and almost too stunned to speak (which takes a lot for me).

"Indefinitely? You mean for the rest of my life?"

"Exactly."

"Will I feel better?"

"Maybe," he replied in a vague, noncommittal tone. Then he asked me a question that surprised me into another moment or two of speechlessness: "How do you think you got this disease?"

"What? Why is he asking me?" I thought, "Isn't it the doctor's job to figure out where diseases come from?"

"I don't know, I mean… How am I supposed to answer that?"

"I think you have a pretty good idea. Why don't you go home and think about it? For now, we'll start you on a low dose of Synthroid and see how you do."

I felt stunned and devastated as I walked out of the doctor's office and got in my car. After years of feeling sick, tired and fat, I finally find out what's wrong with me, there is no cure, and my doctor is insinuating that it's my fault!

On the drive back to Santa Cruz, I went through a range of emotions from sadness to feeling like a victim to rage. How could this doctor just throw a diagnosis at me and send me home with a prescription that might not even make me feel better? An incurable disease for the rest of my life? How could this be happening to me? What did I do to deserve this? I felt helpless and victimized. I felt like running from everything—my life, my job, my husband, and this illness. "How is this my life?" I thought. It's not fair!

What I wouldn't find out until years later was that at the same time, the doctor had run a test that would have revealed a lot about my condition and possible future outcomes, but he never mentioned it to me. The test is called an antinuclear antibodies test (ANA), which documented the presence of antibodies to my own tissues. Positive ANA's are found in many people with chronic inflammation and can indicate a more serious stage of autoimmunity. I know now that my results, along with my symptoms, indicated the beginning of a condition called lupus.

Lupus, like Hashimoto's, is an autoimmune condition but can be life threatening. It can cause inflammation in the joints, the skin, the kidneys, the blood cells, brain, heart and lungs. Lupus is difficult to diagnose until it's full-blown and causing serious symptoms. In fact, many people can suffer with strange symptoms for years before they get a definitive diagnosis.

There are a few reasons why Dr. Wake Up may not have mentioned it. Since many people with Hashimoto's also have positive ANA's and my symptoms weren't putting me in the hospital, he may have decided to "wait and watch" and see if I got worse. He may have been worried that the suggestion of a diagnosis as serious as lupus would throw me into an unnecessary tailspin that would take me down the allopathic road to an even worse condition. He may have intuited that his question, "How do you think you got this?" would stick in my mind.

In the weeks and months that followed, I was physically miserable and emotionally drained. As a practice management and marketing consultant to doctors, I had access to some of the best medical and alternative care in the country. Desperate, I went from specialist to specialist hoping that someone would be able to "cure" me. While I received differing opinions on how to manage the symptoms of my condition, there were two things everyone agreed on:

1. No one knows what causes autoimmune thyroid disease.
2. There is no cure.

I became depressed. I felt sorry for myself. I felt betrayed by my own body. I lost faith in my doctors and the medical system. I even lost faith in God.

I had always assumed that doctors were the experts, the authorities, and only foolish people tried to evade their advice. At least this is what I believed, until I received a diagnosis of a "deadly" and "incurable" disease.

But once I got this incurable diagnosis, a rebellious part of me asked, "Who says this is incurable? What do they mean when they say, 'We don't understand the mechanism of this illness?'" and, most significantly, "If they can't answer these questions, why should I put my health in their hands?"

When I wasn't caught in self-pity or feelings of angry rebellion against medical authority, the surprising question the doctor asked me, "How do you think you got this?" kept popping into my mind.

Deep down, I was unhappy in my work and my marriage. I worked long hours and drank too much coffee and wine. I was chronically depressed and unsatisfied and had lost much of my enthusiasm for life. I did sometimes worry that the stress of it all was making me sick, but I was too scared to rock the boat. After all, my life at the time was a huge improvement over my childhood—at least that's what I kept telling myself. But I couldn't stop the doctor's question from coming up and pestering me for an answer.

One day, I decided to take a three-day weekend alone. I drove south to the little beach town of Cambria and rented a small hotel room. My intention was to stay there and write in my journal until I found the answer to why I was sick. I decided to retrace my whole life—every physical symptom I could ever remember, everything that happened to me that could possibly be the cause. I found myself filling page after page. I was writing so fast that my fingers began to hurt. What I found was that there were possible causes from the earliest age.

The details are not important for this book, but in short, I was the survivor of repeated emotional, physical and sexual abuse throughout my early years. This journaling exercise allowed me to see how those traumas, and my story about them, had influenced literally every area of my life… including my health.

At the end of the three-day weekend, I had filled up an entire journal with things that could be related to my illness. Since all the books I had read said that stress was a major factor in illness, every trauma I had ever experienced was relevant. On the evening of the third day, I looked at myself in the bathroom mirror and asked the doctor's question one more time:

"How do you think you got this?"

I heard a small, quiet voice in my head supply the answer in just three words:

My whole life.

The implication of the answer left me trembling. If I were to heal, I would have to change my life on every level.

Lessons from the Sandbox

If my whole life was the cause, I knew a pill would not be the solution. I decided to see a psychotherapist I'll call the Sandbox Lady. The Sandbox Lady was an overly empathetic, thin, mousy woman with glasses, who had an approach I found frustrating and disappointing. At the start of every session, she would ask me to review, in infinite, graphic detail, another part of my childhood abuse. When I explained to her that I had spent several years in therapy in my twenties dealing with the past, she said that it was clear that I had not processed everything and needed to do more work. Before I even opened my mouth, she would pass me a box of tissues as if encouraging me to cry. As I recounted the episodes, I felt more angry than tearful. But the Sandbox Lady, who had explained at our first meeting that she had been abused too, was always ready to do my crying for me. As soon as I started sharing an episode, and sometimes continuing throughout the entire appointment, her eyes would well up with tears. I began to feel that I was paying her for the chance to be the host of a pity party that was being thrown for her benefit, not mine. My stories seemed to be the background music for her own memories and self-pity. She never offered a word of advice, interpretation or comment of any sort. The only definite thing I got from her was a prescription for Valium.

Right next to the couch I sat on during our sessions was a sandbox with little figurines. In the midst of one session, I broke off her questioning and asked,

"Do you think maybe we could work with the sandbox today?"

She gave me an astonished look, as if I were a first-year nursing student who had just asked if I could give brain surgery a try.

"Oh my goodness!" she replied in an incredulous tone. "You're not even close to being ready for the sandbox!" I found her answer so absurd that I couldn't help but laugh out loud.

"Well, how long do you think it'll take before I am ready?"

"Oh my, I have no idea. Processing these sorts of memories takes a very long time, and the sandbox is an advanced therapy."

I instantly envisioned a decade of weekly pity parties with tissues and Valium in place of tea and crumpets. I didn't have a decade to spend before graduating to the sandbox—and so I decided to stop working with her.

I did, however, learn a very valuable lesson from the Sandbox Lady that has great relevance for everyone reading this book.

> **What You Need to Know:**
> You have the right and the duty to evaluate the quality of care you are getting from a therapist or health care professional of any kind. If you don't feel you are being helped, find someone else!

The realization of this principle, invaluable as it is, wasn't all I had gotten from the Sandbox Lady. The sessions I spent with her resulted in my getting fed up with my "story" and the dramas of the past. She also caused me to become permanently exasperated with self-pity. My days of tearfully gazing into the rearview mirror were over. To heal myself, I had to look at where my life was now and then take actions to keep moving forward.

A Very Deep Adjustment

One day, during the time I was still working with the Sandbox Lady, I was feeling really lousy and at the end of my rope emotionally. A large part of this was the downward spiral of my marriage. I called my mother and said, "I just don't know if I can take this—I can't stay in this marriage anymore!" My mother was silent for a moment, and then, as if looking into a crystal ball, she said in a somber tone,

"If you choose to stay in this marriage, it will make you sick, tired and old."

My mother knew firsthand how an unevenly yoked marriage can drain both partners, so I knew she was talking about herself. I also knew she was looking into my future. The clarity in her voice sent chills down my spine, because I knew she was right.

Then one morning, about a week or so after my final session with the Sandbox Lady, I woke up feeling foggy and exhausted. I staggered to the bathroom and found that my mother's words were running through my head: "Sick, tired and old. Sick, tired and old." I looked in the mirror—and I really looked sick, tired and old. I felt desperate. It was a real "dark night of the soul." I went back into my bedroom and I curled up in a ball on the floor and totally broke down. I found myself praying for the first time in years. I REALLY prayed. "I give up!" I cried. "I'm so tired of fighting. I can't live like this anymore. I can't do this alone. I need help. God, I really need your help! I don't know how to do this alone. Please help me!"

And sure enough, it happened. Later that day, while I was working with my chiropractor, I experienced nothing short of a miracle.

I had been seeing a network chiropractor, Dr. Ian Chambers, and the work that I had been doing with him was pretty profound. It involved somatic integration exercises where you breathe into different parts of your body. This work helped me get in touch with my physical body. I hadn't realized it before, but my consciousness had been floating around and above me instead of being grounded inside my body, which is very common for someone who has been sexually abused. I wasn't in my body, so it was very easy when I was in pain to push myself through the day because I was so divorced from what was happening physically. From the neck up, I was "in," but from the neck down, I wasn't.

What was so remarkable about the work I was doing with Dr. Chambers is that it allowed me to drop into my body. What I noticed right away, within the first month, was that I was more aware of physical sensations and of how my emotional state was affecting my physiology. I could feel things in my stomach that I hadn't felt before. I was making a crucial connection between my emotional state and my physical state. It was rewarding, but at the same time it was a bit scary.

I remember that on that morning, right after I prayed, work seemed to go painfully slow. I felt heavy, and it took an effort of supreme will just to make a few phone calls and do paperwork. It felt like I was frozen in time, like a fly caught in amber or an unlucky space explorer stuck in some sort of time warp. Psychiatrist Carl Jung once described this state as one where, "The life giving rhythm of the aeons becomes the dread ticking of the clock." It felt like the only thing I had to look forward to was the hour-long chiropractor appointment I had scheduled at the end of the workday.

Dr. Chambers seemed to take in my exhausted and dispirited condition with a single glance and asked me to come into the treatment room. I lay down on the table and we began the somatic breathing exercise. I'm not sure how long I was doing it, but suddenly there was this incredible release. It felt like heavy iron plates that had been constricting my chest all my life were falling off. The feeling is almost impossible to convey in words, because it has so many layers or dimensions that all unfolded at once. It felt like space opening up and sunlight breaking through heavy cloud cover. All the colors in the room became so vivid, and I felt a deep love for everything, for every part of my life, even the worst parts, and there was this sense of a deep and everlasting meaningfulness to everything—even to the little things. In my ecstasy, I wept.

As I left the appointment, I was struck with this incredible sensation that I was connected to everything and everyone. I didn't feel alone anymore. I felt a depth of love that I had never experienced before. I wanted to bring the love I felt back to my husband. I wanted to heal our broken relationship. But the feeling had humbled me, too. I knew that despite the great love I felt, we couldn't do it alone. We needed help, a counselor who had great skill in putting broken marriages back together.

My prayers had been answered with a spiritual epiphany that day. One of the benefits, right off the bat, was a sense of empowerment. I felt more empowered than I had ever felt, and it was coming from a very grounded place. I was finally in my body. *I'm here,* I thought. *I'm experiencing this experience of life right now.*

> **What You Need to Know:**
> Be ready to accept help from unexpected people and in unexpected ways during your healing journey. Healing is a process that is often driven by intuition and serendipity, as well as by reason, analysis, research and treatment protocols.

What Can Be Healed, and What Must Pass Away

At the end of this life-changing session, I asked Dr. Chambers if there was anyone he could recommend to counsel my husband and me. He went to the front desk of his reception room and came back with two business cards.

"There are these two wonderful life coach women, Grace Caitlin and Diana Chapman, who work together. We've worked with them in our marriage, and both my wife and I highly recommend them."

It took me a week's worth of convincing and cajoling to get my husband to agree to a session. I told him that I thought we really needed the help, but he was very opposed to any kind of counseling. He didn't like the idea of opening up to strangers.

He said, "I don't trust these people. What are they going to do, and how are they going to help us? I don't buy it. Besides, you're the crazy one. You're the one who needs counseling." I had to practically beg him to agree to a one-hour session.

The session occurred in the home of one of these two vibrant women. They were into acting things out…playful stuff. They wanted us to move around with our bodies. My husband and I were both kind of taken aback by that. At that time of my life, for me to be able to dramatize things through spontaneous movement required medication, or some strong drinks at the very least. I just couldn't feel that uninhibited, cold sober on a Tuesday afternoon. They drew an imaginary triangle on the floor of their living room and then put big yellow flash cards at the three corners of the triangle labeled, "Victim," "Villain," and "Hero." We were asked to stand on a particular point and play out each of these roles as we did in our marriage. Needless to say, this didn't work for my husband. He acted like he had been taken captive by a particularly embarrassing Nickelodeon reality show.

At first, it felt like the exercise was a spectacular failure, but in the midst of it—as I stood on the Victim card and my husband reluctantly slouched on the Hero card—I could suddenly see how we both danced between all three archetypal roles in our marriage. We were stuck in a codependent triangle of shaming, blaming and rescuing one another. Somehow, the exercise had captured the essence, not only of our marriage, but also of all of my relationships!

After a short while, my husband was over it, so we left. Later that night, curious about his feelings, I started to ask, "So what did you think of…" but he cut me off.

"That was the most ridiculous thing I have ever seen in my life. Those people are crazy. They're kooks, and I have no intention of ever going back to see them again, or anyone like them."

"Okay, we don't have to ever go back to those women, but are you willing to meet me half way and work on this relationship?"

"No. I'm tired. I don't want to work on a relationship. A relationship shouldn't be this hard."

That was exactly what I didn't want, but needed, to hear. My husband couldn't have stated his position more clearly. He was not interested in meeting me halfway or doing the work it was going to take to repair our relationship. We had a lot of struggles—financial, emotional and sexual—but I never gave up hoping and trying until that night. The exercise and my husband's own words were like a high-contrast X-ray of our marriage. There was no mistaking the fracture. It was like another incurable diagnosis, but this was not one I could find my way around. I know now that neither one of us was ready to commit. But at the time, I felt abandoned, devastated and scared. I didn't know what I was going to do. My career was devoid of meaning and fulfillment. I was already battling an incurable medical diagnosis, and now I had to face the grim reality that my marriage was terminal. The only thing I knew for sure was that everything would have to change, but I didn't even know where to begin.

> **What You Need to Know:**
> Healing is impossible without willing, committed participants. What doesn't want to be healed has to be allowed to pass away.

Taking Control—From Catastrophe to Conviction

Nine months after my diagnosis, I knew that my life would require massive changes, and that half measures would not suffice. So I did what any smart woman does. I got a divorce, I quit my business and I moved a block away from my mother to a cute little beach cottage in Oxnard, California. I took a look at my life and realized that almost nothing was working the way I needed it to—so I changed everything at once.

It might sound like I'm saying I threw in the towel, but the feeling was different. It was a feeling of surrender. I thought, *I don't know what I'm doing, but whatever I have been doing isn't working, so I'm going to try something else.*

Even though I was alone, and my career and my husband were gone, there was a sense of new possibilities in the air. I began to dream again and felt enthusiastic about my future. They say there are no do-overs in life, but this felt pretty close.

I'm not in any way suggesting that individuals who are diagnosed with a chronic illness quit their jobs or divorce their spouses. Every healing journey is different. For some people, a beloved spouse or enjoyable job may be a key source of support or a major catalyst of change for the better. But for me, I felt like I had no choice, because the life I had created was a lie.

I was living alone by the beach and feeling happier due to the new possibilities in my life, but I still couldn't lose a pound, despite taking two thyroid medications (Synthroid and Cytomel), running for 45 minutes on the beach every morning and eating less than 1,500 vegetarian calories a day. I still had terrible night sweats, rashes and crying spells, my eyebrows were half gone, and I could have woven a rug with all the hair that was falling out of my head. I was starting to feel like independence was somewhere on the horizon, but feeling truly at peace with my body and beautiful in my own skin was still a long way off.

After a few months off I decided to work on an Internet start-up company with my brother, and went back into the "comfortable," stressed-out mode I was used to. The new project had me sleeping an average of six or seven hours a night, waking up, commuting an hour each way to the office, drinking a lot of caffeine, and then coming home and drinking 2-3 glasses of wine to fall asleep. I see now that I was addicted to adrenal hormones and found it impossible to rest and stay still.

Then my mother suggested I see an OB/GYN who was learning about something called functional medicine. My mother had read a book called *The Schwartzbein Principle* by Dr. Diana Schwartzbein, an endocrinologist from Santa Barbara, who had cured her own chronic fatigue. This particular OB/GYN (who I'll call Dr. Edgy) had gone through Dr. Schwartzbein's training, so I made an appointment with her.

I showed Dr. Edgy all my labs and presented her with the diagnosis of Candidiasis and Hashimoto's. I explained that I had tried different combinations of thyroid medication but none had made a real impact. I still had the weight gain and the night sweats and all my other symptoms. I also told her that I was recently divorced and that although it was a good thing, I was still very emotional.

After reviewing my lab work Dr. Edgy said, "You need to be taking at least 3000 mg a day of omega-3s, some DHEA and we need to get you on a compounded T3/T4 thyroid medication."

Like Dr. Wake Up, she had all my labs, but never said anything about the positive ANA results.

Then she said, "I want to get you on a medication for depression." All the hairs on the back of my neck went up. Literally. I didn't want to do that. She explained that she felt that I had a condition called polycystic ovarian syndrome (PCOS) and that an antidepressant was in order. My response was, "I'm not crazy—I'm going through major life changes! And besides, what does depression medication do for cystic ovaries?"

My comment deeply offended her. "I'm on an antidepressant," she snapped, "and they're NOT just for crazy people!" Then she angrily explained that PCOS often causes depression, and that the medication would help. When I asked if it would help the cystic ovaries, she looked at me like I was nuts and said, "No!"

Dr. Edgy wrote me a prescription for the compounded T3/T4. This new thyroid replacement regimen was a game changer! I went from 160 lbs. to 148 lbs. within 6 weeks. Almost overnight, I experienced a huge improvement in all my symptoms. I was still overweight, but this was the first time the scale had budged in years. I should note that I made no changes to my diet whatsoever and we never discussed food sensitivities, gut health or detoxification. I now know that my gut and liver were a mess and wasn't converting T4 to T3 properly.

Dr. Edgy's description of the antidepressant she wanted to prescribe, Cymbalta, scared me. "We have to do some liver tests on you before you can take this because it's very hard on the liver," she told me. Given that I was a heavy wine drinker at the time, I put two and two together and realized that a drug that stressed the liver probably wouldn't be the best choice for me. I also had a hunch that my liver wasn't doing such a great job anyway, and wondered if it was contributing to my symptoms. I also knew that I wasn't ready to stop drinking wine and coffee. I figured that with the stress I was under, having just gone through a divorce, moving, and changing my career, there was no way I could deal with cutting out alcohol and caffeine. So, after researching the side effects of the drug, I decided not to fill the prescription.

When I started feeling better due to the T3/T4 hormone combination, I decided to research the work of Dr. Diane Schwartzbein, so I read her first book. I was beginning to connect the dots about the physical reasons I had developed my condition! I had suffered from chronic stress since I was a baby, and continued a pattern of stress into adulthood. Because I was on a low-calorie, low-protein, low fat, vegetarian diet that included a lot of wine, I had developed a condition called insulin sensitivity, and I had burned-out adrenal glands. The result was a damaged metabolism and an autoimmune condition.

I tried to follow Dr. Schwartzbein's recommendations for my condition, but her nutrition program made me gain ten pounds in two weeks and my symptoms got worse. She explained in her book that some people would gain weight and feel worse before they felt better. The weight gain freaked me out completely, and I felt like I was heading in the wrong direction. I know now that I had a very damaged metabolism, because I definitely felt worse. I didn't do the functional testing for GI inflammation she recommended because I wasn't sure I really needed it—after all, it was not covered by my health insurance, it was expensive and, at that time, considered controversial. I know now that I would have benefited tremendously from that testing and it would have saved me a lot of time and money down the road.

I went off Dr. Schwartzbein's program and back on my very low-calorie (starvation) vegetarian diet and lost the ten pounds. I was able to maintain a moderate level of health on the new T3/T4 thyroid combination. I still had all of my symptoms, although they were not as severe, and I was still 18 pounds overweight, but I figured that it was as good as it was going to get.

After a year of living by the beach, I decided to start dating. Almost immediately, I met a wonderful man named Andrew. After a few months of dating, I moved in with him. Not long after that, he proposed. We decided to move to Taos, New Mexico, and get married.

The decision to get married prompted me to try harder to lose the 18 pounds I was carrying around, so I tried a diet called The Fat Flush Plan by Ann Louise Gittleman. Ann Louise's program is an elimination diet where you remove all grains including corn, legumes, dairy and toxic substances like caffeine, alcohol and over-the-counter drugs for two weeks and then add foods back, one at a time. She emphasizes the importance of eating tons of non-starchy vegetables, a few low-glycemic fruits such as berries, and small amounts of organic lean-animal proteins and omega-3 enriched eggs. The program is designed to improve liver and kidney function, as well as find out what foods are contributing to unwanted symptoms.

Up to this time, I had been a strict vegetarian for over fifteen years and 60 percent of my calories came from whole grains and legumes, 30 percent from vegetables and fruits and 10 percent from fats. The idea of adding animal protein scared me to death! I loved animals and considered the act of eating them immoral, but her rationale made sense so I did Phase One. I lost 9 pounds in two weeks, putting me at the lowest weight I had been in years. I was thrilled! What was weird was that my debilitating hay fever symptoms improved, and my rashes were clearing up as well.

I walked down the aisle at 139 pounds (I'm 5'7") and felt pretty good! After the wedding I did not add foods back one at a time like she recommends. I added them back all at once—and gained all the weight back, plus 2 pounds more, in just four days of my normal, organic, vegetarian grain/legume-based diet! My allergies and rashes came back with a vengeance, and I felt lousy. At this point I was starting to connect the dots between my symptoms, my weight and the types of the foods I was eating versus the quantity or calories in/calories out.

I continued to go on and off Phase One of Ann Louise's program every time I wanted to lose some weight. I sometimes wondered if I was just the kind of person that should stay off grains, corn, legumes and dairy for life, but that seemed unreasonable and unfair. I found myself feeling very angry and frustrated that I couldn't just "eat like everyone else."

Living in Taos was a dream come true. When I was 13 years old, I had read about Georgia O'Keefe and the wide-open spaces of the Land of Enchantment. I had come to visit Taos on many occasions throughout my twenties, and had always dreamed it would someday be my home. Here, at the base of the Sangre de Cristo (blood of Christ) mountains, Taos welcomed me home to heal.

Andrew and I purchased an old adobe home and spent nine months restoring it. I had the job of being the designer on the project, a position I enthusiastically embraced. This was the creative outlet that was so desperately missing in my life. I still didn't feel perfect physically, but I was too excited about life to pay that much attention to my symptoms.

In December of 2007, Andrew and I were vacationing in Mexico, where we decided to sail a catamaran in the Tamarindo Bay. Andrew is an excellent sailor and it was a thrilling experience as we followed a whale and her pup for hours.

Later that evening, I developed painful, fluid filled blisters on every part of my body that was exposed to the sun. The resort docs had never seen anything like it. I tried oral and topical antihistamines with no relief. After four days, the rash was still there, I was extremely fatigued and my joints were beginning to ache. I was getting worried that there was something really wrong with me.

I should point out that my entire diet in Mexico consisted of corn and wheat tortillas, beans and tons of foods made with vegetables from the nightshade family, such as tomatoes, potatoes and peppers.

A week later, when I arrived back in the States, the rash was still there. I went to a dermatologist I'll call Dr. Cavalier, who took one look at me and said, "Well, you probably have lupus." He didn't have lab work to make that diagnosis, so I felt his statement was totally unwarranted. Ironically, the positive ANA results indicating lupus from 2004 already existed, but I had yet to have anyone interpret them for me. So I felt this doctor was making a cavalier assumption about my health, and I was angry!

"Is that your actual answer? There is no way I have lupus! But if I were a different kind of person, I might go home and actually get sick just from your diagnosis alone. You shouldn't tell people things like that, it's irresponsible!" (I have a tendency to be a bit fiery at times.)

He just smirked and said, "Well, your symptoms don't warrant serious medication, so we'll just wait and see what happens. Go home and wait until your symptoms get worse."

Go home and wait for my symptoms to get worse? Really?

He gave me a prescription for a heavy-duty steroid cream, and I went back to Taos. We had just finished the remodel of our adobe home and started the process of moving in. At least I had that to look forward to.

Tending to the Mind, Body and Spirit

I wasn't sure what I was going to do in Taos and had been seriously considering a career in real estate. I went through the real estate licensing program and was offered a job by a broker. I was heading towards another unfulfilling career and I knew it. A couple of weeks before I was supposed to start, I had nothing short of a nervous breakdown. In one weekend, I pretty much lost it and fell apart. I told my husband, "There is no way I can do this—no way! My heart is just not in it. I can't enter into another career that doesn't fulfill me: it will kill me!"

My husband said, "Why would you ever consider doing something that you don't want to do? You should do exactly what you want to do and nothing else."

Who does exactly what they want to do? I had never heard of a concept like that especially related to career. I had always thought that work was work; that's why they called it work!

Andrew's remark was a major turning point in my recovery. Up to that point, I had spent most of my life accepting the unacceptable and, in essence, Andrew had said, "Why would you accept what doesn't make you happy?" The realization that I had the power to opt for something different had never occurred to me.

Dr. Cavalier's flippant diagnosis of lupus had left me pretty distraught. Years ago, I'd had an aunt who had died of lupus. I was sick and tired of feeling like crap, and I was angry that this was happening to me. My intuition told me that there was more to the story. I would not accept the fate of an incurable and deadly diagnosis. I told myself that if even one person had challenged the diagnosis and cured herself, I had hope. A healthy rebellion awakened in me. I was not going to be another statistic! I could not imagine sitting around and waiting to get worse and I refused to accept the diagnosis as my fate. If the doctors didn't know how to cure this, I would figure it out on my own. I was going to have to take charge! I wondered if I could find a way to make it my full-time job to get to the root of what was causing my condition.

Thanks to Andrew, I was able to make my study of autoimmune disease a full-time job. Instead of staying in the victim/martyr role, I leaned on him, and for the first time in my life, I felt that someone was really on my side. I am forever grateful for him and he continues to be one of my biggest supporters.

Over the course of about a year, I spent ten hours a day researching everything I could on autoimmune disease, from medical journals and textbooks to stories of people who had healed their illness. Finally, I came across the work of Dr. David Brownstein. His book, *Overcoming Thyroid Disorders*, made sense, and for the first time ever, I had a hope of actually reversing my condition. All the other books that I had read at the time talked about all of the different therapies and things you could do to "live well" with autoimmune disease. There was no mention of it being curable. In fact, everyone was saying the same thing: "It's incurable." It was really quite depressing to hear, over and over again, "You'll never be able to heal this completely, so the best you can do is live with it." Dr. Brownstein was actually saying, "No, of course you can reverse this absolutely!"

I need to point out how important it was to my healing that a doctor was saying that autoimmune disease could be reversed. It gave me hope, and for the first time in a long time, I was genuinely enthusiastic about healing my body. I believed that I could heal, and that belief system was critical to the process.

In his book, Dr. Brownstein makes the connection between chronic infections, heavy metal toxicity, environmental toxins, adrenal fatigue, other hormonal imbalances, gluten allergies and sensitivities, and nutritional deficiencies. These were concepts that I had come across in Dr. Schwartzbein's and Ann Louise Gittleman's books, but now I was convinced that my overall "body burden" was high and that I would need to detoxify.

I had been working with an excellent medical doctor in California I'll call Dr. Open-Minded, who was familiar with Dr. Brownstein's work and was very open to the suggestion, too, that I could reverse my condition, which gave me even more hope!

I said to Dr. Open-Minded, "Look, I have a feeling that the root cause of my autoimmune disease has been chronic emotional stress, which has caused poor coping mechanisms, adrenal fatigue, a systemic Candida infection, mercury toxicity and a leaky gut. I also think I might be sensitive to gluten." To which he said, "Sure, why not?" I told him that I thought I could completely reverse my disease. He said he didn't see any reason why I shouldn't give it a shot.

Having read almost every book on managing autoimmune disease, including Donna Gate's book, *The Body Ecology Diet*, I was starting to connect the dots between a leaky gut, toxicity, infections and autoimmunity. I wasn't sure how to do it all, because there wasn't a clear road map for success. Nobody had written a book explaining exactly how to cure an autoimmune condition. So I was kind of mixing and matching different protocols and supplements. Essentially, I had become an experimental scientist with my own body.

In March of 2008, I started taking a super nutrient complex and felt better immediately. The supplement combination had all of the important B vitamins that I was deficient in due to chronic stress and a leaky gut, as well as selenium and N-acetyl-l-cysteine, which helped my liver detoxify and boost my body's own glutathione levels. It also had lots of antioxidants and immune system modulators like CoQ10, Alpha lipoic acid, resveratrol, grape seed extract and green tea extract. In addition to this complex, I started taking 3000 mg of an omega-3 complex, an additional 200 mcg of selenium, conjugated linoleic acid and whey protein powder, which included all the amino acids (especially glycine) I was most certainly deficient in.

I started getting to bed by 10:30 p.m. and replaced my high-energy cardio workouts with Pilates, weight training and long walks in nature.

Over the course of a few months, I also had gradually upped the dose of the T4/T3 thyroid hormone until my THS was below .05, which, as I will explain later, was a key factor in reducing inflammation at the site of my thyroid gland.

The change in my energy levels was profound. My skin was clearing up and my allergies were better.

Finally, convinced that rest and healthy nutrition were the answers to healing chronic illness, I wanted to learn more, so I enrolled in a holistic nutrition program at Clayton College of Natural Health. I chose this school because this was where Ann Louise Gittleman (one of my heros) had received her Ph.D.

My independent research in medical journals led me to the connection between gluten sensitivity, gluten allergy, leaky gut and autoimmune thyroid disease, so I did a food allergy test and several food sensitivity tests. Even though I was not clinically allergic to the protein in gluten, I was sensitive to it, as well as many other things like bell peppers, chilies, corn, beans and dairy products. Funny that my diet had consisted primarily of all the foods I was sensitive to!

I decided to cut out grains and nightshades for good, and in 30 days I lost "the last ten pounds" and all my symptoms disappeared completely. My puffy eyes were gone, and I looked and felt amazing!

A New Calling

Soon after, other women started to notice the difference in me and I began to receive requests to help them with their chronic symptoms. So, in September of 2008, I opened a holistic nutrition center in Taos, New Mexico. Based on what I had learned with my own body, I created a program called The Women's Empowerment Program, which is a 12-week nutrition program that helps women discover exactly what foods and substances are contributing to their unwanted symptoms. The program was very successful. In fact, every single one of the women who followed it 100 percent learned what foods they were reacting to, and all were able to lose weight and eliminate their chronic symptoms.

The remarkable success I witnessed with my clients inspired me to found Vibrant Way Inc., a women's nutrition company. In my research of nutritional supplements I had the opportunity to delve deeply into the supplement manufacturing industry and what I found was that a lot of the products on the market were junk at worst and at best had suboptimal levels of nutrients from sources that could not be identified. Some were even made in China! I rarely saw a product that had on the label "manufactured in a GMP, NSF facility." These are designations that guarantee the manufacturer is in compliance with Good Manufacturing Practices and maintain strict manufacturing guidelines set by NSF/ANSI Standard 173, which is the only accredited national standard in the dietary supplement industry. The manufacturers who comply with these standards have their products routinely tested to verify the identity and quality of the active ingredients on the label and ensure the supplements are free of contaminants such as bacteria, molds and heavy metals. I was shocked to learn that not all supplement manufacturers abide by these standards.

I wanted a top-quality super nutrient formula with ingredients sourced from only the U.S., Canada and Europe. I wanted one I could trust for the health of my family, friends and myself. This led me to partner with one of the largest, most well respected supplement manufacturers to create my own custom super nutrient formula called the Women's Empowerment Formula. I modeled my formula after the supplement that I took while I was healing and I added some other important nutrients that had worked for my clients and myself. Since that time, hundreds of women (including my mother, and my 103-year-old-grandmother) take my supplement every month.

Turning the Corner

In February of 2009, I had my thyroid antibodies tested—and they had gone from 237 to 37! This was a significant drop in antibody levels, just from lowering my TSH, changing my nutrition and taking the nutrients I was deficient in.

Dr. Open-Minded was impressed.

"That's amazing," he said. "Look at what you've been able to do with lifestyle changes alone."

"Yeah, I think I have made a connection between mercury toxicity and Candida and I think I can completely eradicate this autoimmune process by completely clearing the Candida and doing a heavy metal detox."

Dr. Open-Minded agreed and told me about a patient of his who had done a heavy metal cleanse and completely reversed her Hashimoto's. This was only one case, but it gave me a lot of encouragement.

In March of 2009, I made an appointment with an integrative doctor in Santa Fe who specializes in detoxification. We talked about the connection between Candida, mold and mercury, and I asked for a heavy metal challenge test. The results indicated that my mercury levels were very high.

This was not a very surprising result in my case, because I had worked clinically in dentistry for years. Back in 1989, we would use old machines called amalgamators, where we added mercury to a metal amalgam powder and then turned a switch on to start the spin cycle, which released who knows how much mercury vapor into the room around it. We inhaled all that mercury and then handled the filling material with our hands!

I researched different ways of clearing Candida and mercury. I had read that you can mobilize mercury with different types of heavy metal chelating agents, but if the liver is sluggish and the gut barrier is compromised by a condition called leaky gut, you can potentially pass this mercury on to other organs, like the brain, where it can do even more damage. Needless to say, I wasn't very excited about the concept of moving mercury to my brain. At this point, I was living on a healing diet, and I had already done a lot to heal my gut by removing aggravating foods, but I knew I had to do more for my liver and gut to completely heal. Keep in mind that I was doing this on my own, so I didn't really know which products were going to work. I had read about glutamine, probiotics, and digestive enzymes, and there were so many products on the market, and so much information to navigate! I ended up trying just about every Candida cleanse and gut healing protocol I could get my hands on.

I started taking grapefruit seed extract (GSE) drops every day, as well as probiotics in the form of acidophilus and bifidus. I took berberine, black walnut and olive leaf supplements. I also started taking a medical food supplement powder called, "Sustain," that is designed to heal the gut. I found this product to work so well that I now include it in my Thyroid Emergency Repair Kit for my clients. Within three months of this protocol, I saw noticeable improvements in my digestion.

I had my silver amalgam fillings removed and replaced with composites by a dentist who specializes in biocompatible dentistry.

I also purchased a far-infrared sauna for my clinic, because there was a lot of research suggesting that these saunas can safely mobilize and excrete heavy metals through the process of sweating. The doctor in Santa Fe had recommended that I use a product called "Beyond Clean," which is an Ethylenediaminetetraacetic acid (EDTA) powder that you add to bath water. I used the sauna and Beyond Clean daily.

I began researching functional medicine testing and started working with functional laboratories like Metametrix and Genova because I wanted to try everything on myself before recommending it to a client. Through functional testing on myself I found that I had an H. pylori infection, as well as a parasitic infection. The good news was that both the Candida and the mercury were gone, so I was on the right track! I used an herbal formula for the H. pylori and I did a parasite cleanse to clear up the infection.

I did a few liver cleanses that included fresh live juices and homemade herbal teas. (I give more details about these treatments in Chapter 17: Restore Your Liver.) I revamped my personal care products and removed anything with parabens or other toxic chemicals. I stopped using toothpaste with sodium lauryl sulfate and fluoride. I stopped using harsh cleaning chemicals such as bleach, disinfectants, and anything I could smell in my home. I started using only organic garden supplies and got rid of all pesticides, including the ones I used on my dog. I got rid of all plastic food storage containers and stopped buying prepared foods and water packaged in plastic.

During my healing process, I tried many things to manage my stress and cultivate enthusiasm. For instance, I cut out ALL NEWS and media consumption and even set my browser to my company's Web site instead of Google News. It has remained that way ever since. I was never a TV person, and I never watched horror movies—even before I got sick—but I wanted to cut out everything that wasn't uplifting, so I turned off my cable

TV. I stopped listening to music that triggered sad memories or reminded me of my sad past. I chose only uplifting, healing music that got me in touch with happy and joyful feelings.

I listened to inspirational CDs from teachers like Eckhart Tolle, Carolyn Myss, Louise Hay and Gay Hendricks. I went to healing workshops and attended lectures by inspiring teachers like Katie Hendricks and Marianne Williamson. I participated in many healing circles with teachers, healers and Native American elders and shaman.

I read books by leading scientists, researchers and doctors such as Bruce Lipton, M.D., Lynn McTaggart and Candace Pert, who write about the new sciences of psychoneuroimmunology and new edge biology, which scientifically prove the "empowering truth that our perceptions and responses to life dynamically shape our biology and behavior."[2] I began to see that I had the ability to consciously respond to the situations in my life, rather than living in a default state of reaction.

I continued to work with a Conscious Loving coach who helped me take 100 percent responsibility for the roles I play in relationships. Looking back on this period of my life, I can now see more clearly that there were some people in my life who felt uncomfortable around me as I started getting healthy. Some would try and sabotage my success, and like "crabs in a bucket," they would try to drag me back down, but I was able to lovingly withdraw my energy, and consequently some of my dysfunctional relationships fell away.

Attitude took on a new importance for me. I stopped complaining, and I stopped listening to the complaints of others. I wanted to surround myself with people who supported my new life and my new thought process, and so I found new friends.

I practiced forgiveness for others, and for myself. I repeated affirmations over and over, such as, "I approve of myself" and "I love myself," until they replaced the negative tape loops in my head. I worked with EFT and Quantum Healing Techniques, as well as flower essences. I developed a daily spiritual practice and a connection to the Divine that continues to fill my heart with joy and inspiration!

By July of 2010, I was clinically free of Hashimoto's and autoantibodies. At long last I was cured! I've been able to maintain a level of health that looks and feels amazing. I have tons of energy, my hair is thick and full, and I no longer have rashes, allergies, night sweats or GI symptoms. My weight stays consistently between 130 and 134 pounds on my 5'7" frame. My skin is clear, and I look much younger than I did six years ago. I never feel hungry or deprived. My periods are regular and I never experience PMS symptoms. My moods are stable and I feel happy most of the time. I don't need an arsenal of supplements or treatments to feel good. I take a good multivitamin, digestive enzymes and probiotics, and I'm on a third of the dose of thyroid medication that I started with.

In 2010, I enrolled in a two-year course at the Academy of Functional Medicine & Genomics, where I gained in-depth knowledge of how to apply functional medical testing and integrative supportive therapies into my nutrition coaching practice. Now, aside from running Vibrant Way, I have a fulfilling vocation as writer, speaker and patient advocate.

So I'm walking into the sunset happily ever after, right? Well, almost.

Even though I'm free of the symptoms that plagued me for years, I have to work to maintain this level of health. I must take care of myself. I can't afford to allow toxins back into my life in any form.

But toxins aren't always physical. Negative thinking is a toxin. Negative emotions are what Alejandro Junger, M.D., calls "quantum toxins." It's easy to identify junk foods because they have the ingredients listed on the label. But junk thoughts and toxic people are sometimes another story. Emotional toxins are not labeled, and they come in the form of any—and I mean ANY—chronic negative thoughts you allow to run through your mind.

In the last two years, I've allowed emotional toxins to affect me. Even though I don't pay attention to the news, I've been affected by the financial crisis. I've also found myself on more than one occasion struggling with relationship issues. I've had times when I've dropped into an unconscious state and allowed what Eckhart Tolle calls my "pain body" to take over. I call it my "unhappy habit," and although it's much easier to catch now, it's been a challenging one to break.

I'm only human after all...

> **❀ What You Need to Know:**
> No one has the right to tell you that you can't heal your life—because you can!
>
> While each of us is unique, I have found that people with autoimmune disorders have certain stressors in common such as chronic negative thoughts, poor coping mechanisms, poor dietary choices, food sensitivities, compromised livers, leaky gut, inflammation, low-grade infections or viruses, and chemical or heavy metal toxicity.
>
> In order to reverse your condition, you have to determine if you have any of these stressors and then work to heal them.
>
> There is one thing I know for sure: no matter how sick you are or how bad your life situation may seem, things can get better. Every day presents you with the amazing response-abilty to make new choices. I'm not suggesting that making life changes is easy, because I know it's not. What I am saying is that you don't have to accept the prognosis of an incurable disease.

You Can Have Vibrant Health!

What came between my before-and-after pictures was years of research and thousands of dollars spent on experimenting with treatments, medicines, supplements and healing modalities. The good news is you don't have to spend years and a fortune to get well, as I did! What you have that I didn't is this book! This book is the distillation of everything I've learned about how to cure (and yes, I mean cure, not symptomatically treat) autoimmune thyroid disorders. If you want to permanently reverse an autoimmune disorder, I am on your side and encourage you to read on.

Introduction

"As with many life-altering events, an autoimmune illness is almost guaranteed to cause you to re-evaluate your priorities."
– Joan Friedlander, *Women, Work, and Autoimmune Disease*

The American Autoimmune Related Diseases Association (AARDA) estimates 50 million Americans have an autoimmune condition.[3] Roughly 75 percent of these people are women.

The American Association of Clinical Endocrinologists (AACE) estimates 14 million people in this country have Hashimoto's thyroiditis.[4] The number is undoubtedly far higher owing to the countless people who remain untested.

Clearly, autoimmune disease has reached epidemic levels. But who's asking the big question: *Why?*

In 2003, the National Institutes for Health, the major funding agency for biomedical research in the United States, allocated $591.2 million for research into all autoimmune conditions. Their budget for cancer research was $5 billion and they spent another $2 billion on heart disease. These numbers are disproportionate, considering the statistics: one in 12 Americans will develop an autoimmune disease, while one in 14 will develop cancer, and one in 20 heart disease.

I'm not, however, suggesting we raise the budget for research in any of these areas. Why? Because lack of funds is not the problem—lack of consciousness is. The modern world is dying of chronic illnesses directly related to man-made toxins, stressful lifestyles and nutritional deficiencies, and we're still trying to find a "pill" to make it go away.

We've been claiming "better living through chemistry," but instead we've created a toxic environment that has cost us our health and our resources.

We cannot expect to continue to dump toxins into our bodies and our planet, and survive. The time has come to wake up to the insanity of our process and use our brains as they were intended—to love, to create beauty and to take care of our planet. We must learn to live in harmony with nature, or perish at the hands of our own egos.

This book is the culmination of six years of personal research, trial and error, and a lot of prayers to find a cure for my autoimmune condition. It is the story of my recovery from Hashimoto's thyroiditis and the beginning stages of lupus by taking responsibility for my health, honoring my body and changing my life. By changing my diet, detoxifying, practicing self-forgiveness, living more authentically and connecting with Spirit, I was able to reverse my "dis-ease."

I am not a doctor. I am a person like you, who was diagnosed with an "incurable" autoimmune condition that was progressively getting worse despite the "standard of care" treatment I was given. I was not satisfied with the results of my treatment or the resignation and complacency of the doctors from whom I sought help.

I wanted to go beyond "living well with my autoimmune disease," and I could not imagine needing a lifetime of support protocols to keep the condition at bay. I wanted to be cured. I wanted to find the cause of my illness. If I could do that then I knew, theoretically, that I could tackle whatever that cause was and reverse the process.

I was curious and became a scientist, as well as my own physician and healer. By researching everything I could on the precursors to autoimmune conditions, I was able to identify the many factors that led to my cluster of symptoms. I was overwhelmed at first because I literally had every single one of the underlying causes. I was the poster child for autoimmune dysfunction!

Like a little kid in a room strewn with toys, I wasn't sure where to start, but I was determined to clean up my mess. I made it my full-time job. Over the course of those six years, I changed everything about my life and discovered how to reverse the autoimmune process in my body. I believe that EVERY person diagnosed with an autoimmune condition can get better, and I am devoted to sharing my breakthroughs with you so that you can do the same.

The journey to recovery is simple, but it's not easy. You don't "catch" an autoimmune condition overnight. Reversing the process begins with going back to a time when you were well, and then creating a timeline that links life events with the appearance of symptoms. Essentially, I want to help you connect the dots between traumas, certain emotions, exposures to toxins and allergic foods, and the onset of uncomfortable symptoms.

Imagine every negative event, exposure, and trauma as splinters that have been festering in your body and causing irritations. Your work will be to gently remove the splinters one by one and let your body heal.

The notion that chronic illnesses, such as autoimmune thyroid conditions, are incurable is ludicrous. The very nature of the autoimmune process should tell us that it's reversible.

Autoimmune conditions are essentially caused by risk factors such as chronic stress, high carbohydrate diets, poor gastrointestinal health, nutrient deficiencies, compromised liver function, infections and toxins. We simply cannot expose ourselves over and over to these "body burdens" and expect ourselves to thrive.

For most of you, the protocols I suggest will be a breeze as you realize the many factors that led to your diagnosis. For others, it may take some serious time and effort, but the payoff is a level of health you may have never thought possible for yourself!

I was reluctant to use the word "cure" in the title of this book, because according to many medical experts, autoimmune thyroid conditions cannot be "cured." For clarification, when I use the word "cure," I am referring to the complete reversal of an autoimmune process and its symptoms by healing the underlying causes of the disorder.

As I mentioned in the prologue, I no longer have clinical Hashimoto's thyroiditis or positive autoantibodies, nor do I have any of the symptoms that plagued me for most of my adult life.

Research indicates that roughly 10 percent of patients diagnosed with Hashimoto's will go into spontaneous remission; my recovery, however, was not spontaneous. It was not accidental. It was directly related to the steps I took to find out what the underlying cause(s) of my

> **cure** (kyoor), n.
> 1. a means of healing or restoring to health; remedy.
> 2. a method or course of remedial treatment, as for disease.
> 3. successful remedial treatment; restoration to health.
> 4. a means of correcting or relieving anything that is troublesome or detrimental.
> 8. to restore health.[5]

illness were and following a holistic treatment program to heal each one. I am certain that I would have continued to progress to an even worse autoimmune state had I ignored my body's signals and followed the conventional "wait and watch" approach. I have since helped several other people reverse similar chronic conditions. Those who have followed the program 100 percent have seen a complete reversal of their antibodies and their symptoms. This is not a coincidence, and falls far, far above the 10 percent remission rate.

The functional mind/body approach I am introducing is a results-based holistic healing program that blends the sciences of functional medicine, psychology, epigenetics and nutrigenomics with the classic principles of detoxification and mind/body awareness.

My goal is to help you to put an end to the confusion of chronic illness, drop the struggle, and step into a more powerful, healthy version of yourself.

What you will learn in this book are the exact steps to take to uncover the underlying causes of the autoimmune process in your body. This program will help you to heal your physical body first so that you can identify and transform the chronic stress cycles and negative emotional patterns that contributed to, if not directly caused, your illness in the first place.

If you've read this far, I know you are one step closer to healing yourself. I'm asking you to step into your power and your truth today. Thank you for your strength and determination. You can get better, and together we can make a difference in our world.

PART ONE: AWARENESS

The Autoimmune Condition

*"Truth is not something outside to be discovered,
it is something inside to be realized."*
– Osho

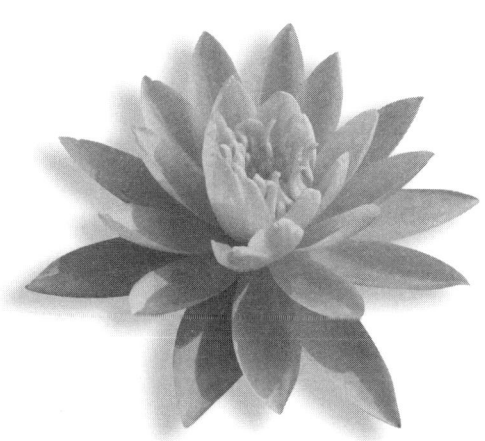

CHAPTER 1

Take Charge of Your Health

"A journey of a thousand miles begins with a single step."
– Lao Tzu

Become Empowered

I begin this book with the topic of empowerment, because becoming empowered is the first step in your healing journey. By definition, if you are not empowered, you are a victim—a victim of circumstance affected by the outside world, where everything feels out of your control. This chapter focuses on ways of becoming empowered and taking back control of your body. My journey to empowerment was at the root of getting better and ultimately reversing my autoimmune condition.

When I was first diagnosed with "autoimmune thyroid disease," I was devastated. *"Why me? How could this be happening to me?"* I wondered. *"What did I do to deserve this?"* I felt helpless and victimized. I was physically miserable and emotionally drained. As a marketing and practice management consultant to doctors, I had access to some of the best medical and alternative care in the country. I desperately went from specialist to specialist, hopeful that someone would be able to "cure" me.

Over and over the answer was the same: "We don't know the cause of autoimmune disease and there is no cure. Let's just 'wait and watch' and see what happens."

It took two years of worsening symptoms for me to finally get angry. After a flippant guess-diagnosis of lupus by a dermatologist, I was outraged: I was not going to be another statistic! I knew I was worth more than this, and simply could not imagine being sick for the rest of my life. If the doctors didn't know how to cure this, I would figure it out on my own. I was going to have to take charge!

I began to read everything I could get my hands on about my condition. I looked into the treatment options and whether or not ANYONE had ever overcome the disorder. If so, who were the doctors who had had success in helping people reverse the condition, and how did they do it?

In my research of chronic illness and its causes, I began to connect the dots. I discovered that nutrition, detoxification, and lifestyle played a huge role in reversing the condition. I read stories about people who had recovered from autoimmune conditions and cancer, and in them I began to see a common thread:

Healing from chronic illness is complex and always involves a deep passion and taking responsibility for getting well. It also involves experimentation, thinking outside the box, personal advocacy, dietary changes, detoxification, medication (in some cases), nutritional therapies, emotional/spiritual work, forgiveness, gratitude, cultivation of happiness and other lifestyle adjustments. The majority of people who had success in reversing their illness are empowered people who made <u>major</u> lifestyle changes and then stuck with them.

I started to see that I was going to have to take some responsibility for my health. I became aware that I was at least partially responsible for my condition, and I needed to make some major changes. In the beginning it seemed like an insurmountable task, but I really wanted to get better! I could imagine myself in a healthy, beautiful and vibrant body. My dream of health was reflected back to me each time I saw a healthy, vibrant woman in the store, in a yoga class, or walking on the beach. I didn't realize it at the time, but I was dreaming a dream of health that would some day become a reality for me. I was on the path to becoming empowered!

Over a five-year period, I became passionate about wellness and borderline obsessed with finding the cause of my condition. I questioned the "standard of care" being offered to me and researched everything I could about how to reverse chronic illness. I became a scientist with my own body, testing different treatments, medications and supplements on myself. I became my own health advocate and sought treatment from medical doctors, as well as alternative practitioners who valued my intuition and were willing to collaborate with me in my healing process. Finally, I made the necessary lifestyle and dietary changes that allowed me to heal.

Let's look at the stages of empowerment and why we must become empowered if we are to get well.

The five stages of empowerment in health are:

Stage One: Get passionate about getting better;
Stage Two: Step out of the victim role and take responsibility;
Stage Three: Take action by challenging the system;
Stage Four: Become your own health advocate; and
Stage Five: Make the necessary lifestyle adjustments to heal!

In the following section I'm going to explain why these stages are necessary. My hope is that you will become inspired, become your own health advocate, and go on to follow the steps in the clinical section.

Stage One:
Get Passionate About Getting Better

"Passion is energy. Feel the power that comes from focusing on what excites you."
— Oprah Winfrey

If I had to identify the most important element in reversing my condition, I would have to say it's passion. Without passion and enthusiasm, I would not have had the emotional strength to stick to the changes I needed to make to get better. I truly believed that I deserved vibrant health and that I would get better, but there were some rough times and disappointments along the way. On the days when I didn't feel so well, or was tempted to throw in the towel, I would open my healing journal and review my reasons for embarking on this journey in the first place. I needed to remind myself of what I really wanted for my life.

In the beginning pages of my journal, I made a list of what was working in my life and what wasn't. I wrote down all of my accomplishments, no matter how insignificant they seemed, and how I had achieved them. My list of past successes reminded me of how capable I was and gave me the confidence I needed to keep going.

In the areas that were not working as well, I made a list of the negative belief patterns that were responsible for how those areas looked, and then rewrote my beliefs. I replaced each negative thought pattern with a new positive one.

I painted the picture of a healthy, vibrant and committed woman who had enough self-love to eat the foods that would heal her body. I envisioned a woman who spoke her truth and knew how to stand up for herself and say "no" when it was appropriate. I saw a woman who was compassionate but strong—physically and emotionally. I saw a woman who was inspired and inspiring. I saw myself in a vibrant, capable body that looked and felt amazing!

The beginning pages of my healing journal reminded me of what I wanted in life so that I could hold steady through the difficult times.

The Empowerment Exercise

There may be days, especially in the beginning, when you will have less energy and may not feel very well. You may even be tempted to fall off the wagon or give up completely. On those days, you will need compelling reasons to stay on track. You will have to remember your passion for getting well.

The following exercise is designed to inspire your passion for getting better. It's also designed to help you uncover the unconscious patterns or belief systems that may be acting as roadblocks to your healing.

Answer the following questions in your healing journal:

- What is your burning desire for your life?
- What gives your life the most meaning? What are you born to do?
- What are your compelling reasons for reversing your autoimmune condition and attaining optimal health?
- How will your life change when you reverse this condition in your body?
- Are you afraid of how your life will change? If so, why?
- What are the areas working well in your life, and how did you accomplish that?
- What are the areas that aren't working?
- Can you identify the negative belief patterns that contribute to the areas that aren't working?

For each negative belief pattern, transform it and write down a new positive thought pattern!

Now write a paragraph that perfectly illustrates the most beautiful vision you have of yourself.

Stage Two:
Step Out of the Victim Role and Take Responsibility for Your Health

"To be in hell is to drift; to be in heaven is to steer."
– GEORGE BERNARD SHAW

If you completed the Empowerment Exercise in the last section, you have identified what your burning desires are for your life and why you want to get better. Perhaps you have even uncovered some negative thought patterns and are in the process of turning them around.

Now it's time to take responsibility! While your spouse, family, friends and doctor may want the best for you, no one is coming to save you. You're going to have to save yourself.

Are you ready to take charge of your health?

You didn't develop an autoimmune thyroid condition overnight. Unless you suffered an acute trauma such as a toxic exposure or radiation, chances are it took years to develop. Many people diagnosed with autoimmune conditions have endured years of living a chaotic lifestyle, suboptimal nutrition, inhuman levels of stress, huge amounts of toxins (both physical and emotional), and in many cases, crippling medications to mask their symptoms.

I know you want a quick and easy cure to make it all go away, but unfortunately there is no magic pill that's going to make your body immune to a lifetime of unrelenting stress in all of its forms.

In order for you to get better, you're going to have to get honest with yourself and take responsibility for where you are now. This is typically where I hear the most resistance: "I know, but… I have such a stressful job, there are so many people depending on me, my mom just died, my teenager just got a DUI, my husband is cheating on me…" The list goes on. I understand the resistance, because I know how it feels to feel "sick and tired" and overwhelmed by your circumstances. I understand how hard it is to get out of the habit of putting everyone's needs before your own. I know how it feels to have low self-esteem and feel the weight of the world on your shoulders. I used to have all the excuses in the world for why I couldn't take care of myself. I was caught in a cycle of dwelling on the negative, giving up, making unhealthy choices, and then feeling guilty and blaming myself for being a loser.

What I have learned is that in order to heal, we must focus on the positive aspects of our lives, forgive ourselves (and others), and learn to love ourselves enough to make our own needs a priority.

There's no getting around it, dear, you just can't give from an empty cup. In order to really love and support others, you have to love yourself first.

Stage Three: Take Action by Challenging the System

"There are two primary choices in life: to accept conditions as they exist, or accept the responsibility for changing them."
– Denis Waitley

Have you ever thought about who decides whether a "disease" is curable or not? Does anyone question what causes the illness? Who decides how a particular "disease" will be treated? I was in the health industry, but it wasn't until I got sick that I asked these questions. Prior to getting sick, I didn't think about it. I figured that scientists and doctors in medical schools and hospitals were looking for the answers to these questions.

I fully trusted that "They" had it under control. If "They" hadn't come up with a cure for chronic illness, they were at least working frantically toward one. Right?

That is what I believed, until I received a diagnosis of a "deadly" and "incurable" disease. Suddenly I asked the questions, "Who says this is incurable?" and "What do they mean when they say, 'We don't understand the mechanism of this illness'?" Even better, "If they can't answer these questions, why should I put my health in their hands?"

My intuition told me that there was more to the story. I could not accept the status quo, and knew there had to be an alternative. I told myself that if there was even one person who had challenged the diagnosis and "cured" herself, I had hope!

Why Am I Asking You to Challenge the Belief That Your Condition Is Incurable?

I'm asking you to challenge the idea that your condition is incurable because "They" don't have all the answers, and very few people are questioning the system. Let's take a look at the health of our nation. According to statistics by the American Association of Clinical Endocrinologists (AACE)

and other medical organizations:
- Approximately 27 million Americans are experiencing a thyroid disorder. This includes the estimate that about half of these cases remain undiagnosed.
- An estimated 50 million people in the United States suffer from some type of autoimmune disease.[1]
- Seven out of ten deaths among Americans each year are from chronic diseases.
- Heart disease, cancer and stroke account for more than 50 percent of all deaths each year.
- In 2005, 133 million Americans—almost one out of every two adults—had at least one chronic illness.[2]
- According to the World Health Organization's June 2000 report, Health Systems: Improving Performance, "The U.S. health system spends a higher portion of its gross domestic product than any other country but ranks 37 out of 191 countries according to its performance."

We are one of the wealthiest nations, with access to excellent medical care, and we are still getting sick and dying from chronic diseases! When we do get sick, why don't the standard treatment protocols make us better? Billions of dollars are being spent in search of a cure. What about the search for the cause?

Understanding What Goes Into a Diagnosis

The diagnosis of an incurable autoimmune "disease" is scary, but realize that it's merely a cluster of symptoms that have been given a name and categorized by a medical coding system. Diagnostic codes are important. Without them, doctors would have no way of naming a condition, but naming a "disease" alone is not enough and it does nothing to uncover its cause(s). Many times, we are simply viewed as a diagnostic code, prescribed drugs and sent on our way without anyone ever asking the question, "Why is this person getting sick in the first place?"

Dr. C.E. Gant explains it this way: "In a good dictionary, you will discover two distinct definitions of the term "diagnosis." One is an educated guess based on the symptoms, and the other is based on identifying the actual cause of the illness (through either hard clinical test results, or symptoms that unmistakably indicate a certain condition).

In other words, until a condition's true cause is identified, it sometimes is known and understood by its symptoms alone. Pneumonia was called pneumonia for thousands of years based on the appearance of certain symptoms such as cough, sputum production, fever, chills, etc. Then, we discovered germs and moved to the scientific level, identifying the cause, and started diagnosing streptococcal pneumonia by the presence of streptococcal pneumonia germs.

With autoimmune conditions, this can become very complicated, because there is no one single cause for chronic autoimmune disorders, as there is with an infectious disease. So, we must resort to what we call "risk factor analysis." For example, when diagnosing heart disease, the risk factors a doctor looks for include cholesterol elevation, hypertension, smoking, etc.

That's why many doctors classify autoimmune disorders (and other chronic or psychiatric disorders) as "incurable." Clinicians basically throw their hands up in exasperation and say, "If there is not one simple cause that can be studied using double-blinded, controlled experiments, it's just too complicated—so we'll just throw drugs at the symptoms, until someday (a day that will never come), when someone will discover the one and only cause of thyroid disease."

But the good news is that these conditions are only "incurable" if we look at them the prescientific way. If we advance to the scientific era and use the risk factor method, we can not only reverse many of the symptoms by targeting those causal factors, but also actually "cure" most patients by doing so.

To get a complex understanding of all these factors, the doctor must be willing to look for and accept a lot of information about lifestyle, nutrition, mental health, and life history from the patient.

In the current system, we aren't asked to look at our stress levels, our lifestyle choices, our nutrition, or the toxins we are exposed to. Instead, we are given toxic drugs to mask the symptoms caused by the toxins and other risk factors that are making us sick in the first place. What's even more ridiculous is that when the medications cause more symptoms, we are sometimes given additional medications to counteract those.

Autoimmune thyroid conditions such as Hashimoto's and Graves' are said to be incurable, and can only be treated with specific drugs approved by the Food and Drug Administration (FDA). When doctors say "incurable," what variables are they taking into consideration? Peer-reviewed evidence, published in reputable medical journals suggests that autoimmune conditions are caused by risk factors such as chronic stress, food allergies and sensitivities, gastrointestinal imbalances, nutrient deficiencies, infections, heavy metals and toxic burdens that ultimately stress the immune system so much that it gets confused and attacks healthy tissue. It would make sense then that if you kept those risk factors in place and took drugs to mask your symptoms, you would have a "disease" that remains incurable.

I had a doctor say to me once, "You haven't cured your disease. If you went back to eating and living the way you did before, like everyone else does, it would come back." This is like saying that if you are getting sick from taking poison, and you continue to take poison, you won't get better. Duh!

What happens when you detox your body, treat any infections and reduce your overall body burden? Has anyone funded studies looking at the lifestyle variables that are responsible for your current cluster of symptoms? No…and under the current system, no one will.

Understand the System Making the Rules

The first part of my journey to empowered health involved getting very clear about the state of our current health care system. Some of my opinions in this section may surprise you, but it is absolutely critical to your journey that you understand the information I present here.

Consider the following analogy: As children, we naturally trusted our parents to know what was best for us in any situation, especially when it came to illness. They were older than we were and more knowledgeable. In essence, they were our medical experts and we listened to them and acted on their advice without question. As adults, we now often place our faith in our doctors instead of our parents to know what is best for us when managing illness. They are, after all, the experts…right? Not exactly.

It is important to understand that doctors operate within a system that dictates how they learn to approach illness and treatment recommendations. Unfortunately, these recommendations fail miserably when it comes to chronic illness! To better understand the health care system that the doctors work within, we have to recognize the powerful role that the pharmaceutical industry (Big Pharma) plays when it comes to health care. Entire books have been written on this subject, but I'm going to offer you the key points.

Big Pharma is motivated to sell patented drugs for maximum profit. In order to achieve its goals, the industry needs help from doctors. Doctors are, after all, the only individuals in our society authorized to prescribe the drugs that Big Pharma manufactures and sells. To get the help it needs, Big Pharma provides huge amounts of money in the form of grants to universities, doctors, hospitals, and research scientists. Everyone in the current health care system depends on this money, and nobody wants to risk being cut off from it. The following excerpt illustrates how Big Pharma dollars shape the entire medical model in this country:

> "It is in the interests of big business to teach this moneymaking protocol and from a business standpoint they have the perfect template in place: fund the students who will administer their medicines, fund the hospitals to administer their medicines, lobby in Washington, D.C., for a standard of care that revolves around their medicines, make it illegal not to use their medicines, and ostracize doctors who don't tow the company line, calling them quacks, charlatans and frauds and running them out of town."
>
> — SUZANNE SOMERS, author of *Knockout: Interviews with Doctors Who are Curing Cancer—And How to Prevent It in the First Place*

Don't get me wrong: I am not trying to vilify our hardworking health care providers. They operate in a flawed system. Doctors learn how to treat symptoms with drugs and are not encouraged to be curious about why we're getting sick in the first place. What I want you to understand is how this all affects you!

> 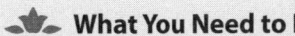 **What You Need to Know:**
> Most chronically ill patients are mismanaged with surgeries and pharmaceuticals that don't help and in many cases make them worse in the long run.

To return to our original analogy, when you visit your doctor with the hope of reversing your autoimmune condition, you simply cannot put your complete trust in them to steer you in the right direction. They don't even know a language that involves addressing the underlying, causal risk factors, so it's like trying to discuss a cure in Russian with a doctor who only understands English. Doctors can help you overcome many medical conditions but you have to understand that our current system does not yet understand the underlying causes of autoimmunity, nor does it have a vision of how to reverse it. *You* need to have this vision to navigate your healing path. That's what this book is for.

You must get outside the system, become your own health advocate and learn about what your doctor may not even know and could not begin to understand without rigorously studying a whole new way of understanding health and disease. This is analogous to what physicists went through over a hundred years ago when the Newtonian model gave way to the theory of relativity and quantum physics.

Stage Four: Become Your Own Health Advocate

"The... patient should be made to understand that he or she must take charge of his own life. Don't take your body to the doctor as if he were a repair shop."
– Quentin Regestein

Getting Outside of the System and Getting Better

The information in the last section is not intended to add more stress to your life, and I'm not suggesting that you run out and become a health care activist. Now is not the time to get political. Now is the time to get well! When you have reversed your condition you can be an advocate for change, but right now all of your energy must be focused on healing your body!

Our health care system has some serious problems. Billion in profits are made each year covering up symptoms with drugs that never address the underlying risk factors for chronic illness. But chances are there is not much you can do about our broken system from where you are right now.

Like the spiritual teacher Byron Katie says, "Love What Is," which, translated means: Accept What Is!

If you look at the case studies of people who have reversed their autoimmune condition, you will find that they had to accept the limitations of conventional care and get outside of the system to get well. When you step out of the current system you can demand a higher level of care—one that will help you to identify the factors that made you sick in the first place. Then you and your open-minded doctor, not Big Pharma, can decide how to proceed with a healing program.

Become Your Own Health Advocate

The idea of becoming your own health care advocate may be foreign to you, but I can't tell you how necessary it is to your healing. We've already discussed what you (and your doctor) are up against with Big Pharma dictating the standard of care in medicine. I'm sorry to break the news, but nobody is going to fight for your cause with the same passion and determination that you can. Who else has the time—and who could possibly care more about your health than you?

While we're on the subject of passion, I'd like to talk about a very important aspect of your healing: building a team of health care providers who enthusiastically support you in your healing process.

Build a Supportive Team

One of the first things you will have to do as your own health advocate is build a team of health care providers who enthusiastically support you in reversing your condition! I do not recommend wasting your time and money with anyone who does not believe that you can get well.

Why do I feel so strongly about finding someone who really believes you can heal?

There was a well-known Harvard research study conducted in the mid-1960's where a group of teachers were informed that some of their underperforming students were just "late bloomers." As teachers "believed" their students were soon to blossom in their academic achievement, these "special" students actually gained significant improvement in their test scores. What was the ultimate finding of this "expectation effect" study? Where they expected success, they found it!

Even Hippocrates, the father of Western medicine, who provided the "Hippocratic Oath," believed in the power of positive thinking within the doctor-patient relationship.

> "Some patients, though conscious that their condition is perilous, recover their health simply through their contentment with the goodness of the physician."   HIPPOCRATES

Aside from excellent clinical knowledge, the most successful practitioners have an open mind, an empathic disposition, a genuine curiosity and a true belief in the body's natural ability to heal. They value efficacy and have an attitude of "the best answer wins" when it comes to choosing treatment options. They are more concerned with the outcome of wellness than they are with proving a particular perspective on "science," which can be as subjective as opinions on anything else. They value their patient's intuition and have enthusiasm and desire to see their patients get well!

This expectation of success—the intention to heal and a belief in the body's natural ability to heal—is sometimes scorned by conventional practitioners as a "placebo effect," when in fact it has always been one of the tools of healing and could be summed up in one word: love.

Your Doctor's Faith in You and Your Ability to Heal

When I first reversed my Hashimoto's autoantibodies, I remember bringing my blood work into an alternative practitioner. He thought it was remarkable that I was able to stop the autoimmune process in my body by cutting out inflammatory foods, healing a chronic infection and detoxing from heavy metals. As he looked over my blood work he began shaking his head and said, "No one is as disciplined as you are, so don't bother trying to tell other people how to do this—besides, you never really get rid of Hashimoto's. It just goes into remission."

I could have felt deflated, but I knew I had truly healed my condition and I was not going to let him take the wind out of my sails!

I said to him, "You know what? I have most certainly permanently reversed this condition, and barring any environmental circumstances out of my control, I will maintain excellent health! And I will bet that there are thousands of people who have the discipline that I have and are willing to change their lives—they just don't know how. I'm going to tell everyone. Watch me!"

He just smiled and said, "Good for you."

On my way home I started to wonder if he had lost his faith in the body's miraculous ability to heal itself, or if he just didn't want to appear to be too optimistic or give me false hope.

I believe that many practitioners who have been working in the health care field for a long time know deep down that chronic illness can be reversed, but they may be intimidated by the system and worry that if they express such notions, they will be accused of quackery, or of giving people false hope. Instead, they are trained to convey false pessimism. As I will cover later, these accusations can have devastating consequences for the practitioner. Others may simply have lost the faith that people will be motivated to follow the steps necessary to heal. Either way, these scenarios don't leave us with many opportunities for successful healing outcomes.

Become a Scientist with Your Own Body

When I ask you to "become a scientist with your own body," I'm not suggesting you go to medical school or become a chemist or biologist. Nor am I asking you to learn how to interpret complicated lab results or spend hours researching the "mechanisms" of disease. What I am asking you to do is develop the genuine curiosity of a scientist.

Ask questions such as:

- How did I develop an autoimmune condition?
- What are the underlying reason(s) my immune system is attacking my own tissues?
- What physical, environmental, and emotional factors may be contributing to my illness?
- What can I do on my own to begin to heal my condition?

I always tell my clients that they are their own best healer. Remember, no one has as much personally at stake in recovery as you do. My guess is that you already have the answers to many of the critical questions that will arise during your healing process. Don't be afraid to bring these up with your doctor; nothing is insignificant. Just because your doctor hasn't mentioned something, doesn't mean it's not relevant.

Becoming a scientist with your own body involves examining every aspect of your body, mind and spirit. You will need to do a sensitivity discovery diet to determine food allergies and sensitivities, and find out what foods are causing symptoms and contributing to your body's immune burden. You may have to heal your GI tract and bring your gut flora into balance if necessary. You may have to test yourself for heavy metals and remove any silver amalgam fillings, root canals and dental implants if necessary.

You may have to address any underlying infections such as gum or bone infections in your mouth, as well as other low-grade infections and viruses that may be lurking. If you have used dermal fillers, gotten breast implants or had other cosmetic procedures such as Botox, you may have to determine how much they are contributing to your overall body burden.

You may need to take inventory of your personal care and household products to determine what chemicals they contain and replace them if necessary. You may need to examine if some of your stress is caused by toxic relationships or unhealthy working conditions. You may need to examine your thought patterns and reverse as much negative self-talk as possible.

You may have to learn about your physical environment, such as where you live and where you choose to go on vacation. Some places have unusually high rates of chronic illness due to environmental factors such as mold contamination, mills, power plants, radon and other toxins, which are all factors to consider when looking for the cause of an autoimmune condition.

Even though the clinical steps outlined in this book are the same for everyone, the results of the tests, treatment protocols and personal outcomes will vary. We each have our own unique biochemistry, lifestyle and history. Becoming a scientist involves collaborating with your health care provider, asking questions, sharing ideas and working together to determine the right treatment for you.

The questions you bring up to your doctor may be foreign to her. Perhaps she has not yet connected the dots linking chronic stress, food sensitivities, and exposure to toxins to the autoimmune process. Many of my clients find that they know more about reversing autoimmune conditions than their doctors do. That's a good thing! Keep asking questions and developing your intuition. Becoming a scientist with your body will not only help you get the care you need to heal, it will also pave the path for others to do the same.

If your health care practitioner(s) expresses a willingness to work with you, that's a gift. Be patient and try not to belittle them for not understanding the autoimmune risk factors as well as you will after studying the information in this book. You may need to become a diplomat, as well as a scientist, in order to guide your doctor in helping you. You need them to keep monitoring your progress and lab results. If you fall off the wagon and your autoimmune process flares, or if you have an accident or an acute problem and need them to support you in more critical care, your doctor or health care practitioner can be an important advocate. Your recovery will open their eyes and perhaps inspire them to go on and heal hundreds of patients with autoimmune disorders in their career.

Stage Five: Make the Necessary Lifestyle Adjustments to Heal!

"Whether you believe you can do a thing or not, you are right."
– Henry Ford

Once you have found the "splinters" underlying your autoimmune condition, you will have to follow a healing protocol that will take anywhere from 3 to 18 months to heal your body. Most of you will have to stick to those changes for life in order to stay well. Change can be challenging but many of us have forgotten how good it feels to be healthy. Feeling happier and healthier will be a generous reward for creating positive changes in your life.

By now I hope you feel inspired and ready to make those changes. Success will never come unless you take action!

I have provided you with an action-planning journal on *The Thyroid Cure* Web site so that you can keep track of every aspect of your healing process. Please use it to stay on track. You can access your personalized online journal at: www.thethyroidcure.com/journal

> **The reason healing can take so long** has to do with the term "epigenetics," which we discuss in Chapter 6: Reframe the Autoimmune Process. When you apply any of the changes suggested in this book, you're causing most of the 200 trillion cells in your body to go into their DNA library, pull out new pieces of your genetic blueprint and make new proteins to adapt to these changes. Therefore, the changes you make don't generally get results overnight, but if you're persistent and consistent with the steps you take, you can radically alter your genetic expression in several weeks. Before you made any changes, your cells were adapted to all the immune stress and inflammation you were subjected to, but as you follow healthier patterns, they will gradually wind down that portion of their genetic adaptation, as the risk factors causing the heightened immunity disappear.

What Can You Expect if You Follow the Steps to Empowerment?

When you take the steps to empowerment and heal your autoimmune condition, you will know what your body needs to thrive. You will have more confidence and vitality.

What does this look like?

First of all, becoming healthy will help you feel great inside. You'll have more energy and your body won't feel like such a burden. Many people lose weight like never before, and secondary health complaints often disappear.

But empowerment and healing also bring transformation on a personal level.

You will know what you need and stay true to yourself no matter what. You will trust your instincts and follow your gut when it comes to food, relationships and your environment.

You will take full responsibility for yourself, honor yourself and be honored by those around you. You will stand up for what you believe in and become a beacon of light for others.

You will have compassion with boundaries. You will be able to give freely, because you have learned to put your needs first. You will forgive others freely, because you will have learned to forgive yourself.

Empowerment means stepping into your truth…and optimal health can only vibrate at the level of truth.

CHAPTER 2

Consider the Real Cost of Wellness

"America's health care system is neither healthy, caring, nor a system."
— WALTER CRONKITE

What I have observed over the years is that most people are initially excited to learn that their autoimmune condition can be reversed—that is, until we start talking about the cost of organic food, supplements, or in some cases, functional medical testing. Many times the first question I hear is, "How much does it cost?" and "Will my insurance cover this?" One of the biggest obstacles standing between many people and vibrant health is their perception that "health insurance" has anything to do with healing.

While there is a lot you can do on your own without seeing a practitioner, some of you may need help from a practitioner. In case you do, I've attempted to open your eyes to the reality of what our health care system offers.

The Limitations of Health Insurance

Health insurance can be helpful in defraying the costs when paying for medical treatment —especially for costly, acute problems, like being injured in an auto accident—but most people don't view it that way. It's common for a client to refuse testing/treatment that is not covered by their health care plan. They feel that it "should" be covered and the idea of paying out-of-pocket for a test or treatment is outrageous. They also may assume, before they fully realize how these things work, that the health insurance company—like their doctor—already knows which diagnostic tests and treatments are truly necessary and which ones are not. So they may also assume that if their health insurance doesn't cover it, it must not be something they really need to get well. For this reason, insurance can be a roadblock to health and wellness, especially when people rely solely on what their "health" plans cover.

Regardless of financial status, most people are just not used to the idea of paying for health care services.

Until the current health care system undergoes a complete transformation from top to bottom, it will keep acting just like an inflamed immune system—it will sometimes harm more than it helps, because it's still full of internal conflicts that don't serve the greater good. For now there may be only one way to get the health care you truly need, and that is to seek it out—and yes—even pay for it yourself!

It's time for health care reform, and it starts with you and me, changing the way we think about who's responsible for our health and who's going to pay for our optimal wellness!

The inconvenient truth is that you get what you pay for in life…and health care is no exception. If you have been diagnosed with an autoimmune condition, chances are you will need office visits, tests, supplements, and perhaps even medication that your plan will not cover. In most cases, you will need to see a health care provider that is outside of your network who probably doesn't even bill insurance. The reason is that doctors and other health care providers who have success with chronic conditions have gone far and above the "standard of care" insurance companies are willing to provide, and refuse to allow insurance companies to dictate how much time they can spend with a patient and how they will treat a particular condition.

Dr. Robert Kornfeld sums up how health insurance companies have been allowed to dictate the standard of care in medicine in his December 2011 article for *The Huffington Post*:[1]

"It always has been physicians themselves that set the standard of care in medicine. Yet, that no longer seems to be the case. And this sets a very dangerous precedent for medical care in this country going forward.

Health insurance companies have been able to take over control of medicine through contracted arrangements with doctors. When a doctor agrees to 'participate' with a health insurance company and become a part of their provider panel, he also becomes beholden to the terms and limitations set forth by the insurance company. Realize that an insurance company is not in the health care business. They are in the 'keep the premium dollars' business. That means that they have a vested interest in keeping down the costs of medical care so that they can maximize their profits. By contrast, the doctor must hold to his oath of providing the best possible medical care while also doing his/her best to do no harm. Clearly, the insurance company/physician relationship can become contentious and adversarial because of these factors.

The truth of what is now happening in this country is that diagnostic tests and certain treatment protocols are being 'denied' by insurance companies as 'not medically necessary.' In other words, they refuse to pay because they simply do not want to finance tests or therapies that cut into their bottom line more than they want them to. In addition, physicians face audits of their records by insurance companies and Medicare in which their records are scrutinized to see that every 'i' is dotted and every 't' is crossed. If not, physicians are subject to demands for 'recovery' of funds for services that were 'inappropriately billed.'

In addition, physicians who incorporate more progressive therapies are being subjected to withholding of payments, bogus peer review and licensure review boards. These 'scare' tactics are working better than they should be. To avoid all of these uncomfortable and potentially damaging threats that are now looming over physicians, many are now fully 'cooperating' with whatever the insurance company dictates as the 'new standard of care' in medicine. In order to do this, physicians look for the quickest and cheapest way to address their patients so as not to stand out and become a sitting duck for an audit. Who suffers are both the patients and the doctors."

Initially this whole health care crisis may seem "unfair," but only because we've been brainwashed into thinking that our health and wellbeing are someone else's responsibility. Unfortunately, it's this kind of thinking that keeps us sick and enslaved by a broken system.

> **What You Need to Know:**
> You want a health care practitioner who works for you, not for an insurance or drug company. You have the greatest stake in your own wellness. Your doctor has the next greatest stake, as they want to fulfill their life's mission and successfully heal patients. Drug companies and insurance companies only have a stake in increasing their own profits!

The Silver Lining

Your insurance company may not be your ally most of the time, but insurance companies have recently begun to notice the fact that total recovery from autoimmune disorders is now possible using the advanced technologies of integrative and functional medicine. Luckily, sometimes your recovery can be compatible with their desire to maximize profits. Insurance companies are slowly realizing that they can spend tens of thousands of dollars in the next decade on conventional care, managing all the complications of your autoimmune disorder as you gradually march towards dysfunction and early death, or they can spend a few thousand dollars upfront on integrative/functional care and realize enormous profits in the years ahead as you continue to pay your premiums and hardly ever need to see a doctor at all. They are beginning to understand the economic benefits of their members taking responsibility for getting themselves well, and they are becoming increasingly willing to cover the lion's share of the diagnostic testing and other costs to help them get there.

Consequently, more and more PPOs are paying for functional testing and treatments. Not only that, specialty laboratories, such as Genova Diagnostics, are offering special programs that allow you to enjoy the benefits customarily associated with traditional insurance-reimbursed medical services. For more information on this, please see the Resources section under the heading "Laboratories."

I predict a trend in this direction, as more and more consumers become educated and demand this level of care.

Fee-for-Service Providers

The difference between choosing a fee-at-time-of-service provider versus going to one who is contracted with an insurance company is simply the difference between comprehensive and basic care. Most doctors who have taken the risk of becoming independent of insurance companies have done so because they know that providing quality care takes time—much more time than any health insurance company has been willing to pay in the past.

Many of these doctors have been successful in treating and reversing chronic illness because they have taken their power back and broken away from what licensing boards call "the accepted standards of care." What this means is that they have refused to allow insurance companies, drug companies, or regulatory agencies to tell them how much time they can spend with and how to treat their patients.

This choice gives them the freedom to spend as much time as is necessary with you—really listening, taking comprehensive health histories, ordering and reviewing comprehensive tests and then carefully prescribing customized complex treatment protocols that actually work!

Functional and integrative medical doctors who have had experience with autoimmune conditions can help you get to the bottom of what's going on quite fast, which will save you time, money and aggravation down the road.

You can expect to have a larger out-of-pocket expense, as these practitioners generally cannot take your insurance as payment without risking economic, professional and regulatory penalties. They will charge you for their services upfront and at the time of service. They work much like other highly trained, specialized professionals such as lawyers and architects.

Your insurance company may pay you back for a portion of your visit and tests but this payment will be based on what they feel is "usual and customary"—not on what the actual fee is. It's important to keep in mind that "usual and customary" has no basis in reality; it's just a number that works for the insurance company's bottom line. Remember that "usual and customary" care is not designed to get you well, but is designed to cover up your symptoms and "manage" your illness in the most cost-effective way.

Other things not considered "usual and customary" might be the cost of any nutritional supplements or bio-identical hormones that may be necessary for your body to heal. However, if your insurance is a high-deductible HSA (health savings account), your doctor can write and sign a one-sentence statement that all out-of-pocket costs such as nutritional supplements and bio-identical, compounded hormones are "medically necessary."

Working Within Your Health Plan

If you have health insurance, there is no doubt that choosing providers within your health plan will help save money. There are many excellent doctors who have made the decision to contract with insurance companies. What you need to remember is that many of these doctors and other professionals simply don't have a lot of time to spend with you at each appointment. They may have just enough time to medicate your symptoms so that you can function in life—most don't have adequate time to get to the reversible risk factors underlying your autoimmune condition. In fact, they typically have less than ten minutes per patient and most are seeing over twenty patients a day. I call this medicine on roller skates!

As your own health advocate—especially if you can't find a functional or integrative medicine doctor to do the time-consuming work, or you can't afford their upfront fees—you will need to acknowledge the limitations of this level of care and do all of your own footwork in advance of your appointment. You must be ready with a list of questions and specific requests for functional tests, etc. You will have to be patient and understand that your doctor is in a hurry, and even though she probably wants to spend more time with you, she has a waiting room full of people.

Be prepared to educate your doctor—yes, you read that right—on the nature and importance of the tests you're asking for. You may be requesting things that she is not familiar with, and in some cases hasn't even heard of, which may catch her off guard. Explaining these things quickly may not be easy, but it may be necessary in order to get your doctor to order the tests you need. Now is not the time to get snappy or demanding. We all know the stressful feeling of not having enough time to do a job right, so keep this in mind and do your best to be clear and to the point, asking for exactly what you want.

It is possible to maximize your health benefits and get well within this type of system, but you must be willing to take on most of the responsibility and guide the process.

Even if you do find a practitioner within your plan who is willing to order the tests and prescribe a treatment plan and help you work with your insurance company, you must still be prepared to pay for supplements and bio-identical hormones, as most health plans do not consider them a covered benefit.

Make Your Health a Top Priority

When you make your health a top priority, you direct the process of getting well and everything becomes *your* decision. You become an educated consumer of services, and you expect your doctors to help you identify the cause of your illness and to help you get well. You expect your health insurance company to serve that journey wherever possible—not to dictate your treatment.

In essence, you demand a higher level of care and you're willing to pay for it.

This might be a new way of thinking for you and it may be hard at first to justify spending money on something that "should" be paid for. You probably already pay for all or part of your health insurance every month with the expectation that it will insure your health. Unfortunately, as you know, that expectation is rarely met, especially in the case of chronic illnesses such as autoimmune conditions.

If you find yourself struggling with this concept, consider reframing the situation as loving yourself enough to put part of your discretionary income toward getting well.

From a more practical standpoint, getting and staying healthy will actually save you thousands of dollars over your lifetime.

Let me put things into perspective….

Consider the cost of dining out, or what you spend on items such as alcohol and coffee each month. The average North American spends over $1000 a year on coffee alone and another $2000 a year on going out for lunch during the week. This doesn't even include alcohol or more expensive dinners on the weekends. In fact, statistics show that Americans spend over $90 billion per year on alcohol alone.

Then we turn around and spend another $320 billion on prescription and over-the-counter drugs to manage the chronic symptoms caused in part by our unhealthy lifestyles!

Take a look at the statistics, according to *The Use of Medicines in the United States: Review of 2011*, a report by IMS Health:[2]

In 2011, U.S. consumers and their insurance companies spent:
- $23.2 billion on oncologics (cancer drugs)

- $21.0 billion on drugs to treat asthma and chronic obstructive pulmonary disease (COPD)
- $20.1 billion on lipid regulators (cholesterol lowering drugs)
- $19.6 billion on drugs to manage diabetes
- $18.2 billion on antipsychotic drugs for disorders such as bipolar disorder and schizophrenia.
- $12.2 billion on drugs to manage autoimmune conditions
- $11 billion on antidepressants

The same report revealed that in 2010, U.S. consumers and their insurance companies spent an astonishing $7.2 billion on the cholesterol-lowering prescription drug Lipitor. We spent another $6.8 billion on Nexium, one of several proton-pump inhibitors (PPIs) to treat heartburn and acid reflux. These are two disorders easily reversed by following a healthy lifestyle.[3,4]

The report did not include spending on over-the-counter drugs and other temporary fixes. Spending for non-durable medical products, such as over-the-counter medicines, reached an astonishing $44.8 billion in 2010!

Not a single one of these drugs address the underlying causes of illness, and in most cases just add to our toxic burden; have uncomfortable and possibly dangerous side effects; and cost us billions of dollars.

In conclusion, making your health a top priority may involve shifting some of your values about how you spend your money, but in the long run it will save you money and pain down the road. Your health is an investment and you're worth every penny. Pay a little more now to get the long-term optimal health you deserve, and the extra energy and vibrant health will be more than worth the extra expense in the prosperous years to come!

CHAPTER 3

Explore Different Medical Approaches

When medicine shifted from the art and science of "healing" to the "business of trying to understand the mechanisms of disease," much of the feminine, more intuitive, wisdom of the ancient ways was lost. If we are going to succeed in healing chronic illness and our world, we must bring the feminine back.

"Every patient carries her or his own doctor inside."
— ALBERT SCHWEITZER (1875 - 1965)

As I began my own recovery, I realized that one key part of my journey would be an in-depth exploration of the current medical modalities and approaches we have for treating autoimmune disorders in the United States. I carefully investigated each one, probing deeply into their respective limitations and potentials, and the following is what I discovered.

Western / Conventional / Orthodox / Medicine

The dominant medical model in this country is called Western, conventional, orthodox, or allopathic medicine. The term "allopathic" (from the Greek "allo" meaning "other") medicine was coined by Samuel Hahnemann, M.D., in the late 18th century in reference to the use of therapeutic modalities to treat symptoms. This type of medicine is based on a view of the world (and the body) that is very mechanical. Allopathic medicine operates under the belief that in order to understand something complex, such as the human body, you have to take it apart and reduce it to its simplest parts. Then, you directly address the part(s) of the body that seem to be malfunctioning with surgery or drugs (often without identifying the larger source of the problem). Basically, since the time of Pasteur's discovery of germs causing disease, allopathic medicine has looked for the single causes of specific diseases and targeted treatments accordingly.

Allopathic medicine excels in acute and emergency care. There is no argument that without this model many people would die unnecessarily from infections, wounds and other traumas.

But it has its limitations…

When we present a set of symptoms to our doctor, she imagines our bodies as a machine with a bunch of independent parts (organs) that work together, much like the parts of a clock. If we present her with symptoms such as weight gain, cold hands and feet, constipation and hair loss, she is trained to see that the "part" that needs fixing is probably the thyroid. She'll run a few tests to confirm or refute her diagnosis and then if necessary give us a prescription to "replace" the thyroid chemically. This is very satisfying because the approach is measurable and predictable.

But this approach doesn't take into consideration why the thyroid stopped producing optimal amounts of thyroid hormone, and, in most cases, the reason(s) it stopped will go untreated and lead to further health issues down the road.

In the case of autoimmune conditions, conventional Western doctors will say something like this: "We can observe how the immune system works, and we can track what happens to the different parts when things start to go wrong, but we don't know why things go wrong. The body just starts attacking its own tissues and we can't figure out how to effectively stop the process and get the immune system to work properly again."

The question of why the immune system is attacking "self" is not asked, and the patient is given immunosuppressive and anti-inflammatory drugs designed to suppress the immune system, which is only responding aggressively to the challenges presented to it.

These drugs may be necessary in acute situations and can help the person to feel more comfortable. However, pronged use of anti-inflammatory drugs can injure the immune system and cause other uncomfortable symptoms. Since the underlying challenges are not looked for and treated, the condition is likely to progress even if the symptoms are lessened.

As you have learned, the well-meaning physician is only allowed a short time with each patient. If you are sensitive to gluten, in a stressful job and bad relationship, and have also had exposure to heavy metals and you have a stealth infection affecting your immune system, she won't have the time to connect those triggers as contributing to your condition.

Because of our current medical model, allopathic medicine has a poor record treating, much less curing, autoimmune conditions. I believe this is because the singular disease model of illness fails when the body's entire system of wellness is disturbed by multiple aggravations (I call them "splinters" in this book). There is no single cause or a single cure.

Treatment should be a quest to uncover the roots of the illness with the curing or reversal of the autoimmune process as the goal – all while making the patient as comfortable as possible. Pain in and of itself is toxic to the body, mind and spirit, so I feel it is important for alternative practitioners to explore what conventional medicine has to offer in the way of acute pain management and anti-inflammatory drugs. It is up to the practitioner and patient to determine which is worse for the body – the pain, or the toxicity of the drug.

> **The Value of the Conventional Medical Approach**
> The conventional approach to autoimmune conditions is not without merit. The use of immunosuppressive drugs can be very helpful in managing acute inflammation. For example, if you have a patient with lupus, rheumatoid arthritis, or any type of acute flare up of an autoimmune process, the use of anti-inflammatory drugs can be extremely appropriate and help the patient achieve a better quality of life in the short term. Where conventional doctors miss the mark, is stopping here without looking for and treating the underlying cause of the illness.

For example, there certainly isn't anything wrong with taking aspirin when you have a headache but if you have a headache that goes on for six months, the aspirin ceases to be the most appropriate treatment and the question should be: *Why do I have this headache?*

I feel that pharmaceuticals can be appropriate and I definitely rely on the skills and wisdom of western medical doctors, especially in times of acute illness. Without them we'd wind up like Humpty Dumpty and in pain to boot!

Alternative Medicine

"Alternative Medicine" is an umbrella term used to refer to any treatment not taught by U.S. medical schools or offered at any U.S. hospital. The term is a bit misleading because by definition, alternative medicine is not a particular system or practice of medicine. In fact, it can refer to everything from natural and chiropractic to Ayurveda and traditional Chinese medicine…and everything in between.

> "Alternative medicine has come to mean a treatment, which is not the standard of care in conventional medicine. Basing a whole area of medicine on something which it is not, rather than on what it is, suggests that there is no theoretical foundation to the field of alternative medicine." — ANNA MACINTOSH, PH.D., N.D.[1]

I feel this term disrespects the individual philosophies and systems of valid healing modalities by lumping them into one category.

This is a situation that arises from the legal, political and societal dominance that conventional medicine enjoys, at least in the United States. Practically by definition, if the healer isn't a conventionally-educated and licensed practitioner of allopathic medicine, they are "Alternative" and what they can claim and practice is severely limited by law. They can be charged with "practicing medicine without a license" without regard to whether their patients are getting better or not.

Complementary and Alternative Medicine (CAM)

A common inclusive term for "Alternative" medicine these days is "Complementary and Alternative Medicine (CAM)." "Complementary Medicine" is any treatment outside of standard conventional medical practice that is used *in addition* to allopathic treatments. An example would be using herbs or meditation in conjunction with pharmaceutical blood pressure medications for treating hypertension. An alternative treatment becomes "complementary" when used in conjunction with an allopathic treatment, even if it may be used by itself and called simply "Alternative."

> "By using complementary as a synonym for alternative medicine, allopathic doctors are comfortable with alternative treatments

used in conjunction with, but not instead of allopathic treatments. This inappropriate interchange of terms creates unwarranted assumptions and dilutes the credibility of alternative medicines in the mind of health care consumers. It suggests that all non-synthetic agents (i.e. nutrient, herbal, other supplements) are unproven in efficacy and have all been compared to synthetic drugs for their overall safety and effectiveness."

— Anna MacIntosh, Ph.D., N.D.[2]

The Federal Government established the National Center for Complementary and Alternative Medicine (NCCAM) in 1998 with a mission to "define, through rigorous scientific investigation, the usefulness and safety of complementary and alternative medicine interventions and their roles in improving health and health care."[3] NCCAM is funded by about $128 million per year. In comparison, Matthew Herper of Forbes recently totaled R&D spending from 12 major pharmaceutical companies from 1997 to 2011: they had spent $802 billion to gain approval for just 139 drugs—that's a stupendous $5.8 billion per drug![4] It's clear that we can't expect a revolution in "rigorous scientific investigation" for "alternative interventions" when the government agency funding research operates on about 1/50th the amount of money it takes to test and approve one conventional drug.

On one hand, conventional medicine and government are concerned that unregulated, snake oil salesmen may divert patients who need serious medical intervention into unproven treatments that might not do any good. On the other hand, our system is rigged so that unproven treatments that can't be patented and sold for large profits will never get a chance to be "proven."

Many alternative and CAM healing approaches address the "symptoms" of chronic illness in the same way conventional medicine does. The therapies can help an individual manage pain or "live well" with their condition while avoiding the long-term use of toxic pharmaceuticals. These treatments are often quite helpful; however, many practitioners rely on intuition and guesswork rather than scientific testing. Thus, all of the underlying causes of the autoimmune process are rarely found, and the disease progresses.

Traditional Medicine

The term "traditional medicine" encompasses the vast field of knowledge acquired from ancient cultures. It is not the same as "orthodox medicine," which is the dominant paradigm in our current society. "Traditional" is defined as opinions, doctrines, practices, rites, and customs handed down over time by different cultures, especially by oral communication. Correct word usage would dictate "traditional medicine" to designate Chinese, Ayurvedic, Tibetan, or other ancient indigenous medical systems. All of these have centuries-old philosophies and practices, which are heavily rooted in the traditions of each society. Cultural, spiritual and societal beliefs have often influenced traditional medicines although many systems are complex and integrated. Many of these traditional medicines aim at creating a state of personal wellness that is less vulnerable to disease, and when disease happens, they have treatments aimed at helping the body heal itself.

Traditional medical systems fall under the category of alternative medicine.

Many states license acupuncturists and numerous insurance companies have begun to pay for acupuncture in applications where it has been proven effective. In fact, even the United States Army is employing acupuncture as a much needed alternative to pain medication for troops coming back from combat.

Natural Medicine

Natural medicine, also a form of alternative medicine, is a system of medicine that originated in the early 1900's. Natural medicine is defined as the "science and art of preventing, curing or alleviating ill health using treatment modalities in harmony with the laws of nature."[5]

Natural medicine is also called naturopathy and practitioners are called naturopaths.

Naturopaths are licensed in a number of states to practice medicine within certain limits. Naturopathy focuses on the use of nontoxic healing methods derived from the world's traditional healing systems. Natural medicine focuses on the individual rather than the disease.

Integrative/Holistic and Functional Medicine

Integrative, also called *holistic*, medical approaches to chronic illness, such as autoimmune disease, have been very successful because they address the body, mind and spirit, targeting the root causes of illness and aiming at restoring wellness. The patient is invited to collaborate in the process. Integrative medicine is informed by empirical evidence and focuses on the whole person—not just the "dis-ease." Integrative practitioners make use of all appropriate healing modalities, which can include both alternative, traditional, and conventional treatments, to achieve the goal of wellness. A good integrative practitioner may use the best tools of allopathic medicine for any given condition, but will also keep the entire state of being of the patient in mind, aiming to restore them to a healthy, disorder-resistant state of wellness.

> "Integrative medicine seeks to incorporate treatment options from conventional and alternative approaches, taking into account not only physical symptoms, but also psychological, social and spiritual aspects of health and illness." — THE OSHER CENTER FOR INTEGRATIVE MEDICINE AT THE UNIVERSITY OF CALIFORNIA

The emerging field of functional medicine may hold the most promise for curing chronic illness, because it takes the integrative approach one step further by incorporating cutting-edge, advanced scientific testing. Genetic information from specialized testing may also be utilized. It is grounded in scientific principles and information widely available in medicine today, combining research from various disciplines such as toxicology, biochemistry, physiology, psychology, anatomy, and genetics.

Dr. Elizabeth Lipski, a certified clinical and holistic nutritionist who has been working in the field of holistic and complementary medicine for over 25 years, describes it this way:

> "In older systems of medicine it was believed that the body was self-regulating and that disease occurred when this self-regulation became disrupted. In more contemporary terms we speak of feedback loops. When these feedback mechanisms get stuck or disrupted, imbalances and disharmony occur. We call this being "sick." The aim of functional medicine is to help your body

to come back into dynamic alignment.

"Functional medicine focuses not on endpoint or pathological state, but on the dynamic processes which underlie and precede it. While acknowledging the existence of pathology as well as a need to understand it, functional medicine focuses on the underlying processes and seeks a path of therapy that engages these underlying events. Functional medicine is used in combination with contemporary medicine for the best possible approach."

In other words, functional medicine chooses from the best available treatment methods by their merits alone. Many functional medical practitioners value a variety of ancient and traditional ways of healing, as well as conventional treatments. Functional medicine may employ a wide variety of healing methods, tailored to the individual situation, according to the experience of the practitioner. From there, doctor and patient collaborate over which treatment methods are most appropriate. A good practitioner is open to numerous modalities, but will look to science and empirical testing to determine the diagnosis and which treatments will be the safest and the most effective for a particular person.

In the case of autoimmune disorders, an effective practitioner looks for the underlying cause(s) of why the immune system is attacking the body, and then chooses from the full spectrum of healing modalities to address each factor until the immune system quiets down and the body heals.

Typically, when there's a choice, the least invasive treatment is chosen from the full spectrum of healing modalities, taking into consideration patient compliance—meaning the patient's willingness to believe in it, pay for it, follow through with it, and then maintain their health.

You may be interested to know that many "alternative," natural, traditional, integrative and holistic practitioners have been using functional testing in their practices for over 20 years with much success!

The Foundation for Alternative and Integrative Medicine states on their Web site:

"The Foundation for Alternative and Integrative Medicine believes that functional medicine is the bridge that will unite allopathic medicine (Western medicine) and alternative and integrative medicine as we move into the future. Functional medicine looks at the symptom as a sentinel, telling the patient there is an imbalance in the body. This can then be investigated to see what organ system needs to be addressed to restore health to the body rather than simply treating the symptom."

A New Vision is Needed to Heal

Each practice of medicine that I've outlined possesses a vast body of knowledge and power for helping and curing a great number of illnesses. Most practitioners care about their patients and intend to serve them. The problem that I see is that the majority of these medical systems do not recognize that chronic conditions can be completely reversed. This innocent lack of vision is not limited only to those trained in medicine: society has also trained patients to be passive consumers of medical treatments. Most of us feel that we do our part by showing up for appointments and taking recommended drugs, herbs or supplements. We go through the motions of treatment without setting out to really heal. Since we don't believe full reversal is possible, we don't try.

We didn't sail around the world when we thought it was flat. Even the bravest and most knowledgeable sailors were intimidated. Once people realized the world was round, it became commonplace.

I believe that in the future—hopefully the near future—the roots of autoimmune conditions will be universally recognized and medicine will routinely aim at reversing the autoimmune process. Until that time, it is up to the individual to be an intrepid explorer and seek the best help that's available for their healing journey. You can help prove the autoimmune world is round.

Art Versus Science

Whatever practice of medicine is concerned, there is both art and science that goes into healing. Some practitioners have too much of one but not enough of the other. The difference between practitioners is told by patient outcome. Do the patients get better? Different practitioners of the same style of medicine can get very different results. Look for practitioners with a record of success in the art and science of healing.

Heal Faster While Saving Time and Money

Reversing an autoimmune condition is a time-sensitive issue. Cutting out the guesswork is critical, because you need to get to the root cause before the condition progresses.

Functional testing allows the practitioner to know exactly what is going on nutritionally, how the gut is functioning, and if there is toxicity, food sensitivities or infections that are part of the problem. You are not left running from practitioner to practitioner "trying on" different treatments and supplements for what someone intuits "might" be causing your condition. Instead, you and your doctor are armed with knowledge and the power to act quickly and efficiently.

The Ingredients of a Successful Model of Healing

Integrative/holistic medicine, with the addition of the functional medicine technology and treatment modality, more closely resembles some of the ancient models of healing such as Ayurveda. These ways of healing reach beyond palliative and emergency care to bring the body into optimal balance.

The successful treatment of autoimmune conditions always includes:
- Recognizing the individual as having a unique biochemistry and life circumstances
- Strengthening with nutrition (whole foods, correcting deficiencies, probiotics, etc.) exercise and proper rest
- Enhancing the body's natural detoxification by supporting the liver and healing the gastrointestinal tract
- Finding and removing toxins (i.e. bacteria, fungus, viruses, heavy metals, and chemicals)
- Cultivating happiness and a sense of purpose!

> **What You Need to Know:**
> The body knows how to be healthy and will naturally move toward vibrant health if given what it needs, such as happy thoughts and fulfilling relationships; vibrant food and proper nutrients; healthy GI and eliminatory systems; good detoxification pathways; and healthy environments.

Finding a Practitioner

If you already have a diagnosis of an autoimmune thyroid condition, you will need to have a heart-to-heart conversation with your practitioner to ask her if she will support you through the process of reversing your condition. If she is willing, great! If not, you MUST find a new practitioner!

If you do not have a practitioner or you need to find a new one, you have two options:

1. Find a functional or integrative practitioner who has had success in reversing autoimmune conditions.
2. Find an integrative, functional or conventional practitioner who is at least open to the concept that your condition can be reversed, is willing to order the required tests, and will support you 100 percent in your quest for health.

Finding a practitioner who has had success with reversing autoimmune conditions is an obvious first choice. At the very least, your practitioner must recognize the value in eliminating the stresses that weigh on your immune system and be willing to order appropriate tests to reveal where those stresses come from.

Most practitioners are not trained to uncover and treat the many underlying factors that cause chronic illness. Finding the right practitioner often takes time, effort and determination, but your choice will profoundly influence your ability to heal. You can find a functional medical doctor by visiting the Institute for Functional Medicine's website at www.functionalmedicine.org. Click on the tab "Functional Medicine Resources" and choose "Find a Functional Medicine Practitioner" to find someone in your area. If you find a practitioner in your area, be sure to ask if they offer functional medical testing and have experience treating and reversing autoimmune conditions. Alternatively, we have compiled a list of practitioners on *The Thyroid Cure* Web site at www.thethyroidcure.com/practitioners

Besides medical doctors (M.D.), there are other types of practitioners who can facilitate your healing process, if they understand the principles of reversing the autoimmune process detailed in this book:

- Doctor of Osteopathy—D.O.
- Natural Doctor—N.D.
- Doctor of Chiropractic Medicine—D.C.
- Doctor of Oriental Medicine—D.O.M.
- Physician's Assistant—P.A.
- Nurse Practitioner—N.P.
- Holistic/Integrative Nutritionists—degrees vary

Screening Candidates

Regardless of which route you choose, here are some questions to ask prospective candidates before you schedule your first appointment:

I have been diagnosed with _____. Do you feel my condition can be reversed?

Ideally, you'd love to find a practitioner who responds with an enthusiastic "Yes!" But if a practitioner is familiar with integrative or functional medicine, speaks from the perspective of addressing the cause of your symptoms, and is open to the possibility of a complete reversal of your condition, that's an excellent place to start.

I believe it's important not only to supplement Thyroid hormone, but also to find and eliminate the underlying triggers that are causing my immune system to destroy my thyroid gland. I have research backed by progressive physicians that will help guide us to identify different infectious, allergenic, and toxicological factors that may be driving the autoimmune response. Are you willing to work with me and advocate tests and treatments to identify and eliminate these factors?

The answer to this question should be "Yes!"

Do you have experience helping other people reverse similar conditions?

Ideally the answer should be "Yes!" There are practitioners in the country who are experienced in helping people reverse their autoimmune conditions. We have compiled a list of practitioners on *The Thyroid Cure* Web site at www.thethyroidcure.com/practitioners

If you are unable to find a practitioner who has direct experience, you will want to find someone who has an open mind and is willing to help you find and treat all of the underlying triggers in your autoimmunity.

What type of diagnostic testing do you utilize in your practice to get to the root of the condition?

Ideally you will want to find a practitioner who has access to a lab that can run a complete serum (blood) thyroid panel. In addition, you will want a practitioner who utilizes functional medical testing from functional laboratories such as Metametrix and Genova (who have now merged), Spectracell, Doctor's Data or Diagnos-Tech's. Functional testing goes into greater detail and covers more ground than traditional doctors are used to looking at. This testing is based on strict science but most doctors are not yet aware of their existence or how to use their findings.

Do you utilize therapies for detoxification and healing the GI tract?

The answer to this question should be "Yes!" The practitioner should tell you that the therapies will depend on your test results and individual needs.

Do you take insurance, or are you fee-for-service?

If you have health insurance, it's good to know up front what your plan will cover and what you will be expected to pay. Many functional and integrative practitioners have made the decision to break free of insurance company dictates and will not accept insurance as payment. This is typically a good thing, because they have the freedom to spend more time with you and can utilize advanced testing and treatments that will address the root of your condition fast. Many practitioners will help you maximize your benefits by providing you a super bill to submit to your insurance company.

Keep in mind that the cost of getting well is always ultimately cheaper than the long term costs of being sick. In the short run, healing may cost you more money, but staying sick will eventually lead to more pain and costly illness, perhaps even unnecessarily losing years of your life.

What is the cost for the initial office visit, and how long will the practitioner spend with me? What is the cost for a follow-up appointment, and what is the time I'll be allotted with the practitioner?

There is no "correct" answer to this question, and practitioners' fees will vary. The most important thing is to find a practitioner who will spend at least 45 minutes with you on the first visit and at least 30 minutes on follow-ups. Only you can decide whether the fees are within your budget.

Does the doctor correspond via e-mail or take after-hours calls? If so, what is the fee for these services?

Again, there is no "correct" answer to this question, but it's worth it to ask upfront so that there are no surprises.

Do you have a Web site? Can you send me some more information about your practice and the practitioner's clinical training?

Not every practitioner's office has a Web site, bio or brochure to send to patients, but many do. It's a good idea to learn as much as possible about the person you are entrusting your health with.

There is a lot you can do to feel better and begin healing on your own without the help of a medical practitioner. Still, many people will need access to detailed testing, advanced medical knowledge, and the medicines required to treat infections and the other factors exacerbating their autoimmune response. The bad news is that good practitioners for reversing autoimmune conditions are still hard to find. The good news is that you are determined to succeed and will do what it takes to find the right one.

CHAPTER 4

Discover Your Thyroid

"It doesn't matter if you're a killer whale or a human or a mouse or a guinea pig — you've all got thyroid hormones. You've all got the same kind of immune system." – PETER ROSS

How a Healthy Thyroid Functions

The thyroid is a small, butterfly-shaped gland that sits just below your larynx, or Adam's apple. It weighs less than an ounce and is made up of two halves called lobes that lie along the trachea. It's controlled by a small, peanut-shaped gland in the brain called the pituitary.

When the levels of thyroid hormones drop too low, the pituitary will produce thyroid-stimulating hormone (TSH), which in turn stimulates the thyroid to make more hormones. As the levels of thyroid hormones rise in the blood, the pituitary senses the elevation and decreases TSH levels. Conversely, when thyroid hormones lower in the blood, TSH levels rise.

The pituitary gland is controlled by the hypothalamus. It's the hypothalamus that tells the pituitary to produce TSH. It does this by producing thyroid-releasing hormone (TRH)

Once stimulated, the thyroid gland takes up iodide from the foods we eat and converts it into iodine to make the thyroid hormones thyroxine (T4) and triiodothyronine (T3). The thyroid cells convert iodide into iodine inside of the gland using a process that requires hydrogen peroxide (H_2O_2) With the help of an enzyme called thyroid peroxidase (TPO), it combines the iodine with the amino acid tyrosine on the backbone of thyroglobulin protein molecules, and thyroglobulin splits and forms the thyroid hormones T4 and T3. These hormones are then released into the bloodstream where they are essential to the development of literally every cell in the body.

The thyroid produces both T4 and T3, but T3 is approximately three times more potent than T4 and is the active form of the hormone. In order to get more T3, a healthy body will convert roughly 60 percent of the circulating T4 into T3. This process occurs mostly in the liver by an enzyme called iodothyronine 5' deiodinase. The remaining T4 is converted to T3 in a healthy GI tract. If you have a healthy liver and GI tract you'll be optimally converting T4 into T3 and feel great! If your liver and GI tract are compromised in some way, the conversion will not take place at adequate levels, and signs of hypothyroidism will be present.

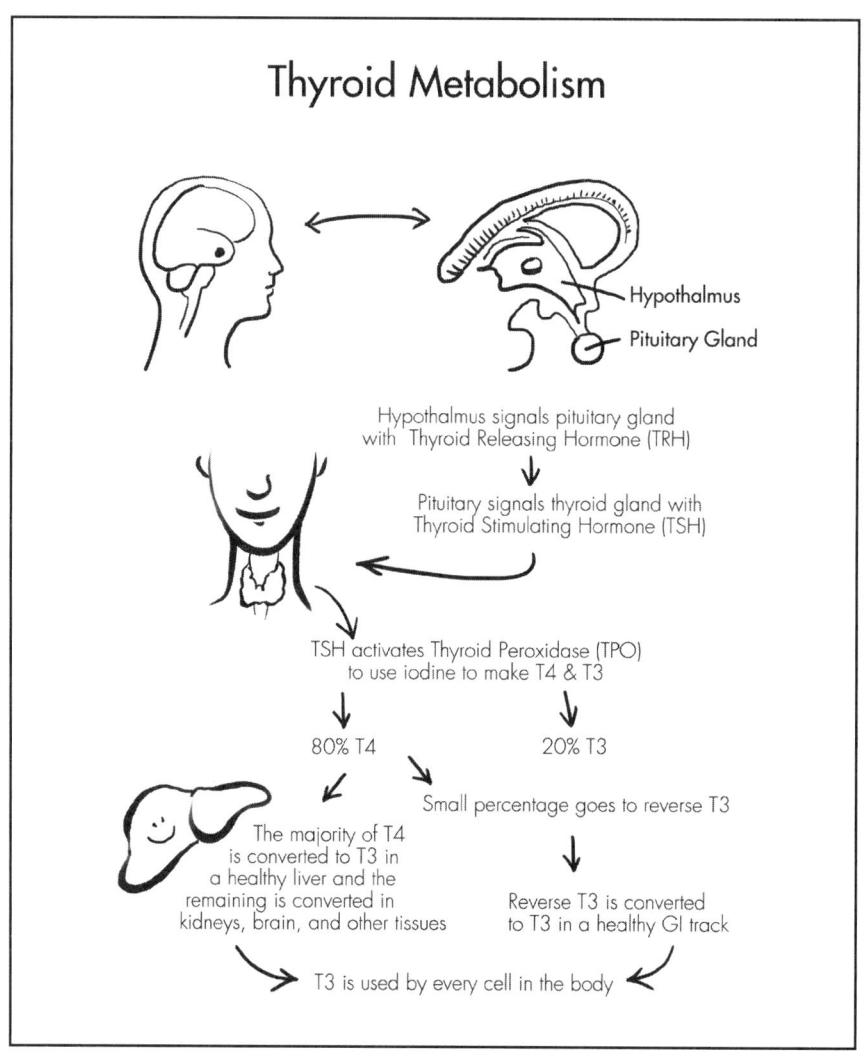

> **Your Liver and Your Thyroid:** Your liver is responsible for converting the thyroid hormone T4 into the active hormone T3, and it needs the mineral selenium to do it. If your liver is stressed-out and overloaded, it can't do the job of converting these hormones and you'll be called a "poor converter," which means you don't have enough of the active thyroid hormone circulating in your body. The results are you'll feel sick and tired even if you're taking T4 hormone replacement.

Some common reasons your liver might not be converting T4 to T3:

- Stress
- Alcohol
- Sugar
- Trans fats
- Advanced glycation end products (AGE's)
- High carbohydrate diet
- Leaky gut and selenium deficiency
- Heavy metals
- Petrochemicals and other toxins
- Infections such as Candida

If you have been diagnosed with an autoimmune thyroid condition, in fact any autoimmune condition, supporting your liver is critical to recovery!

> Think of your thyroid gland as your body's furnace, and your pituitary gland as its thermostat. When the furnace (thyroid) gets too cold, the thermostat (pituitary) will sense it and produce TSH to stimulate the production of thyroid hormones, which effectively turns up the heat. When the levels of thyroid hormones rise and the furnace gets hot, the pituitary slows the production of TSH, which turns the heat down.

Why We Need Optimal Thyroid Hormone Levels

Just Google "the role of thyroid hormones" and you will find thousands of scholarly articles that have been written on the functions of thyroid hormones. Thyroid hormones regulate the metabolic functions of literally every cell in the body—from brain chemistry to digestion.

Maintaining optimal thyroid hormone levels are important to achieving and maintaining vibrant health.

Let's take a brief look at some of the areas where they play a key role:

Body Weight and Metabolism: Ultimately, your body temperature and metabolism affect your body composition. If the hormones are too high, you feel hot all the time, and you may become too thin. If your hormones are too low, you feel cold all the time, and you will burn fewer calories and gain weight. Thyroid hormones assist in the conversion of food into energy and heat. Low thyroid hormones slow down the conversion of glucose and fat into energy, which results in a slow metabolism and weight gain—even on restricted calorie diets. It also impairs the production of human growth hormone (HGH), which is needed to make lean muscle mass.

Stress: Optimal thyroid hormones are needed to produce the adrenal hormones cortisol and DHEA, which help us to manage stress. Both hyperthyroidism and hypothyroidism play a role in adrenal fatigue and exhaustion, resulting in low levels of these protective hormones.

Sex Hormones: Low thyroid hormones can cause an imbalance of testosterone, estrogen and progesterone leading to many conditions such as infertility, low libido, weight gain, menstrual problems, symptomatic menopause, polycystic ovarian syndrome, hair loss and the risk of certain cancers that are associated with imbalanced sex hormones.

Aging: Thyroid hormones regulate the production of human growth hormone (HGH). Low thyroid hormones depress this important hormone leading to accelerated aging, osteoporosis, skin wrinkles, increased body fat, low energy levels, and decreased lean muscle mass.

Immune System: Thyroid hormones play a crucial role in the development and regulation of the cells involved in both humeral and cell-mediated immunity, thus protecting the body from infections and viruses. This is why individuals with low levels of thyroid hormone suffer from chronic infections.

Brain Function: Hypothyroidism depletes pregnenolone, which is often called the "mother" of all hormones because it is a key building block in the production of all steroid hormones. It acts to improve memory and combat depression, and it also has powerful anti-inflammatory properties. Thyroid hormones also affect brain chemistry by stimulating and regulating the action of neurotransmitters such as serotonin, norepinephrine, and GABA (gamma aminobutyric acid). These neurotransmitters are important in the regulation of anxiety, mood, sleep, appetite and sexuality.

Cardiovascular System/Cholesterol Levels: Optimal thyroid hormones protect against heart disease by normalizing homocysteine levels in the blood. They regulate circulation, increasing blood supply to the hands, feet and surface of the skin. Increased blood supply delivers essential fatty acids and nutrients, which keep the skin soft and healthy. Hypothyroidism slows metabolism, which decreases the liver's ability to clear cholesterol from the blood, resulting in high cholesterol and triglycerides. Low thyroid levels are frequently associated with hypercholesterolemia and may increase the risk of atherosclerosis. Low thyroid hormones can cause an enlarged heart and impair the heart's ability to pump efficiently.

Digestion: Low levels of thyroid hormones cause constipation, and slow the production of stomach acid by depleting the hormone gastrin. Hyperthyroidism can cause diarrhea and rapid transit time of food through the GI tract. Both of these conditions increase the risk of chronic GI infections from harmful yeast and bacteria and can lead to inflammation, malabsorption, nutrient deficiencies, leaky gut, food allergies and uncomfortable GI symptoms such as gastroesophageal reflux disease (GERD).

Liver and Gallbladder Function: Thyroid hormones help the liver and gallbladder to function optimally, which affects detoxification, hormone production and the conversion of T4 to T3.

Anemia: Hypothyroidism can cause a decrease in the number of red blood cells that carry oxygen to the body's tissues. This condition is called anemia, which produces symptoms of pronounced fatigue.

Blood Sugar Regulation: Thyroid hormones regulate the absorption of glucose into the cells as well as the elimination of excess glucose. Hypothyroidism slows the rate of absorption and elimination, resulting in symptoms of hypoglycemia or dysglycemia.

Ideal Body Temperature: According to researchers at Albert Einstein College of Medicine, "98.6 degree body temperature strikes a perfect balance: warm enough to ward off fungal infection but not so hot that we need to eat nonstop to maintain our metabolism." Thyroid activity is directly related to body temperature as thyroid hormones govern your basal metabolic rate to generate energy (or heat). A classic indicator of poor thyroid function is feeling cold (or hot for hyperthyroidism). This may be why so many people with low thyroid hormones suffer from chronic fungal infections!

> **Why Do You Lose Hair with a Thyroid Disorder?**
> Hair growth has three phases: the *anagen* phase, the *catagen* phase and the *dormant* phase. When a person suffers from an imbalance in thyroid function—either too much thyroid hormone (hyperthyroidism) or too little thyroid hormone (hypothyroidism)—the mechanism of the hair growth process can be disturbed or shut down. Changes in metabolism due to thyroid function can cause hair follicles to remain in the dormant phase for longer than normal, which leads to stunted hair growth and hair loss. Think of it this way: under times of stress the body works to conserve energy for the repair and regeneration of essential body functions, and since you can live without your hair, it diverts energy away from hair growth. Many times, thyroid imbalance exists with GI imbalances such a leaky gut so the absorption of nutrients the body needs for hair growth is compromised, as well as the optimal temperature needed for chemical reactions. Many people enjoy the pleasure of hair regrowth when they optimize their thyroid hormones, reduce stress, heal their GI tracts and optimize their nutrition.

As you can see, the body needs optimal thyroid hormones to be healthy. When thyroid hormones become imbalanced and are too high, or, more commonly, too low, we begin to experience some pretty severe symptoms.

There are many reasons our thyroid hormones can become imbalanced—from nutrient deficiencies and adrenal fatigue to conditions of the pituitary gland and other illnesses. While the principles in this book are applicable to many autoimmune disorders, our primary focus is to address thyroid dysfunction caused by the autoimmune conditions known as Graves' and Hashimoto's. We will discuss each of these conditions in detail in Chapter 7: Autoimmune Thyroid Conditions. First, however, I'd like to give you a basic overview of the immune system.

CHAPTER 5

Understand Your Immune System

"In an autoimmune condition the immune system's white blood cells are attacking normal body tissues in a state of chaos and confusion. Therefore the less confused and the more certain and educated you are, the better it is for your immune system." – Dr. Alexander Haskell

You've made the commitment to reverse your thyroid condition and you're ready to get started. So how much do you really need to know about the immune system to get better? The truth is, not that much; however, a basic understanding of the cells and organs of the immune system and how they function will help you to become more empowered in your health. I found that as I learned more about my immune system, I was able to connect the dots as to why I was experiencing an autoimmune response in my body. I also found that I was able to communicate intelligently with my doctors about my diagnosis and treatment. After all, when you know what's going on you can ask good questions and you can decipher which treatments will make the most sense for you. We are our own best healers and it's our responsibility to educate ourselves. Who knows, you may even find yourself enlightening your doctor about a few things!

In this chapter, I will give you a brief overview of how the immune system functions.

Immune System Basics

The immune system is a complex web of interdependent cell types that protect the body from bacteria, viruses, parasites, molds, environmental toxins, and the growth of cancer cells. To put it in basic terms, the immune system has the job of identifying the cells and organisms that belong in the body and eliminating or neutralizing anything that doesn't belong. This miraculous system is made up of protective barriers, bone marrow, white blood cells, lymphatic vessels and organs, and various specialized cells and substances that work in harmony to keep us healthy.

Immunity

At birth, our immune system is functional but immature. This is what is called our innate immunity. As we mature and get exposed to a variety of harmful invaders, our immune system becomes more sophisticated. This is called our adaptive immunity.

Our immunity is influenced by many factors beginning with our mother's body, her emotions, her nutrition, her personal relationships and her environment. When we are born naturally through the birth canal, we are exposed to our mothers vaginal and bowel flora, which helps establish our own balance of healthy microbes. When we are breastfed, our mother passes her healthy flora on to us in the colostrum and breast milk. This helps the colonization of our gut flora and sets the stage for a strong immune system. It's important to know that 60 to 80 percent of the body's immune system cells live in the tissues of the gastrointestinal track to keep potentially unfriendly flora in check.

> **What You Need to Know:**
> Our immune system is influenced by all of our interactions with the world. Literally every thought, emotion, personal relationship, food choice, as well as our surroundings, has an influence on this incredible mass of cellular information. If we are to be healthy, we must do our utmost to make every encounter with the world around us as positive as possible!

The Barriers

The skin is your body's largest organ, and arguably the first line of defense in the immune system's barriers. It wraps our entire body in what is probably the most magnificent packaging the world has ever seen.

The skin allows our body to detoxify through sweat glands, and it does a great job of keeping large organisms and toxic molecules from getting in our bodies and causing harm, but many of us don't realize how porous it actually is. We absorb a lot through the skin. Just think about it: transdermal skin patches and creams are often used to deliver hormones, nicotine, pain killers, and other drugs directly into the bloodstream simply through application to the skin. From contaminants in our water supply to toxic chemicals in our lotions and cosmetics, everything our skin comes into contact with has the ability to affect our immune systems.

Apart from being a protective barrier, our skin is our largest sensory organ, with millions of tiny nerve endings just below the surface. These receptors interact with the world through the sensations of heat, cold, pain, pressure and contact. Our immune systems are influenced by these sensations—especially contact with other living beings. A hug, the gentle caress of a lover's hand, therapeutic massage…we all need to be touched consistently for our immune systems to thrive.

> **What You Need to Know:**
> Your skin absorbs a lot. A good rule to follow while you're healing: If you wouldn't eat it, don't put in on your skin! You need to sweat to be healthy! You also need positive physical contact in order to thrive, so start hugging and loving, get a massage, hug a friend or a pet—whatever you do, get some love right now!

The mucus membranes of the GI tract, the lungs, mouth, nose and urogenital tracts make up your "internal skin," or secondary protective barrier. Throughout the entire length of the small intestine are patches of lymphoid tissue called Peyer's patches, which make up what is called "gut-associated lymphoid tissue," or GALT for short.

The GALT is home to as much as 80 percent of the body's immune cells and represents the largest mass of lymphoid tissue in the human body. The health of our GI tract is paramount to our wellbeing and you can bet that if you are experiencing an autoimmune condition, your GI tract is suffering.

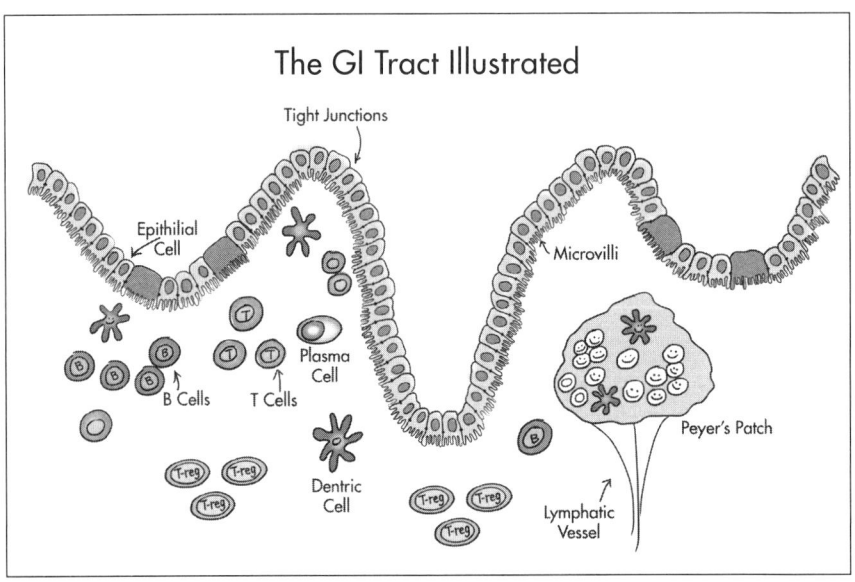

> **What You Need to Know:**
> The gastrointestinal tract is derived from the same embryonic cells as our skin. In fact, you can think of the GI tract as your skin on the inside. We are literally shaped like a doughnut with a hole down the middle! If you include the lining of the respiratory tract, it's easy to understand why the vast percentage of immune system cells live in and around the tissues of these areas. Everything you eat, drink, and breathe comes into contact with this inner tubing!

The GI Tract Illustrated

Think of your GI tract as the neighborhood your immune system lives in. Imagine it as a peaceful, clean neighborhood where the inhabitants take care of their homes and yards. The clean streets are lined with beautiful trees and flowers. The sky is clear blue with no pollution. Everyone is happy and healthy — it's a safe place, where you see children playing in the park and people walking their dogs and having a great time. There are happy caretakers in charge of caring for the trees and plants, and repairing cracks in the pavement and buildings. There is beautiful, uplifting music playing from the town center and sweet smells of greenery fill the air.

There is a synergy among the inhabitants, and everyone feels secure. The police force is strong and always ready to protect the inhabitants from any intruder who threatens the peace. The police captain is well-informed and has trained his force with precision. If an intruder comes into town causing unrest, he knows exactly how to direct his force to capture the invader and remove him before he causes harm. The police are not stressed-out and don't overreact to every little upset.

Now imagine your GI tract as a bad neighborhood. The homes are broken down or condemned. The sky is grey with pollution. There are no trees or flowers. The streets are dirty, and the residents are sickly and weak and have been mostly starved out by aggressive gang members. There are trucks that come through regularly to dump loads of corrosive material onto the streets, killing whatever is left of the living plants and even burning holes in the pavement. The only music playing is loud death metal and gangsta rap. There are daily riots and shootings, which cause the inhabitants to exist in a constant state of confusion, paranoia and hostility.

The police captain is completely stressed-out and on edge. There are emergency calls coming into the station every second of the day, resulting in officer dispatches around the clock. The entire force is always on high alert, waiting for the next attack. Because the police never get any rest from the turmoil in the streets, they become overworked and confused. After so many years of fighting, it gets to the point where they can't tell the difference between the innocent inhabitants and the bad guys. They become trigger-happy and shoot everything that moves, including the innocent.

In case this wasn't clear, the innocent inhabitants are the healthy tissue and cells, and the trees and flowers are beneficial bacteria like lactobacillus and bifidus. The happy caretakers are health-enhancing foods and nutrients, and the trucks dumping corrosive material are the unhealthy, chemical-laden, allergy-causing foods, drugs, and toxins that constitute an unhealthy lifestyle. The music, beautiful or toxic, equates to positive or negative thoughts. The gang members are opportunistic infectious agents such as harmful bacteria, parasites and fungus. The police force is your immune system—either strong, precise, rational and capable of protecting you when the bad guys strike, or overworked, confused and irrational, adding to the chaos in your body, attacking anything that moves, including your own tissue.

If you have an autoimmune condition, there is no doubt that your immune system is living a bad neighborhood! Just how bad, is hard to say and depends on many factors. It will be up to you and your practitioner to access the situation and determine what will be needed to clean it up.

While you can't move your immune system to a new neighborhood, you can clean up the one it's in…and you can do it fast. I will guide you through the process in Chapter 16: Heal Your Gut.

> **What You Need to Know:**
> Most of the cells of your immune system live in your gut. Research indicates that only 10-20 percent of patients with an autoimmune condition have a completely normal GI tract. If you have an autoimmune condition, your GI tract should be the first place to look for clues as to what's triggering your illness!

The Liver

The liver weighs about three pounds and sits on the right side of the abdomen just under the rib cage. It performs over 400 functions vital to life. The liver filters about three pints of blood every minute before passing it on for circulation in the body. The liver is responsible for detoxifying chemicals, metabolizing drugs and hormones, breaking down fats, and regulating blood sugar.

The liver removes toxins in two phases, known as Phase I and Phase II detoxification, which require a number of vitamins, minerals, amino acids, and phytochemicals found in foods in order to work properly.

Phase I processes the toxins through an array of chemical reactions involving P-450 enzymes. They are either neutralized or converted into intermediate forms and passed on to Phase II for further processing and elimination. Oxidation and/or hydrolysis are important parts of Phase I.

Phase II continues the neutralizing process by further transforming toxins so that they can that can be excreted via urine from the kidneys or by bile through the gut. Phase II involves six different pathways: glucuronidation, acetylation, sulfation, methylation, glycine conjugation, and glutathione conjugation.

Some substances are actually made more dangerous during Phase I. Dangerous free radicals are produced in the process. Proper nutrition, vitamins, and optimal liver function are thus particularly important so that Phase II is able to finish the job and neutralize the harmful byproducts of Phase I.

In addition to detoxification, the liver is critical for many aspects of digestion (breaking nutrients down) and assimilation (building up body tissues). It stores many essential vitamins (B12, A, D, E, and K) and minerals such as iron and copper. The liver produces the red blood cells that carry oxygen around the body. Specialized immune cells in the liver called Kupffer cells, destroy bacteria, small foreign proteins, and old blood cells, helping the body fight infections.

A number of prescription drugs, household and environmental chemicals, not to mention alcohol, are tough on the liver and may even cause lasting damage.

With its multitude of biochemical roles, it is easy to see how the liver can get into trouble either as a result of nutritional deficiencies or an overtaxing of its detoxification functions.

The Cells of the Immune System

Don't let the following scientific explanation glaze your eyes over and tempt you to put this book down. If you must, skim this part and return to it when your interest has piqued. It's important that you make it to the sections on autoimmune splinters and how to remove them.

All the cells of the immune system are formed in the bone marrow through a process called hematopoiesis. During this process, white blood cells called leukocytes change into either mature cells of the immune system or into precursors of cells that will continue their maturation elsewhere. The cells of the immune system live primarily in the GALT (gut-associated lymphoid tissue) and the organs of the lymphatic system.

There are over two dozen types of white blood cells produced in the bone marrow.

A comprehensive overview of them all is far beyond the scope of this book. To simplify things, I'll review the ones that play the most prominent roles in the immune response.

Our immune system effectively learns how to identify and "tag" potentially harmful foreign substances, identifying them as "antigens." It then "remembers" these antigens, so that if they're encountered again they can be effectively dealt with.

The immune system does this by two separate responses called cell-mediated immunity and humoral immunity.

Lymphocytes are the cells that make up both of these responses and they include B-cells and T-cells.

On the surface of each lymphocyte are cell receptors that enable them to recognize only one specific antigen. Imagine each of these cells are handed a picture of a different criminal and they each roam the body in search of their own "bad guy." This might seem crazy, but don't worry: your body makes up for this by producing so many lymphocyte cells that your immune system is able to recognize almost all antigens!

Cell-mediated immunity involves T-lymphocytes or T-cells. The "T" stands for thymus, a lymphoid immune system organ located just below the sternum and above the heart. T-cells mature and are "educated" in the thymus gland and then circulate throughout the bloodstream, the lymphatic system and the GALT. They are in charge of initiating, directing and stopping the fight against the foreign invaders (antigens). The initial T-cell response is called a Th1 response.

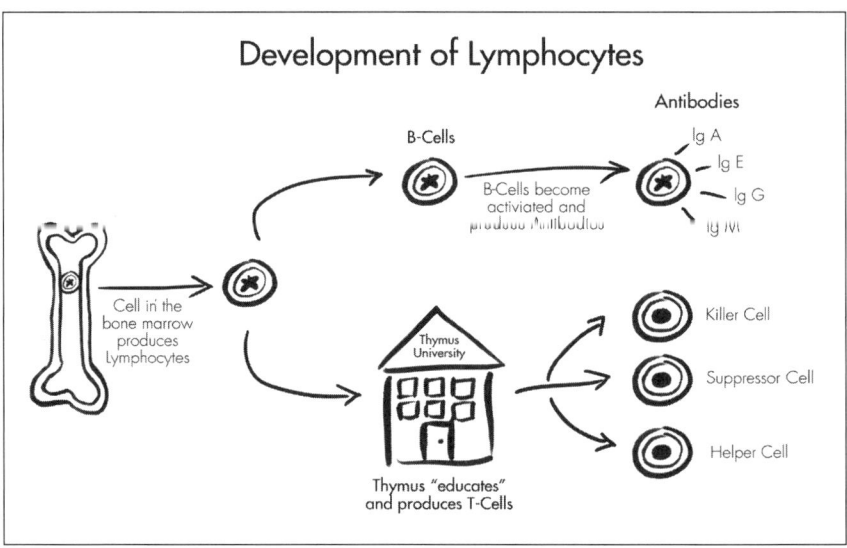

T-lymphocytes are called by different names depending on their function:

- Cytotoxic T-Cells/CD8+ T/Killer T-Cells:
  These cells are important in directly killing certain tumor cells, viral-infected cells, parasites, bacteria and fungus.

- Memory T-Cells (can be either CD4+ or CD8+):
  Memory T-cells are derived from normal T-cells that have learned how to overcome an invader by "remembering" the strategy used to defeat previous infections. They can live in the body for up to twenty years.

- Helper T-Cells, also called CD4+T:
  Once "activated," these cells play a major role in controlling and regulating the immune system by communicating with other cells by the secretion of proteins called cytokines that activate other white blood cells to fight off infection. Cytokines include interleukins, growth factors, and interferons. Cytokines are responsible for controlling inflammation in the body and are triggered by stress, infections, toxins, poor nutrition, and a sedentary lifestyle.

- Regulatory T-Cells/CD4+reg:
  These are the peacekeepers who tell the immune system when the battle with the infectious pathogens is over and to stop fighting. They also suppress the activity of "self-attacking" T-cells that may have escaped destruction in the thymus. These are the cells that are very important in healing an autoimmune condition because they regulate (turn off) the immune response!

- Natural Killer Cells:
  Natural killer cells, often referred to as NK cells, are similar to the killer T-cells and directly kill certain tumors such as melanomas, lymphomas and viral-infected cells, such as herpes and cytomegalovirus.

Humoral immunity involves B-cells, which are also known as antibody-producing lymphocytes. B-cells proliferate and differentiate into plasma cells. Their job is to look for the invaders and then "tag" them with proteins called antibodies, which stick to *antigens* on the surface of parasites, bacteria and fungi. The invader is thus identified as a pathogen marked for destruction. Each B-cell produces a specific type of antibody called an immunoglobulin. If you've ever been tested for allergies or for the presence of antibodies to a particular bacteria or virus then you may recognize some of these. The "Ig" before the capital letter stands for "immunoglobulin."

This secondary B-cell antibody response is called the Th2 response.

The main types of antibodies are:

- Immunoglobulin A (IgA) is the chief antibody found in the mucous membranes, particularly those lining the respiratory passages and gastrointestinal tract. IgA makes up the first line of defense against microbes and antigens and is directly affected by the stress hormone cortisol, which we will talk about in later chapters. A lowered or suppressed IgA increases our risk for infections and allergies.
- Immunoglobulin G (IgG) is the most abundant type of antibody found in the blood and other body fluids. It protects against bacterial and viral infections.
- Immunoglobulin M (IgM), which is found mainly in the blood and lymph fluid, is the first to be made by B-cells to fight a new infection.
- Immunoglobulin E (IgE) is associated mainly with allergic reactions to environmental antigens such as pollen, dust mites or pet dander. It is found in the lungs, skin, and mucous membranes.

Phagocytes

This is a group of immune cells specialized in finding and "eating" bacteria, viruses, and dead or injured body cells. When they come across a foreign invader, they surround it, eat it and then die. In some cases, they kill microbes by dumping toxic chemicals on them such as hydrogen peroxide and hydrochloric acid. This action can sometimes damage any healthy tissue in the surrounding area.

There are three main types of phagocytes: the granulocyte, the macrophage, and the dendritic cell.

Granulocytes arrive at the scene of an infection in large numbers to engulf pathogens (antigens) and degrade them, using powerful chemicals. The pus in an infected wound is mostly made up of dead granulocytes. Granulocytes include neutrophils, eosinophils and basophils, which are predominant in the neutralization and removal of bacteria and parasites from the body.

Macrophages are referred to as scavengers or "big eaters," because they roam the body like Pac-Man, gobbling up pathogens. They are slower to respond to infections than the granulocytes, but they are bigger, longer living, and, unlike granulocytes, they "activate" or direct T-cell activity. They do this by displaying fragments of the antigen on their surfaces for T-helper cells to recognize. That is why they are also called *antigen-presenting cells*, or APC for short. Once a T-helper cell recognizes the antigen, it triggers the macrophage to send out a chemical alarm (cytokine) called interluekin-1, which in turn stimulates the T-helper cell to multiply and call for help by secreting a chemical called interleukin-2. Interluekin-2 calls in cytotoxic T-cells and B-cells to the scene to help fight the infection.

Dendritic cells also originate in the bone marrow and, like the macrophage, they function as antigen-presenting cells (APC). In fact, the dendritic cells are more efficient APCs than macrophages. They help lymphocytes decide whether to become T-helper or T-regulatory cells. In other words, they do a better job of activating T-helper cells.

Mast cells are like the body's water hose. They live in the skin, as well as the respiratory and GI tract. Unlike phagocytes, they prefer to flush out infections instead of eating or poisoning them. They produce chemicals such as histamine that signal body fluids from the blood to flush the mucous membranes and wash away the pathogen. Sometimes, they mistake harmless particles like pollen or dust as pathogens, which create an allergic reaction such as hay fever or hives.

The Organs

The Thymus

This wise gland is located just below the sternum and above the heart. It is often referred to as the "master gland of the immune system" because it not only converts lymphocytes into T-cells (which stands for thymus cells), but it also has the wisdom to "train" these cells to do their specific jobs. There is no doubt that in the early stages of our development, the thymus is responsible for "programming" the way we fight infections. Within this important gland is the "code" for making sure the immune system does not turn against itself. Exactly how it does this is unknown, but one thing scientists have observed is that it appears that 95 percent of the lymphocytes that are matured in the gland are actually destroyed there. The probable reason for this is that these cells would have had the potential of turning against the body's own tissues.

The Spleen

The spleen's main function is to act as a filter for the blood and make antibodies. It is made up of B-cells, T-cells, macrophages, dendritic cells, natural killer cells and red blood cells. Not only does it filter out old red blood cells, but it also removes abnormal cells and certain harmful bacteria floating in the blood. In the spleen, macrophages and dendritic cells carry foreign materials or *antigens* to T- and B-cells, and the immune response begins.

The Lymph Nodes

The lymph nodes function as the filter for the body fluid known as lymph. Lymph nodes are found in all tissues of the body except the central nervous system, bone, cartilage and teeth. Similar to the spleen, they are made up mostly of T-cells, B-cells, dendritic cells and macrophages and are responsible for draining and filtering fluid from our tissues. As in the spleen, the macrophages and dendritic cells that capture antigens present these foreign materials to T- and B-cells, consequently initiating an immune response.

The Immune Response Illustrated

When an invader in the form of a bacteria, virus, or fungus breaks though one of our immune system barriers such as the skin, mucus membranes or intestines, the immune response is launched.

For instance, let's say you cut your finger with a knife. The first on the scene are the phagocytes, such as macrophage and dendritic cells, which begin to gobble up any bacteria that may have been on your skin. You put a Band-Aid on, forget about it and in 24-36 hours they have killed any possible infection and the cut is completely healed.

Suppose for a moment that the knife was dirty, and along with the normal bacteria on your skin, there was a tougher microbe like Staphylococcus aureus? In such a case, you could expect a very different scenario.

As the staph bacteria multiply, your finger becomes swollen and hot as the immune cells produce inflammatory cytokines. This response is natural and is called inflammation. The increased blood flow is actually carrying millions of backup white blood cells in the form of phagocytes, macrophage and dendritic cells to the area to help fight the infection. As the battle continues, the casualties of dead microbes and dead white blood cells begin to pile up into a thick yellow fluid called pus. Now your Band-Aid covered finger is throbbing and you notice that your cut is "infected."

Below the surface of your skin, the macrophage and dendritic cells continue to gobble up the staph microbe like little Pac-Man characters and then they display tiny parts of it on the outside of their cells to present to T-helper cells. They communicate with each other through chemical messengers called cytokines, specifically interluekin-1.

Once the macrophage and dendritic cells present the antigen to the T-helper cells, the T-helper cells become "activated" and begin to multiply and call for help by producing cytokines called interluekin-2. These cytokines then signal the immune system to call millions of NK and cytotoxic T-cells to the scene. NK and cytotoxic T-cells that recognize a unique antigen on the surface of the infected macrophage and dendritic cells will produce chemicals to kill these cells along with the pathogen inside of them.

Let's say the staph microbes are too strong or too many. That's when the B-cells are called in to help. The T-helper cells will produce other cytokines called interleukin 4, interleukin 13 and interleukin 10, to stimulate the production of millions of B-cells. Activated B-cells divide and will turn into either plasma cells or memory cells.

The plasma cells' job is to turn into antibody-producing factories and flood the bloodstream with antibodies that can bind to the surface of the antigen on the staph aureus and tag it to make it easier for the other cells to recognize.

For example, imagine T-cells holding up a picture of a red fox. The B-cells will then make antibodies for a red fox and when they find it, they will grab it and tag it so that the phagocytes can come in for the kill.

Once the antigen is effectively destroyed, Regulatory T-Cells/CD4⁺ will come in and stop the fight so that the immune system doesn't go out of control and attack healthy cells.

Meanwhile, memory B-cells will stick around in the bloodstream with antibodies to "remember" the antigen. In other words, they will "record" what strategies worked in the last attack, so the next time the staph is encountered the immune response will be more efficient.

The cells of the immune system work together much like skilled musicians in an orchestra, each playing a special instrument with a specific part, and each equally important to the final performance. Every day, inside of our bodies, our immune system orchestrates compositions as complicated as Beethoven's Ninth Symphony. We take this remarkable orchestra for granted and many times we forget it's there…that is, until we experience a problem.

In the coming chapters, we will be reviewing what occurs in the auto-immune process and the ways an autoimmune response can cause thyroid symptoms.

CHAPTER 6

Reframe the Autoimmune Process

"Our key to transforming anything lies in our ability to reframe it."
— MARIANNE WILLIAMSON

The immune response is designed to run smoothly, and under normal circumstances, it does. However, there are times when the system trips up, makes errors, and harmful invaders are "tagged" as safe. When this happens, the result may be an illness such as cancer.

Other times, harmless invaders such as pollen, dust or pet dander are tagged and the immune system launches into overdrive, causing reactions such as allergies. In the case of an autoimmune condition, the immune system becomes overwhelmed due to a combination of triggers such as chronic stress, poor nutrition, nutrient deficiencies, allergies, infections, and toxins. These triggers can cause the immune system to overreact and produce too many T-cells or B-cells (or both), which can then attack healthy tissue.

Is the Autoimmune Process a Condition or a Disease?

We commonly associate the word "dis-ease" with sickness or illness; on the other hand, the word "condition" implies a "state of being." Conditions can get better or worse depending on circumstances, yet diseases are typically thought of as curable or incurable.

The term "autoimmune thyroid disease" is misleading, because it's not a disease of the thyroid gland and it's not a disease of the immune system. It's the "condition" or "state" of the immune system overreacting to the stimulation of constant inflammation, and the outcome is an attack on the thyroid gland or other tissue.

I'd like you to start thinking of the autoimmune process as a reversible condition instead of a disease. When I began to view the autoimmune process this way, I was able to "reframe" things in my mind and instead of thinking I was the victim of a mysterious illness that had no cure, I was able to observe that my choices could influence my "state of being," for better or for worse, and I began to realize that I could get better!

Stress and the Autoimmune Process

Current medical research shows that all autoimmune conditions are essentially the same process occurring in the body: the inflamed immune system, under the strain of continual cellular stress (triggers), mistakes healthy tissue as foreign and begins to destroy it.[1] The only difference between various autoimmune conditions is which organ is being attacked. With lupus, it can be the skin, the liver, the joints, etc. With type I diabetes, it's the pancreas; with multiple sclerosis, it is the brain and spinal cord; and with ulcerative colitis, it is the large intestine and rectum.

In the case of Hashimoto's and Graves', the thyroid is the obvious target, but it's important to note that it's rarely just the thyroid being affected, and there are typically many conditions happening at the same time.

In the autoimmune process, the cells of the immune system, that ordinarily work to kill harmful invaders and regulate immune response, get overworked, and thus become overproduced, under-produced or confused. They begin, instead, to tag and destroy our healthy cells and tissues.

Throughout history people have known that stress makes you sick. While they may have lacked the "science," ancient healing systems were built upon relieving stress and detoxing the body, thus restoring balance and health. Today, scientists have proven how both acute and chronic stressors directly affect the cells of your immune system resulting in autoimmunity.

Here are just a few examples:

- Acute stress in any form (psychological and physical) can cause a rise in the stress hormones adrenaline and cortisol, which suppress T-cell activity. This is why you may catch a cold after a stressful event.
- Chronic stress in any form can cause adrenal fatigue, which causes the hormones cortisol, adrenaline and norepinephrine to become depleted. This can allow immune system T-cells to get out of control, resulting in inflammation and an imbalance between T-cells and B-cells.[2]
- Chronic stress can impair methylation, which can suppress T-cell production. Impaired methylation of T-cells may be involved in the production of autoantibodies.[3]

- Chronic infectious stress can cause both B-cells and T-cells to be overproduced resulting in autoimmunity.[4,5]
- Gastrointestinal stress, perhaps caused by parasites, yeast or an overgrowth of bad bacteria, affects all the cells of your immune system, and disrupts the balance between T-regulator cells and Th1 and Th2 cells.[6]
- Food allergies and sensitivities, for instance to gluten, can cause B-cells to be overproduced, which may result in an accidental attack on healthy tissues.[7]
- Nutrient deficiency is a form of stress that can be at the root of an autoimmune response; for instance, selenium and iodine deficiencies have been found to cause thyroid inflammation, thus driving up the production of T-cells and B-cells.[8]
- Exposure to heavy metals can cause both T-cells and B-cells to be overproduced.[9]
- Certain medications and vaccinations can be "antigenic," which means that the body produces antibodies to the substance, thus initiating an immune response. In some cases this can trigger an autoimmune response.[10,11]
- Literally thousands of environmental toxins from cleaning products and pesticides to dry cleaning fluids and plastics can become antigenic and trigger an autoimmune condition.[12]

What I really want you to grasp is that the autoimmune process is a "symptom" of several underlying issues that have gone ignored or untreated for so long that the immune system becomes totally overloaded.

Scientists are scrambling to understand the mechanics of the immune system so that they can find a way to chemically manipulate it to function properly while being pushed past its limits. But what if we were to take a different approach? What would happen if the stressors were removed and the immune system was taken off its 24/7 high-alert schedule?

There is no question that modern medicine has made incredible advances in understanding the complexities of immune function, yet experts still don't agree on why the immune system turns against its own body.

Our immune systems are influenced by everything in our environments from our positive and negative thoughts, the good and bad foods we eat, to the toxins and infections we are exposed to. Once we observe these effects, we can accentuate the positive and reduce the negative so the immune system can come into balance. When we reduce the burdens on our body and emotions and restore the conditions for wellness, autoimmunity can be reversed. I know this in my heart, and I have seen it hundreds of times with my clients.

The Th1 Versus Th2 Dominance Hypothesis

There's a lot of talk in both conventional and alternative medicine about Th1 and Th2 "dominance." If you've been researching autoimmune thyroid disease, there is no doubt you have come across these buzzwords in books and blogs on the Internet. This hypothesis arose in the late 1980's when scientists observed the cytokine patterns of T-helper cells in mice. The theory was adapted to the human immune system and has since been considered gospel by many practitioners as well as pharmaceutical and supplement manufacturers who specialize in "immune system modulation."

Experts who agree with this hypothesis will say that anyone with an autoimmune "disease" is either Th1 or Th2 dominant. That means that if we are experiencing an autoimmune response, our T-helper cells are sending out signals, specifically cytokines or interleukins, which drive up the proliferation and activity of either too many T-cells, or too many B-cells.

Some researchers theorize that the over-activation of either pathway can cause an autoimmune attack, and that the only way to fix the problem is to dampen the overactive pathway and boost the underactive pathway, to restore the balance between the two.

This is why some practitioners will suggest that their patients with an autoimmune condition get a medical test called a cytokine panel to see which part of the immune system has become "overactive" or "underactive." By measuring the Th1 cytokines, IL (Interluekin)-2, IL-3, IL-12 and tumor necrosis factor alpha (TNFa), they can determine if you have too much natural killer and cytotoxic T-cell activity. By measuring the Th2 cytokines— IL-4, IL-5, IL-6, IL-10 and IL-13 —they can determine if you have too much B-cell activity. Once they have determined which pathway is dominant, they will prescribe immune-system-modulating compounds in an attempt to quiet the dominant pathway and boost the underactive pathway.

If one part of the immune system is overacting, then it makes sense to calm it down, right?

Well, yes and no. As long as we don't miss the forest for the trees!

The question of why the Th1 or Th2 pathway is overactive must still be asked.

For instance, let's say you have become infected with a chronic bacterial infection, and your immune system is ramped up to fight it. Let's say this goes on for years, as in the case of a stealth mycoplasma infection, and your Th1 response is on high alert but can't kill the infection completely. While it's trying to knock it out, it starts attacking healthy tissues. Doesn't it make sense to find out what pathogen is driving the Th1 pathway to be on high alert and treat that first, or at least at the same time?

Additionally, new studies show that defective T-regulator cell activity due to imbalances in the gut microbiota can lead to an over expression of both Th1 and Th2 pathways resulting in allergies and autoimmune responses. This research makes a clear connection between the health of your GI tract and your immune system![13, 14]

It's important to note that not all experts agree with the Th1 vs. Th2 hypothesis. Some suggest that the human immune system rarely exhibits one dominant pathway over the other. In fact, most people with autoimmune disease will flip back and forth from one pathway to the other, depending on what's "bugging" them at the time.[15]

The table below shows disorders that some experts claim are related to one dominant pathway or the other:

Common Th1 dominance disorders	Common Th2 dominance disorders
Organ-specific autoimmune diseases	Systemic autoimmune diseases
Multiple sclerosis	Allergies: food and hay fever
IBD/Crohn's disease	Asthma
Type 1 diabetes	Eczema
Hashimoto's disease,	Chronic sinusitis
Graves' disease	Many cancers
Psoriasis	Hepatitis B and C (mixed Th1 and Th2)
Rheumatoid arthritis	Ulcerative colitis
H. pylori induced peptic ulcer	Urticaria
	Viral infections
	Systemic lupus erythematosus
	Helminth infections

Like many of my clients, I experienced symptoms from both sides of the table, and at the same time. For instance, I had Hashimoto's, H. pylori, allergies, chronic sinusitis, viral infections, rashes (urticaria) and my lab tests and symptoms were suggesting lupus! Was I Th1 or Th2 dominant? Apparently, I was both! It appears that the autoimmune process is highly individualized, and a person can have symptoms that point to Th1 dominance, Th2 dominance, or both.

Pharmaceutical and nutrition companies are scurrying to develop formulas that will modulate a particular pathway, but if they don't address the underlying reason the immune system is on high alert, they won't help many people prevent or reverse the condition.

> "Michelle Corey has eloquently put into perspective the debate about the involvement of the immune system in autoimmune thyroid conditions. Both ancient systems of healing and modern scientific medicine have taught us that balance, or imbalance, in the body is the result of myriad processes, which are simultaneously complex and beautifully simple. Variable gene expression, protein production, immune up-and-down-regulation, enzymatic reactions, buffering systems, detoxification, and the alignment (or misalignment) of energetic fields are just a few such processes which can lead to a state of homeostasis or one of disruption where the body attacks itself as if its very tissue were an enemy.
> To think that the cause of a given autoimmune disease is the dominance of one of two pathways and/or the submission of the other is to ignore the wisdom of traditional holistic systems of health as well as modern science. The ultimate expression of wellness or disease is a complex interplay of multiple factors — environment, genetics, and exposures (i.e. food, emotions, toxins, lifestyle). Our understanding of autoimmune disease will continue to evolve rapidly, but universal principles will always hold true: go upstream to find the source of the problem, search for and treat the root causes, nourish the physical and emotional body, and do not get lost in the details of the ill condition while failing to remove the "splinter" which stuck the person in the first place.
> — Eric Grasser, M.D., Unity Medicine, Santa Fe, New Mexico

In conclusion, natural immune system modulators such as green tea, white willow, pycnogenol, reishi mushroom and echinacea may help many people feel better while they are healing, but they should not be used like pharmaceuticals to mask or suppress a natural response of the body to heal itself. A good practitioner will always start with removing pieces of the splinter. If she feels that calming the immune system at the same time will help you to feel better and heal faster, that's great…just make sure she's looking for the cause of the immune system flare at the same time!

Your Genes are Not Your Destiny!

We have been taught to think of genes as being set in stone, a determining factor over which we have no control. If someone has family members, or relatives with the same autoimmune disorder, they may assume that "it's in their genes" and there's nothing they can do about it. But your genes are not your destiny; they are "instructions" to build the proteins, hormones and everything else your body is made of.

Many factors influence how well, or poorly, those proteins get built. The emerging science of epigenetics studies the factors that influence, and even control, how our genetic code expresses itself.

Visionary developmental biologist Bruce Lipton in his book, *Spontaneous Evolution*, uses a building construction analogy that I'll expand to illustrate how gene expression works. Your genes are like the blueprints used to construct a house. The blueprints are a crucial source of information that informs contractors how to build the house.

Although the genetic difference between human beings is less than 1 percent, everyone's blueprint is a little bit different although our blueprints do have much in common—doors, windows, floors, ceilings, etc. Some blueprints are designed to make mansions, and others to make a ranch house or cozy bungalow. It's possible to make a shoddy mansion even from perfectly good blueprints if you use poor materials and incompetent workers. Epigenetics describes everything that goes into creating the final result out of the original blueprint in your DNA.

Imagine that you give identical blueprints to five contractors in different parts of the country. Will they build exactly the same house? No, there will be all kinds of variations. The houses may look similar, but one may end up with shoddy plumbing because of an incompetent subcontractor that used old, broken parts. One builder might purchase the finest finish materials, while another buys everything from the discount building center.

One contractor might be distracted, and makes mistakes everywhere, while another is conscientious and creates a beautiful, long-lasting home.

You could use the same analogy for a dinner recipe. If you don't have all the ingredients, or use foods that have begun to spoil, the best recipe could wind up, at the least, not tasting very good and, at the worst, make you sick.

Epigenetics informs us that if we give our body the proper ingredients and a positive, non-toxic, inner environment, it can give us optimum health and the best expression of our unique genetic code.

The foods and supplements you eat are the main ingredients your body needs to fulfill your inner blueprint. If your DNA needs certain amino acids to create your best body, and you don't provide those building blocks, the body has to make do and the resultant weakness makes way for possible illness. Stress and toxins are other important factors that can confuse and distort the process.

In 2010, a paper in *Science Magazine* reported that while risks of developing chronic diseases are attributed to both genetic and environmental factors, 70 to 90 percent of disease risks are probably due to differences in environments.[16] This should be commonsense to everyone with a garden or houseplants. Genetic variations might allow some plants to have bigger leaves or different colored flowers, but if you don't water them, or give them the light that they need, it's going to make a much bigger difference in whether they flourish or wilt. Different plants have different needs and the same is true for people.

> **What You Need to Know:**
> Your doctor might tell you that you have a genetic predisposition that led you to develop your autoimmune condition. My experience has shown that by removing the physical, emotional and environmental factors that trigger autoimmunity, your condition can be reversed. You can get better. The bottom line is that you have a lot of control over your health and your genetic expression.

CHAPTER 7

Autoimmune Thyroid Conditions

"The first step toward a cure is to know what the disease is."
— LATIN PROVERB

In this chapter, I will be discussing the two causes of "primary" thyroid dysfunction in the Western world —Hashimoto's thyroiditis and Graves' thyrotoxicosis. These conditions can cause symptoms of hyperthyroidism or hypothyroidism, and in some cases an alternating between both states. As you have learned, all autoimmune conditions are essentially the same process happening in the body; the only difference is the system or organ being affected.

If you're reading this book you most likely have been diagnosed with a thyroid condition or you think you may have one. The purpose of this section is to familiarize you with the conventional ways in which these conditions are diagnosed and treated.

In the coming sections I will be discussing in greater detail the factors that can play a role in triggering these conditions, as well as how to heal them and reverse the process.

First let's take a look at the most common cause of *hyperthyroid* symptoms—Graves' Thyrotoxicosis.

Graves' (Thyrotoxicosis): Hyperthyroidism

Graves' is an autoimmune condition named after the Irish doctor Robert James Graves, who first discovered it in 1835. In this condition, as the immune system attacks the thyroid gland, it becomes enlarged and produces excessive amounts of the thyroid hormones thyroxine (T4) and triiodothyronine (T3).

It is estimated that this condition affects roughly 2.5 million people in the U.S., and as with most autoimmune conditions, Graves' is more common in women, usually between the ages of 20 and 40.[1] Although Graves' is the number one cause of hyperthyroid symptoms, not all people with Graves' have symptoms, and not all people with hyperthyroid symptoms have Graves'. Sometime symptoms can be caused by a goiter, which we will address later.

Graves' has been recognized as being directly related to trauma and stress.[2] In fact, many people report the onset of their symptoms being precipitated by a traumatic event or acute infection.

How is Graves' Diagnosed?

Graves' may be difficult to diagnose because many of the symptoms come on gradually and mimic other conditions. It's not uncommon for a person to visit her doctor five to six times before the thyroid is suspected.

> **What You Need to Know:**
> Autoimmune thyroid conditions rarely exist alone. There are typically combinations of several conditions presenting at the same time.

When the thyroid makes too much thyroid hormone, a person can begin to experience a variety of uncomfortable symptoms:

Physical Symptoms

- Sensation of feeling too warm, sweating, sweaty hands—heat intolerance
- Feeling hungry all the time and losing weight despite eating more
- Feeling of fullness in the neck, goiter, enlarged thyroid
- A fast or irregular heart rate
- Inner trembling, tremors
- High blood pressure
- Shortness of breath—feeling like you can't catch your breath
- Nausea, frequent bowel movements or diarrhea
- Insomnia
- Feeling "wired but tired," exhaustion, fatigue

- Bulging eyes, painful dry eyes, puffy eyes
- Muscle and joint pain or fatigue
- Hair loss or brittle, dry hair
- Bleeding gums and gum infections
- Chronic urinary tract infections (UTI's)
- Chronic yeast infections of the GI and urogenital tract
- Chronic sinusitis—fungal
- Libido changes—increases for women; decreases for men
- Infertility/pregnancy complications/light or ceased menses
- Skin conditions, vitiligo, rashes, hives, itching, rash on ankles and shins (Graves' dermopathy/pretibial myxedema)
- Swollen lymph glands
- Nail changes—separation of nail bed from skin

Emotional/Psychological Symptoms

- Manic feelings/racing thoughts
- Sleep disorders—difficultly falling and staying asleep
- Mood swings
- Depression
- Anxiety and panic attacks
- Quick temper, uncontrollable anger or rage
- Memory problems
- Difficult concentration
- Trouble making decisions
- Feeling like there is not enough time
- Feelings of being left out

That is a long list of symptoms, and since most doctors have less than ten minutes with each patient, you can see how easy it might be to misdiagnose this condition. The most common symptom is anxiety and irritability; so many people are given prescriptions for depression and anxiety before the thyroid is even suspected.

Once your doctor suspects that your thyroid is the cause of the symptoms, she will usually order a series of blood tests to determine levels of thyroid-stimulating hormone (TSH) and thyroxine (T4).

If the test comes back with a suppressed TSH and a high level of thyroxine (T4), she will most likely refer you to an endocrinologist. This is because most general practitioners, OB/GYNs and nurse practitioners don't feel as comfortable treating hyperthyroid patients as they do hypothyroid patients. This is probably a good thing because hyperthyroid conditions can be dangerous, and it's important that the practitioner has experience in the diagnosis and treatment of acute hyperthyroidism.

The endocrinologist or thyroid specialist will typically do a physical examination and run a full thyroid panel to determine whether your symptoms are due to an autoimmune process such as Graves' or Hashimoto's, a "hot" nodule (also called toxic nodular goiter), or thyroiditis.

Note: There are other reasons your thyroid could be making excessive amount of thyroid hormone. In this book, we are only going to focus on the autoimmune causes, Graves' and Hashimoto's.

Blood Tests

With Graves' the thyroid becomes swollen and starts to produce too much thyroid hormone. When thyroid hormone levels go up, the pituitary gets the signal and stops producing TSH.

People diagnosed with Graves' may have high levels of antithyroid peroxidase antibodies (anti-TPO); Thyroid-Stimulating Immunoglobulins (TSI)—also called TSH receptor antibodies (TRAb); and antinuclear antibodies (ANA).

If you have symptoms of hyperthyroidism and you test positive for anti-TPO and TSI/TRAb, a diagnosis of Graves' is made. But it's important to note that not all people with Graves' have these antibodies, which makes it a complicated condition to diagnose.

Other Diagnostic Tests

The body needs iodine to make thyroid hormones. One way to assess thyroid hormone function is by a radioactive iodine uptake test. For this test, you will be asked to take a small dose of radioactive iodine or radioiodine (iodine 123), and then you are checked with an X-ray a few hours later to see how fast your thyroid absorbs it. With Graves', the entire thyroid become "hot" or overactive, and will take up a higher amount of iodine than a normal thyroid. This causes an elevated RAU-I result.

This test is also used to find out if thyroid nodules are hot or cold. Hot nodules overproduce thyroid hormones, and will show up that way on the X-ray.

If your symptoms of hyperthyroidism are due to a pituitary tumor or you are taking too much thyroid hormone, the results of the uptake will be normal.

Sometimes, your doctor might order a fine needle aspiration of the thyroid, which will show the activity of macrophages and T-cells.

What is the Conventional Treatment of Graves'?

Conventional doctors don't typically question why a person's thyroid is under attack by the immune system. Their main concern is to stop the production of excess thyroid hormones at all costs—even if that means the total removal of the gland itself!

If you've been diagnosed with Graves', there's no doubt that you have been presented with one or all of the following options. These options do not address the cause of the autoimmune condition. Instead, they remove or suppress the target organ and the condition continues in the body resulting in further autoimmune activity down the road.

Antithyroid Drugs (ADT)

Your doctor might initially prescribe antithyroid drugs such as methimazole (Tapazole) or propylthiouracil to block the formation of T4 and T3. While roughly 30 percent of people treated with long-term antithyroid medication will go into "remission" with this treatment, it's important to remember that it's not a cure. Sometimes, beta blockers, including propranolol (Inderal), atenolol (Tenormin) and metoprolol (Lopressor), are prescribed to relieve the symptoms of rapid heart rate and nervousness, but these drugs can potentially cause side effects and do nothing to address the cause of the autoimmune process.

If your hyperthyroid symptoms are severe, the short-term use of antithyroid medications may be indicated, but you and your doctor must search for the underlying cause of your autoimmune condition and treat that immediately in order to heal completely.

RAI (I-131): Radioactive Iodine Treatment

When antithyroid drugs fail to alleviate the symptoms of hyperthyroidism, the next course of treatment is to permanently shrink the thyroid gland with radioactive iodine (I-131). The thyroid needs iodine to make its hormones, so it absorbs the radioactive iodine and the radiation destroys some of the thyroid cells. The treatment is taken orally, either in liquid or pill form in a single dose, and takes three to six months to shrink the gland.

The amount of damage that that this treatment does cannot be controlled, so most people wind up becoming hypothyroid after this treatment and then need to take thyroid replacement hormones for life.

Caution

Since you have radiation in your body during treatment, you will be advised to avoid close contact with other people and pregnant women for two weeks after treatment. This includes sleeping in the same bed with your partner! The radiation is also absorbed by other tissues such as the breasts, the ovaries and testes, the pancreas and GI tract and may lead to DNA damage and increased cancer risks down the road.

This treatment does not address the cause of the autoimmune process, and the condition will likely persist somewhere else in the body. It also sets the stage for other conditions that may be caused by radiation exposure.

Surgery

The most drastic form of treatment is a thyroidectomy, where all or part of the thyroid is surgically removed. As with radioactive iodine treatment, most people become hypothyroid and have to take thyroid replacement hormones for life. The complications of surgery can include paralysis of the vocal cords and damage to the parathyroid glands, which are the tiny glands behind the thyroid gland that control calcium absorption in the body.

Final thoughts on Graves'

If you have been diagnosed with Graves', it's likely that you have had many differing opinions on how to move forward with treatment. Don't worry! In Part Two you will learn how to utilize the least invasive conventional treatment while you work to uncover the underlying triggers in your condition and then heal them.

Next, we will discuss the most common cause of primary hypothyroidism: Hashimoto's thyroiditis

Hashimoto's Thyroiditis

Hashimoto's thyroiditis, also called autoimmune thyroiditis, autoimmune thyroid disease or chronic lymphocytic thyroiditis, is a condition that was first discovered by the Japanese specialist Hashimoto Haruko in Germany in 1912.

In Hashimoto's, the body produces antibodies to the enzyme thyroid peroxidase (TPO). These antibodies are called antithyroid peroxidase, or anti-TPO for short. In some cases there may be antibodies to the protein thyroglobulin; these are called antithyroglobulin, or TgAb. When these antibodies are present, it results in the invasion of the thyroid by cytotoxic T-cells, which attack the thyroid gland and result in inflammation and destruction of the gland. In many cases, the thyroid becomes enlarged and a goiter may develop. If left untreated, it can lead to hypothyroidism with intermittent bouts of hyperthyroidism.

While the American Association of Clinical Endocrinologists (AACE) estimates that 14 million people in this country have Hashimoto's thyroiditis, many experts feel that the number is much higher because millions of people are suffering from symptoms but have yet to be diagnosed.[3]

As with Graves', women are about 20 times more likely than men to develop Hashimoto's disease, and the typical patient is 30-50 years old; however, it can also affect children as well.

How is Hashimoto's Thyroiditis Diagnosed?

As with Graves' and most autoimmune diseases, it may take a few visits to your doctor before she suspects your thyroid is the cause of your symptoms. As you learned earlier, the thyroid affects literally every cell of your body, so when your thyroid hormones are low, the symptoms can mimic many other medical conditions. It's no wonder that millions of people suffer needlessly for years, and millions more go undiagnosed. I suffered with the symptoms of Hashimoto's for over four years before my thyroid was checked. When my doctor finally suspected that my thyroid was the problem, she tested my TSH and T4 levels, which were just out of range. She told me that she would retest in six months and handed me a prescription for an anti-anxiety medication. It took another two years and over a dozen doctors' visits before I was tested for antibodies and given a diagnosis of Hashimoto's.

> **What You Need to Know:**
> Autoimmune thyroid conditions rarely exist alone. There are typically combinations of several conditions presenting at the same time.

When the thyroid is under attack and makes too little thyroid hormone, a person can begin to experience a variety of uncomfortable and debilitating symptoms:

Physical Symptoms

- Weight gain—even on a restricted calorie diet
- Hair loss on the head and the outer edges of the eyebrows
- Digestive problems—typically constipation—but it can alternate between constipation and diarrhea
- Other GI symptoms such as upset stomach and GERD
- Menstrual problems, such as heavy periods, cramping and raging PMS/PMSD
- Infertility and complicated pregnancies
- Sleep disorders—sleep apnea
- A feeling of fullness in the neck or problems swallowing because the gland is enlarged or a goiter, sore throat or hoarse voice
- Chest pain and tachycardia

- Chronic urinary infections (UTI's)
- Chronic yeast infections of the GI and urogenital tract
- Chronic sinusitis—fungal
- Sensation of feeling cold all the time—especially hands and feet
- Migraine headaches
- Muscle weakness and pain
- Feeling "wired but tired"—exhaustion and fatigue that is not relieved by rest
- Bleeding gums, gum infections and periodontal disease
- Water retention, puffy face—especially around the eyes
- Low libido—in men and women
- Skin conditions, rashes, hives, itching
- Hay fever and food allergies
- Swollen lymph glands
- Anemia
- High blood sugar
- High cholesterol
- Brittle nails
- Dry skin

Emotional/Psychological Symptoms

- Depression
- Mood swings—from manic to depressed
- Anger and rage
- Anxiety and panic attacks
- Uncontrollable crying
- Memory problems
- Difficult concentration
- Trouble making decisions
- Feeling of giving up—what's the use?
- Feeling that there is never enough time
- Feelings of "What about me?" "I never get what I want." and "I

never get to speak up."

Here we go again with a long list of symptoms! It takes real detective work to diagnose Hashimoto's. The most common symptoms are depression and weight gain, so many people are given antidepressant medication and told to limit their calorie intake. Other common conditions include high blood sugar and high cholesterol so many times a person is simply told to cut down on sugar and fat and given a prescription for cholesterol-lowering drugs.

If your doctor does suspect that your thyroid is the cause of your symptoms she will usually test your levels of thyroid-stimulating hormone (TSH) and thyroxine (T4).

If your test comes back with an elevated TSH and a low level of thyroxine (T4) she may suggest a "wait and watch approach" before doing anything more. If she is well educated in thyroid health, and has taken the time to listen to your symptoms, she will suggest running more blood tests to investigate further.

Blood Tests

The diagnosis of Hashimoto's involves measuring thyroid-stimulating hormone (TSH), Free T3 (triiodothyronine), and Free T4 (thyroxine) hormone levels, as well as antithyroid peroxidase antibodies (anti-TPO), and/or antithyroglobulin antibodies (TgAb). (Other acronyms are Tg and TGB).

In the case of Hashimoto's, the body produces autoantibodies to thyroid peroxidase and sometimes to thyroglobulin, thus initiating a response from cytotoxic T-cells, which then attack thyroid tissue, causing swelling, inflammation and destruction of thyroid cells. When this happens, the traumatized thyroid slows its production of thyroid hormone. When blood thyroid hormone levels fall, TSH levels rise to stimulate the thyroid to make more hormones. A healthy thyroid will respond to TSH and make more thyroid hormone, but in the case of Hashimoto's it cannot because it's under attack—and so are the enzymes and molecules that are needed for thyroid production.

If a person has elevated TSH, a low T4 and T3 and a positive anti-TPO and/or TgAb, a diagnosis of Hashimoto's is made.

Note: There are many variables with thyroid testing and not everyone with Hashimoto's will test positive for antibodies. Conversely, not everyone with antibodies will have true Hashimoto's. This is for two reasons:

1. The immune system fluctuates, so there may be times when the antibodies will fall within the normal range, even though a person has a full-blown autoimmune thyroid condition and all of the accompanying symptoms.
2. Even healthy people have some autoantibodies to thyroid cells, due to the normal activity of the thyroid gland, but they rarely are elevated too far out of the normal range.

I will talk about optimal versus suboptimal thyroid panel ranges and the different possible scenarios in Chapter 12: Test—Don't Guess!

Other Diagnostic Tests

Your doctor might order a fine needle aspiration (FNA) of the thyroid, which will show the activity of macrophages and T-cells. She may also suggest a radioactive iodine uptake test, which would show an enlarged thyroid gland with diffuse uptake of the radioactive iodine. In some cases, your doctor will do an ultrasound of your thyroid gland, which will show nodules and sometimes even assess how much destruction has taken place.

What is the Conventional Treatment of Hashimoto's Thyroiditis?

I don't mean to keep picking on conventional doctors, but please remember that they are not taught to question why your thyroid has become the target of your immune system. If your hormones fall within, or slightly below, the normal range, your doctor may suggest a "wait and watch approach" and send you home. If she detects a hormone deficiency, she will typically prescribe a synthetic (T4) thyroid hormone replacement called levothyroxine (brand names: Levothroid, Levoxyl, Synthroid) to bring your TSH and T4 back into the "normal" range. This treatment works moderately well for 50 percent of the people who take it. In some cases, it even helps to lower the antibody activity because it reduces inflammation by reducing the activity of TSH and "turning your thyroid off."

However, it does not address the reasons why the thyroid came under attack, and the underlying cause goes untreated and often leads to more autoimmune issues down the road.

It's also important to note that not everyone does well on T4 replacement alone, so even though their lab tests look "normal," their symptoms persist. It's not uncommon for a person to suffer needlessly for months or years before finding the correct hormone replacement. I will discuss the different hormone replacement options in Chapter 13: The First Steps Toward Reversing your Autoimmune Thyroid Condition.

New Studies Show TSH as a Cause of Thyroiditis

In the case of Hashimoto's, there may be another cause of inflammation that's driving cytotoxic T-cells to destroy the thyroid gland. In his book, *Hope for Hashimoto's*, Dr. Alexander Haskell explains how the condition of autoimmune thyroiditis or Hashimoto's is caused by an iodide/iodine deficiency, which in turn causes low thyroid hormone levels. Low thyroid hormone levels then cause TSH levels to go up and hydrogen peroxide is produced in the cells of the thyroid, as it gets ready for the process of making thyroid hormones from iodine. In the case of chronic iodine deficiency, there is no iodine to uptake so the H_2O_2 just hangs around, causing oxidation of cells. He states that it's the H_2O_2 that is causing inflammation of the thyroid, which in turn causes white blood cells (T-cells) to rush to the site to clean up the mess. If they have to stick around for a long time, say months or years, they may become overzealous and begin to attack some of the healthy tissue and cells, including thyroid peroxidase and thyroglobulin. This would explain why antibody levels go down in some people when they begin thyroid hormone replacement and lower their TSH.

The Next Steps

If you have been conventionally diagnosed with Hashimoto's or Graves', please read on to learn about what the new scientific research has determined is at the root of all autoimmune conditions—chronic stress in all of its forms.

CHAPTER 8

Become Conscious of Stress and Body Burden

"The body maintains balance in only a handful of ways. At the end of the day, disease occurs when these basic systems are out of whack."
— MARK HYMAN

The Cause of Autoimmune Conditions: Chronic Stress in All Its Forms!

It only took me a couple of years of research in autoimmunity before I began to see the physiological connections between chronic stress (emotional, infectious, and toxic), and chronic illness. Needless to say, I was dumbfounded at how our medical system could be missing these connections.

We've all heard the saying "Stress kills," but how many of us have really taken that message to heart? Sadly, not many of us even know what it means—that is, until we get sick, and even then most of us will try to ignore, minimize or work around our stresses as if they don't exist.

Our Cup Runneth Over…But Not in a Good Way!

The total amount of toxins your body is enduring at any given time is called your body burden. The total amount of stress you have at any given time is called your total stress load. We each have a limit to how much body burden or total stress load we can take. When I had my nutrition practice, I would explain it to my clients this way: we are each born with a cup: some of us have small cups, while others have larger ones. The amount of stress and toxins we can tolerate depends on the size of our cup. It doesn't matter how big your cup is; there is a limit to how much it can hold before it spills over.

We all have genetic strengths and weaknesses, and each of us has a maximum limit of how much we can take before we get sick. For some, it's the cardiovascular system that breaks down after years of chronic stress, and they might have a heart attack. For others, it's lowered immunity, and there might be a diagnosis of cancer. For those of us with autoimmune conditions, our immune systems become confused and overwhelmed and attack our own tissues.

We live in an increasingly toxic world and most of us—yes, most—are living at or just below our "maximum full" line. We are literally stressing ourselves to death, and we're not even conscious of it. In fact, we take drugs to mask our symptoms so that we don't have to feel how sick, tired, depressed, anxious, and unhappy we really are. We eat foods full of chemicals we can't even pronounce, we work at jobs we hate, we watch terrifying stories on the news, and when that's not enough we watch violent films and TV shows for "fun." We drink too much coffee and booze, tolerate lousy relationships, and slather on personal care products that could kill a cockroach. We clean our homes with poisons, breathe in smog and chemicals and then take prescription drugs to relieve our pain and symptoms. It's a vicious cycle and the more stress we endure, the more unhealthy coping mechanisms we have to come up with, just to keep going!

The human body was not intended to be a hazmat dumping zone, but unfortunately that is what we have become. We are told that we should be able to "handle it," and that if we get sick that there is something fundamentally wrong with our physiology or our genes.

Let's get real about this, people! We are stressed-out and toxic and that is why we are sick. It's commonsense, really…but when did commonsense become so uncommon?

> **What You Need to Know:**
> It is impossible to have an autoimmune condition and not be stressed on many levels. If you have an autoimmune condition, you have reached your personal saturation point for the total amount of stress your body can handle. In order to reverse your condition, you will have to identify the biggest areas of stress and alleviate them!

Before we explore the main areas of stress underlying all autoimmune conditions, let's take a look at the physiology of stress.

Understanding the Physiology of Stress

Any threat to our survival (real or perceived) triggers part of our nervous system called the autonomic nervous system to release a cascade of neurochemicals and stress hormones in our bodies. This is called the fight-or-flight response. The autonomic nervous system is responsible for controlling all of our "automatic" body functions such as heart rate, digestion, body temperature and blood pressure. We don't have to think about these functions—they just happen. Similarly, the fight-or-flight response is beyond our conscious control and just takes over when we're in danger.

The autonomic nervous system has two branches that regulate the fight-or-flight response:

- The **sympathetic** nervous system: Initiates fight-or-flight
- The **parasympathetic** nervous system: Turns off fight-or-flight

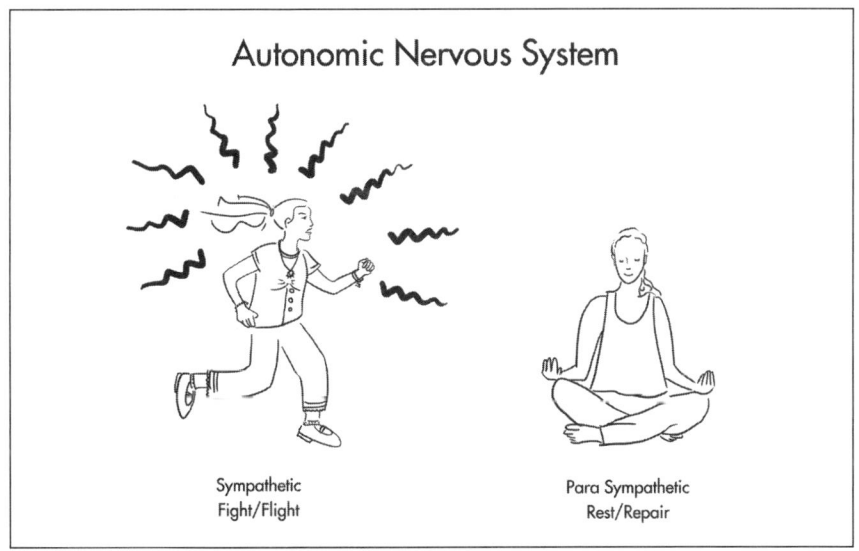

We only need to think of a stressful situation and our sympathetic nervous system is activated. It all begins in a part of the brain called the locus coeruleus. This is where the neurotransmitter noradrenalin, also called norepinephrine, is manufactured. Noradrenalin is the fuse that ignites the explosion of the fight-or-flight response.

Once the response is ignited, another part of the brain called the hypothalamus will produce corticotropin-releasing hormone (CRH). CRH stimulates the pituitary gland to release adrenocorticotropic hormone, or ACTH.

ACTH signals the adrenal glands to release the hormone adrenalin, more noradrenalin and the anti-inflammatory corticosteroid hormones cortisol, cortisone and corticosterone.

The release of these chemicals triggers our bodies to go into super survival mode, and we can experience intense emotions of fear or anger. Our respiratory rate increases. Our senses sharpen, and we become hyper aware of our surroundings. Our pupils dilate. Our digestion slows as blood flow is redirected from our GI tract to our limbs, so that we can either fight or run away. This heightened state can be so powerful that we may become capable of superhuman feats—such as a woman lifting a car off of her child.

Once the threat is over, the other branch of our nervous system, called the parasympathetic nervous system, helps slow down the response to bring our body chemistry back into balance. When the parasympathetic nervous system is activated, our breathing slows and our heart rate returns to normal. Blood flows back to the digestive system; blood pressure and body temperature drop. Our muscle tension decreases, and we become calm and centered. The body can now use its energy to repair and heal.

The fight-or-flight response is healthy and can save our lives when we're facing a physical threat to our survival.

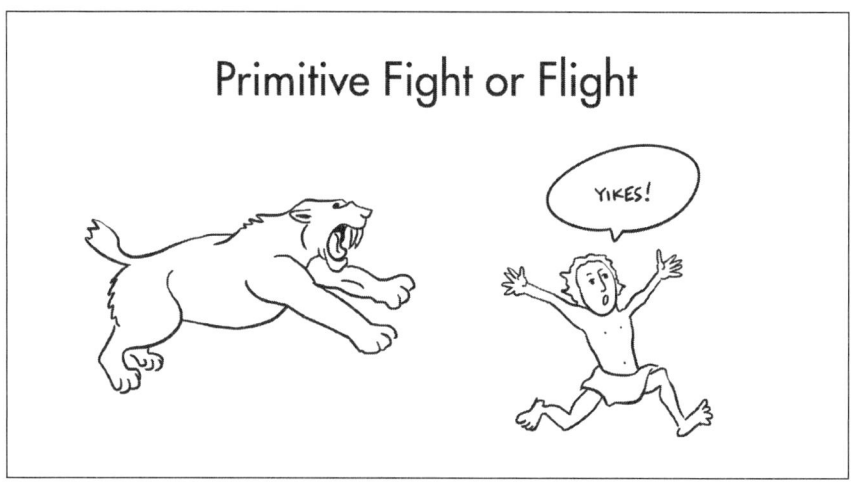

> **What You Need to Know:**
> - The Fight-or-Flight response overrides all other metabolic functions, which means it takes the energy away from our body's normal processes to enable us to move quickly until the danger passes.
> - The Fight-or-Flight response is only designed to last a few minutes.

Our ancestors came across a physical threat or predator every once in a while and either fought back, escaped or were killed. If they survived, the physical act of fighting or running away helped to metabolize the surge of stress hormones in their bloodstreams, and when the threat was over their body chemistry would return to normal.

We experience the same fight-or-flight response that our ancestors did, only our "predators" come in the form of chronic stressors such as missing a mortgage payment, losing a sale, arguing with our spouse or sitting in rush hour traffic. Most of the time, these stressors also have absolutely no physical activity attached. So instead of outrunning a saber-toothed tiger, breaking a cleansing sweat, and then relaxing and completing the cycle as we tell the tale around the fire, we find ourselves trying to find a few minutes on a treadmill somewhere so we can outrun foes like heart conditions, cancer and autoimmunity.

The sad truth is that most of us live in constant fight-or-flight mode, churning out stress neurotransmitters and hormones all day long! Adding insult to injury, we don't have the luxury of fighting or running away like our ancestors did. For instance, we can't really run screaming from the building every time our boss infuriates us (and we probably can't punch him out, either). Instead, we have to learn to "control ourselves" and "deal" with our "predators." But the physical way our ancestors dealt with their stress is now long gone. Since we're not working our large muscles and metabolizing our stress hormones by beating up or running away from our source of stress, these hormones begin to build up and become toxic in our bodies.

When our adrenal glands are forced to produce and sustain higher levels of adrenalin, noradrenalin and cortisol than we are able to metabolize, our bodies become toxic and begin to break down. Our digestion becomes compromised, which affects the cells of our immune system. Our detoxification pathways weaken and we begin to experience oxidative stress. Our muscle and bone break down and we begin to lose our mental sharpness. Over time this causes the depletion of neurotransmitters in the brain and protective hormones resulting in a condition called burnout. The result of burnout is premature aging, and it will also set your body up for serious conditions like autoimmune, cancer and heart disease.

> **Stress and the Thyroid:** In times of acute and prolonged stress the body will naturally slow the process of converting T4 to T3 in the liver and other tissues. In its wisdom the body will render the thyroid hormones to an inactive form called Reverse T3 or rT3. The job of rT3 is to block the active hormone T3 so that you don't totally burn out. The production of rT3 is not a disease but rather a survival mechanism. The body knows that under times of extreme stress more thyroid hormones will be like kicking a sick, worn out horse—if you're not careful it could drop dead!

> **What You Need to Know:**
> Our bodies cannot tell the difference between running from a saber-toothed tiger and an emotional upset such as an argument with our spouse. Chronic sympathetic nervous system activity, or fight-or-flight mode, causes adrenal fatigue and our bodies to break down on a cellular level.

In the next chapter, I'm going to review the underlying causes of autoimmune conditions. I have chosen to format it in a workbook style, so that you can follow along and uncover the areas of chronic stress in your life that may be contributing to your condition.

CHAPTER 9

Uncover the "Splinters" in Your Autoimmunity

"When Life starts to knock on your door, it's best to answer and take a look at where the noise is coming from. Otherwise the knocking gets louder and Life might even knock your door down to get your attention." – KARL BABA

Imagine every negative event, exposure, and unresolved trauma as a splinter that has been festering in your body and causing irritation. Your work will be to identify and then gently remove the splinters one by one and let your body heal.

In this chapter, you will begin some major detective work to uncover the splinters in your autoimmunity. You might be thinking, "Why me? Isn't that my doctor's job?"

The answer to that is, "It's only part her job—the lion's share is your *response-ability!*"

Consider the words of Dr. Jeffrey Bland in the preface of the Institute for Functional Medicine's 2010 textbook:

> "Physicians who focus on the management of complex chronic disease have not chosen an easy path…We can acknowledge that most diseases are rarely the result of a single physiological problem localized to a single organ. Rather, most chronic disease results from the complex interactions of multiple organ systems and multiple physiological and biochemical pathways with environmental influences and genetic predispositions."

What he is saying is that doctors who work with chronic illness have a very difficult job to do, because chronic illness does not have a single cause—it has many.

We can't walk into our health practitioners' offices and expect them to be able to unravel a lifetime of traumas, limited beliefs, chronic negative emotional states, unhealthy coping patterns, poor nutrition, and infectious and toxic exposures. Even if they were all psychic and had all day, without our active participation, they would miss a lot!

Each of us holds the key to our own wellness—the best a practitioner can do is hold the light and walk in front of us when we need a lot of support, and then help us light our own lantern and point us in the direction of health.

The Many Forms of Stress

Before I got sick, I felt stressed-out emotionally, but I hadn't realized that the stress was affecting my health. I was not conscious of the relationships between my many different forms of stress, such as poor nutrition, GI issues, inflammation, infections, and toxins and how they were burdening my body and igniting an autoimmune response.

In this section, I'll review the most common areas of stress and how they each comprise a "splinter" in autoimmune conditions.

Many of these areas overlap, and you'll see certain "splinters" show up again and again, but as you read through this chapter, try to pinpoint where you are currently experiencing the most stress. This process will help you begin to uncover your personal body burden and total stress loads, which will help you decide where to look for the splinters that are having the most serious effects on your health.

I'm referring to these insults to your wellbeing as splinters here, because splinters can be removed. If a splinter is removed soon enough, it probably won't cause lasting damage, but if it's neglected and allowed to fester, there's no telling what might happen.

Be honest, and don't judge yourself for admitting what you have been through and how you feel. This self-exploration can give you the keys to healing. We are all human, and everyone has experienced a share of stress, trauma and toxicity.

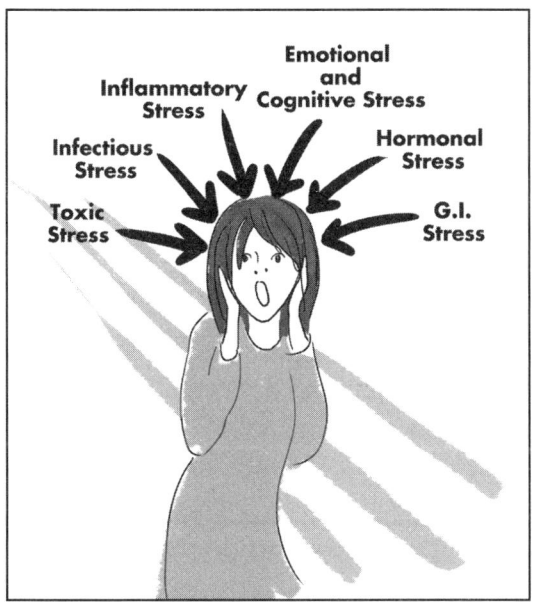

Splinter #1: Chronic Emotional Distress

In the last 20 years, we have seen considerable growth in the science of psychoneuroimmunology (PNI), which explores how our psychology affects our biology. This new science demonstrates how chronic negative emotional states keep us in chronic flight-or-flight mode, which plays a key role in the development and exacerbation of inflammatory conditions such as heart disease, diabetes, multiple sclerosis, Alzheimer's, and autoimmune disorders.

It's important to make the distinction here between the healthy experience of feeling negative emotions as a temporary response to situations in our lives and the experience of *chronic negative emotional states*. At times, intense feelings such as guilt, anger, resentment, and sadness are a normal part of the human experience for all of us. Allowing ourselves to fully feel these uncomfortable feelings seems to be a natural part of our maturation process, one that helps shape our character and teaches us empathy.

However, sometimes we may have a difficult time moving through life's painful experiences, and can find ourselves stuck in chronic negative emotional states that eventually wear us down on a physiological level.

"Hurry Sickness" and Everyday Stress

The pace of modern life has quickened to such a degree that many of us suffer from the accumulated stress of incessant day-to-day challenges. The everyday demands of work, parenting, chores, and obligations eat up our time and wear us down with concerns. Many of us sacrifice not only our time but also our health when we insist on working too long and taking on too many obligations. While some of us are capable of amazing productivity and may relish a busy lifestyle, it's important for us to recognize when the pressure of life is wearing us down. I have observed that many of us who are predisposed to autoimmune disorders also tend to take on the weight of the world while silently resenting our thankless position.

Some doctors and psychologists talk about "hurry sickness." It is the sense of never having enough time.[1] We fill our schedules to the brim and try to adapt to living at a hectic pace, but the stress keeps the sympathetic (fight-or-flight) system on alert. We live in a near panic, as if lack of time were about to overcome us. If one more task or emergency is added to our already full cups, we boil over and our stress hormones explode in turn. Just because an insane pace of life is becoming increasingly common, it doesn't mean it's normal or healthy!

The bottom line is that chronic emotional distress makes us sick. If we are to get well, we must assess how much time we spend "stressed-out" and in negative emotional states.

While the experiential causes are too many to list, below are some of the most classic sources of emotional stress. See if any apply to you.

Causes of Emotional Distress

- Death of a loved one
- Divorce, separation, or bad break up
- Being in an unhappy or unfulfilling marriage or relationship
- Hurtful betrayals, such as finding out your partner is having an affair or that a loved one has been dishonest with you
- Loss of a pet
- Traumas that can cause post-traumatic stress syndrome (PTSD), such as war, childhood abuse (sexual, physical, emotional), abusive relationships, spiritual/religious abuse, or witnessing a crime or abuse

- Unbalanced brain chemistry due to sugar, drug, or alcohol addiction or poor nutrition and toxins
- Estrangement from your family, emotionally or financially
- Loneliness—lack of close relationships
- Lack of fun or play
- Moving
- Trouble with the law
- Problems with your children
- Caring for aging, sick, or mentally disabled parents or relatives
- Loss or change of job, including retirement
- Loss of a close friend
- Feeling exploited or underappreciated
- Experiencing racism, classism, or sexual discrimination
- Vocational stress from demanding bosses and customers, or a job that is boring and/or unfulfilling
- Financial crisis from debt and living beyond one's means, not having enough money to pay the bills, or even bankruptcy
- Being chronically overtired, overcommitted, or rushed by life situations
- Witnessing "state-of-the-world" trauma such as war, poverty, global warming, etc.
- Emotional stress includes such emotional states such as anxiety, frustration, anger, rage, and sadness.

Cognitive Stress is different from emotional stress. Cognitive stress is the way we think about or assess our traumas and experiences; it's how we create the stories that help us understand our reality. These are the stories we tell ourselves (and usually others) about our past and present experiences. Some of these stories are like poison pills we mix up for ourselves, out of toxic ingredients like victimhood and shame.

If we're not careful, our inner dialogue can start to sound something like this: "My life would have been great if not for what he/she/they did to me!" or "I never get what I need. I'm trapped. My life sucks. Nobody loves me. I'm worthless. I'm damaged goods. I don't deserve love. I hate myself. I wish I were dead—maybe then they will miss me."

Toxic stories typically include feelings of shame, martyrdom, irrational demands, lack of gratitude, lack of empathy and compassion, and unrealistic expectations of others and ourselves.

Many of these stories are driven by feelings of abandonment, low self-esteem, deprivation, and entitlement.

Purposelessness Stress has to do with feelings of meaninglessness, inability to live in the now, or lack of inspiration, motivation, serenity, spirituality, or a higher purpose. When we experience these states, we tend to lose our enthusiasm, curiosity, and excitement for life. We may feel depressed and disconnected, and see each day as another hurdle to overcome, instead of a great adventure to explore.

Symptoms of Emotional, Cognitive, and Purposelessness Stress

- Feelings of being "stressed-out" all the time
- Constant worry about the future
- Constant anxiety about the past
- Persistent anxiety about the state of the world
- Feeling spaced out; disoriented
- Memory problems; forgetfulness
- Feeling unsafe or unable to speak one's truth; lying; or withholding
- Constant worry about finances
- Feeling overcommitted or unable to keep commitments
- Inability to say "no" at work, in relationships, or with family
- Inability to forgive, harboring negativity over past events
- Chronic feelings of guilt or shame
- Loneliness, boredom, or isolation
- Frustration, anger, or hostility
- Confusion
- Lack of gratitude; not appreciating the good things in your life
- Lack of empathy; not caring how others feel or understanding their feelings
- Feeling left out, abandoned, or neglected
- Feeling misunderstood
- Feeling trapped, or that you don't have choices
- Feeling hopeless, depressed, or dejected about your life

- Feeling that you have no life purpose, no mission, no reason to go onwards
- Feeling apathetic; not caring for your health and welfare or that of others
- Lack of enthusiasm, curiosity, and excitement for life
- Unrealistic expectations of self and others; demanding perfection, fairness, and approval
- Inability to let go of past hurts—holding a grudge

Which of the symptoms above apply to you? Are there any additional symptoms you have of psychological stress that are not on the list?

_____
_____
_____
_____
_____
_____
_____

Splinter #2: Unhealthy Coping Patterns

Most of us endure high degrees of emotional stress—usually much more than we can handle effectively. According to New York's American Institute of Stress, 90 percent of all American adults experience high stress levels one or two times a week and a fourth of all American adults are subject to crushing levels of stress nearly every day.[2,3]

Unfortunately, many of us have adopted methods to cope with stress in ways that only *add* more stress to our bodies and undermine our health and vitality. From the obvious culprits such as sugar, carbs, caffeine, nicotine, alcohol, and drugs to overspending, overworking and procrastination, there seems to be no end to the unhealthy ways we run from our stress. Many of us are even unconscious of our patterns—until we run into trouble.

Indulgence in sugar, carbs, nicotine, and alcohol leads to major blood sugar imbalances and impaired detoxification. In fact, the unhealthy coping patterns of alcohol and carb addiction are the number one cause of dysglycemia (imbalanced blood sugar), insulin resistance, and diabetes—not only in this country, but worldwide.

Many unhealthy coping patterns tend to run in families. Often, this is not because of any genetic factor; instead, it's caused by the habits and traditions of a particular family. For example, if you grew up in a family that started drinking at 5 o'clock to unwind, that is an unhealthy coping pattern that can be instilled in you by conditioning. Many families have stress-inducing lifestyles and poor eating habits that can be contributing factors to an autoimmune condition.

Examples of Unhealthy Coping Patterns

- Overeating or under-eating
- Drinking too much alcohol
- Drinking too much caffeine
- Eating too much sugar
- Eating too many carbs
- Smoking
- Abuse of prescription, over-the-counter, or recreational drugs
- Serious eating disorders: binge eating, anorexia, bulimia, overuse of laxatives
- Overspending, compulsive shopping
- Gambling
- Withdrawal from friends and family
- Sleeping too much
- Zoning out in front of the TV, video game, or computer
- Filling up every moment in the day to avoid your problems
- Exercising too much
- Procrastination
- Perfectionism
- Violent behavior—"blowing off steam"
- Obsessive-compulsive behavior
- Promiscuity or seeking attention in inappropriate ways
- Love, sex, or relationship addiction

Without judging yourself, can you think of some unhealthy ways you cope with stress?

_____

_____

_____

_____

_____

_____

_____

Splinter #3: Poor Nutrition, "Frankenfoods," Individual Sensitivities, and Food Allergies

How you eat translates directly into how you feel. Nutrition affects the state of your health more than any other single factor. Our bodies don't come with maintenance manuals, so many people just eat what tastes good: foods that are cheap, easy, and addictive. Many of us behave as if food were just for entertainment and sensual pleasure. Our bodies can "tolerate" a poor diet for a while, but the consequences of missing nutrients and consuming toxic or allergic ingredients eventually takes a toll on our wellbeing. Food can be medicine, or it can be poison.

Just one example of the consequences of poor nutrition is the epidemic of diabetes in the United States. The prevalence of diagnosed diabetes increased 176 percent from 1980 to 2011.[4] This is alarming, and profoundly affects thyroid sufferers as well, as up to a third of type 1 diabetes patients ultimately develop thyroid dysfunction.[5]

You are not your genes, but you are what you eat! In Chapter 6, we discussed epigenetics: how your environment, which includes the food you eat, can affect how your DNA is able (or unable) to express itself optimally in your body. Imagine that the food you eat is literally telling your DNA how to behave. The science of nutrigenomics reveals that all food carries information that speaks directly to our genes, influencing every aspect of our health. Your DNA requires the building blocks supplied by proper diet to make your flesh and bones, and as with buildings or any manufactured item, the quality of the components greatly affects the durability of the finished product. Without the right ingredients, you inhabit an increasingly makeshift body that eventually suffers dysfunction.

The fact is that giving our bodies the correct fuel can prevent and even cure chronic illness—including autoimmune conditions!

The buck doesn't stop with you. Dr. Mark Hyman has noted that when the DNA of our ancestors has been tagged by an environmental factor, like mercury in sushi, smoking, or excess sugar, it can become part of our "epigenome," and then can be passed down through generations.[6]

The Standard American Diet and Chronic Illness

Unfortunately, the Standard American Diet (SAD) is filled with bad building blocks in the form of saturated and trans fats, refined sugars such as high-fructose corn syrup, refined carbohydrates, toxic additives, and hormones. The cumulative results of our poor dietary habits are evident in the epidemics of cancer, diabetes, heart, and autoimmune conditions that now afflict westernized countries.

Toxic and dangerous food has had such an impact on our health that New York City banned trans fats from restaurants by 2008, and tried to ban the sale of sugar-sweetened beverages larger than 16 ounces in 2012. These were not popular political moves to garner votes, but rather a reaction to the drastic public health effects that increasingly result from harmful food and drink. Handing a child a 32-ounce soda isn't much better than handing her a cigarette. Ironically, a 2009 Yale study illustrated how the tobacco industry and the big food industry have used similar political tactics to prevent regulation of the harmful effects of their products.[7] It's not just processed sugar that contributes to diabetes, either. Refined carbohydrates also turn quickly to sugar when digested, elevating blood sugar.

There are literally thousands of books, articles, Web sites, and studies on the dangers of processed junk foods, yet many people continue to indulge in these foods and then wonder why they're sick. Many people tend to assume that once science identifies why certain food products and chemicals are bad for you, the government (or someone else) will step in to stop them from being sold, and that the food available for sale at every market is safe and appropriate for them to eat—but that just isn't true. Just because these foods can still be mass-produced, sold cheaply, and marketed everywhere, doesn't mean they aren't the very things that are making you sick, fat, and old!

Poor nutrition, with its attendant toxic, allergic, or dangerous ingredients, will be covered extensively in the sections to come, and I'll offer some solutions for avoiding these common pitfalls in Part Two, but nutrition is *such* a huge splinter for *so* many people that when I talk about nutrition, I want you to imagine me jumping up and down, waving my arms around! Embracing good nutrition *can change your life*, making you feel better almost immediately. You may have to summon the will to change your habits, but it will be worth it. Feeling better means you'll be happier and healthier, which are the conditions your body needs to reverse your autoimmune condition.

Poor Nutrition and Deficiencies

Poor nutrition leads to multiple deficiencies in the many vitamins and minerals we need for optimal health. Many people are surprised to learn that gross nutritional deficiencies underlie their autoimmune condition. Common deficiencies include important antioxidants, such as beta-carotene and other carotenoids, Vitamin C, E, zinc, and selenium, as well as amino acids and important minerals.

Frankenfoods: The GMO Controversy

Imagine there was a substance so unhealthy that dozens of countries, even those in the second and third worlds, had already banned it. Wouldn't you want your own nation to ban it too—or at least label it, so people could choose not to expose themselves to it? And wouldn't you be puzzled (and suspicious) if your government refused to take those precautions? What if that substance became part of the food we eat, and was present in almost everything the entire population of the country ate, every single day?

I'm talking, of course, about America's genetically modified food supply.

At least 61 countries, including all of the European Union, Japan, Russia, and even China, require the labeling of genetically engineered foods. Some countries also have bans and restrictions on genetically modified crops. The United States is by far the world's biggest producer of genetically engineered crops, and naturally there is a powerful industry lobby to prevent any restrictions, testing, or mandatory labeling of genetically modified foods. In 2012, the industry spent $40 million to help defeat a GMO labeling measure on the California ballot.

At this point, unfortunately, the science on the dangers of genetically modified organisms is incomplete and inconclusive. This is partly because companies don't have to prove their genetically modified products are safe (or even provide their proprietary genetic formulas to third parties for study), so studies providing definitive information about GMO foods are few. This is because GMO foods are assumed by both the industry and federal regulators to be "essentially the same" as their whole food counterparts. Paradoxically, these companies are somehow allowed to patent that "something" that is "essentially the same." We have to wonder just how similar it really is.

It may well be possible that some GMO food isn't harmful, but as long as companies are allowed to flood the market with GMOs without proving they are safe, every new "Frankenfood" is an untested risk to your health. Just as it took decades for science to realize that asbestos in the walls of your home was leading to lung damage and cancer, the ultimate effects of certain GMO foods may take years to uncover, and in the meantime, the damage may be building up in the walls of your body itself.

This is not merely theoretical, and autoimmune sufferers are at particular risk. For one very simple example of how genetic modification can make a food more allergenic, let's look at the effects of eating transgenic soybeans that had 2S albumin from Brazil nuts introduced. A study published in *The New England Journal of Medicine* showed that the allergy-provoking qualities of the Brazil nut were transferred to soybeans in the process of modification.[8]

But the changes in GMOs go much farther than mixing in the DNA of other plants, or even the DNA of other animals (as in the famous instances of fish DNA being added to a variety of foods). One of the reasons plant genes are modified is to incorporate the properties of pesticides like Bacillus thuringiensis, or Bt, directly into the plant itself. So instead of spraying pesticide on the plants, farmers can plant seeds that grow up naturally containing genetic mutations that act as pesticides themselves. (And then, instead of spooning pesticide directly from the bag into your mouth, you can simply eat it as part of your cereal…how convenient.) GMO-producing companies say the Bt toxin genetically introduced into GM corn is destroyed in the stomachs of those eating it, but a Canadian study detected Bt toxin in the blood of 93 percent of pregnant women tested, 80 percent of babies, and 67 percent of non-pregnant women.[9]

GMO companies always seem to claim that the genetic information from plants consumed doesn't transfer or incorporate into the bodies of those who consume it. But a recent Chinese study found the MicroRNA from rice in the bodies of Chinese rice consumers.[10] This genetic material from rice actually influenced the uptake of cholesterol from the blood. The possibility of horizontal gene transfer from bioengineered crops to humans is alarming, because we could be making changes to our biology that are untested and can't be reversed.

I'm not going to pretend to have the final answers to the GMO question, and at this point, you shouldn't believe anyone who claims to have them. Unfortunately, the truth is that until GMO-producing companies are forced to release the proprietary genetic information they're using to create the GMOs they are feeding us, third-party research about the issue will be severely hampered. Until then, no one can truly know what the long-term consequences of eating genetically modified foods will be. In the meantime, we are playing with fire. One problem is that our bodies are tuned from millions of years of evolution and haven't adapted to these new foods yet. Many people's autoimmunity is aggravated by allergy-induced inflammation, and evidence is beginning to show GMO "Frankenfoods" may be more allergenic than the unadulterated foods our bodies have eaten for thousands of years.

Individual Sensitivities

Finding your own formula for proper nutrition is also complicated by the fact that we are not all the same. Our genes and natural biology are different, and our chemical exposures, sensitivities, and allergies are all unique. What might be a perfectly healthy food for one person—organic, nutritious, and free from known toxins—might be detrimental to another person and even contribute to their autoimmune condition.

For this reason it's impossible for anyone to come up with an autoimmune nutrition program that works across the board for everyone. The only way to really know if a food is contributing to your condition is to eliminate it for a few weeks and then reintroduce it. I will show you exactly how to find out what foods are triggering your symptoms in Chapter 14: Optimize Your Nutrition.

Food Allergies and Sensitivities

The term "food allergy" is sometimes used to describe all adverse reactions to food. However, more specifically, the term "allergy" refers to food reactions that are mediated by the immune system.

When our immune cells identify a foreign invader or antigen, they try to prevent it from causing harm in the body. For example, when antigens from bacteria or viruses get into our bodies, we can get the flu, or the common cold. We don't get the flu from food antigens, but we can get a wide range of immune-related symptoms that range from the sniffles and hives to anaphylactic shock (a life-threatening condition in which the throat swells and blocks the passage of air). Immediate hypersensitivities affect only a small percentage of the population and autoimmune conditions.

Food Allergies

Allergic reactions to food, also called food hypersensitivities, can be either immediate or delayed. Immediate hypersensitivity reactions occur within hours or even minutes of eating a food. The foods that people are most commonly allergic to include milk, eggs, peanuts, tree nuts (walnuts), soy, strawberries, wheat, fish, and shellfish.

Many people with immediate food hypersensitivities must completely eliminate the offending food from their diet to avoid symptoms—and these symptoms can be severe and noticeable. They include swelling, a rash, hives, or a headache. In rare cases, immediate hypersensitivity reactions can cause anaphylactic shock.

Food Intolerance and Delayed Reactions to Food

Food allergies are pretty straightforward. If you have one, you know who you are. And you probably know which foods to avoid so you don't wind up looking like the Pillsbury doughboy or end up in the ER.

When it comes to delayed reactions to food, however, things can get a little more complicated. This is because many of the same foods, such as milk or eggs, that are known to cause immediate hypersensitivities in a small number of people have also been implicated as a cause of delayed or "masked" food sensitivities in much larger numbers of individuals. In fact, some physicians have suggested that as many as 60 percent of all Americans suffer from masked food sensitivities!

When someone has a food intolerance, this means that they have an abnormal physiological response to a food and that response is not caused by an antibody/antigen reaction. For example, some food intolerances are caused by enzyme deficiencies, while others are caused by poor function of the digestive tract or sensitivity to a natural or synthetic chemical.

Lectins

In the following sections, you'll discover that many healthy-sounding foods can disturb your GI tract. One reason is that many plants we commonly eat contain proteins called lectins. Plants use these lectins as a natural defense against pests and fungus. They tend to be bitter and difficult to digest. Lectins can stick to the walls of the small intestine, causing inflammation and obstructing the natural healing process of the GI wall, leading to cell death and contributing to leaky gut syndrome.[11] There is evidence that lectins can contribute directly to autoimmune responses, particularly rheumatoid arthritis.[12]

Lectins are everywhere, but it's important to know the foods that contain the most lectins: grains, dairy, legumes (particularly soy), nightshade vegetables (tomatoes, potatoes, eggplant, peppers, and more), and nuts. To make matters worse, some foods are genetically modified in a way that adds to their lectin content.[13]

Lectins are generally reduced (but not completely eliminated) by soaking, sprouting, and cooking. The lectins in red kidney beans, for instance, are toxic unless cooked. Soaking and then pressure-cooking is the most effective means of reducing lectins (and phytic acid, another anti-nutrient).[14] I soak and then dehydrate my almonds to neutralize some of the lectins. While moderation may work for some people, many are more sensitive and need to assertively minimize lectin exposure to give their gut a chance to heal and to reduce inflammation and immune system aggravation.

Wheat and Gluten

One of the most common food sensitivities is to gluten. Gluten is a protein found in wheat, rye, barley, oats, kamut, and spelt. Gluten remains after all the starch is washed away from the flour of these grains, and is made up of two protein groups called gliadins and glutenins.

Some researchers note that humans have only been eating grains for around 10,000 years, a fraction of the time that we have been eating other foods, so we haven't had the evolutionary time to adapt to grains being a staple in our diet.

Modern wheat has also changed dramatically since the 1940's, when it began being extensively hybridized, backcrossed, and mutated with chemicals, creating a form of wheat that human digestion is even less prepared to cope with. It was around that same time that we began eating more wheat in processed foods. Because of this combination of factors, it can be even tougher to tell where our sensitivity to gluten comes from.

As of 2013, genetically modified wheat (by the strict definition of GMO) is not being sold anywhere in the world, although a rogue field of unapproved GMO wheat was recently discovered in Oregon.[15] Also contrary to rumor, an analysis has shown that modern wheat does not contain more gluten than previous varieties; the wheat of biblical times had even more gluten.[16] These are technicalities that I am including for the sake of accuracy, but wheat has been greatly changed by conventional means in recent times. According to Dr. William Davis, cardiologist and author of *Wheat Belly*, the problems with modern wheat may result from alternations in the structure of the proteins gliadin and agglutinin, and from new forms of alpha amylase inhibitors and other proteins provoking allergies and sensitivities thus aggravating the immune system.[17]

Again, we are all different. Some people don't seem to be bothered by gluten at all, but others are extremely sensitive to it. It's also difficult to rely solely on testing, as it's common to find people who test negative in the common AGA-IgA and AGA-IgG tests for gluten allergy, but who nonetheless show dramatic improvements when they take gluten from their diet. Doctors who work with autoimmune clients have found that many of their patients report major improvements when they remove grains from their diets.

Dairy

Milk and dairy products can cause problems for people if they are lactose intolerant or have casein or whey sensitivity.

Lactose is the naturally occurring sugar in milk. We use the enzyme lactase to digest lactose, but many people produce far less lactase after the age of three or four. This makes sense in nature (milk digestion enzymes disappear around the age when children naturally stop breastfeeding). If you drink milk or consume certain dairy products and you lack enough lactase, it can cause gas, bloating, cramping, or diarrhea. Lactose intolerance is strongly linked to your genetic heritage; people of Asian or African descent are highly likely to suffer lactose intolerance, while those of northern European descent are less likely.

Casein and whey are milk proteins that can cause an allergic reaction in some people, and studies have implicated both proteins in autoimmune conditions.[19] People with leaky gut syndrome are also more likely to have trouble with the milk protein. Besides gas, bloating, and other digestive symptoms, dairy sensitivity can also cause skin rashes, hives, headaches, runny nose, itchy eyes, gastroesophageal reflux (GERD), and coughing. Serious complications like anaphylaxis can happen in the worst cases.

Corn and High-Fructose Corn Syrup

Corn sensitivity can provoke a variety of symptoms, including headaches, fatigue, moodiness, joint and muscle pains, nausea, and diarrhea plus gas, bloating and cramps. Allergies to corn are less common, but can also include hives, rashes, swelling of lips, upper respiratory problems, stuffy nose, and even more severe reactions. Corn sensitivity is hard to test for, but an elimination diet can show if corn sensitivity is an issue for you.

According the United States Department of Agriculture (USDA), the percentage of genetically engineered corn grown in the U.S. went from 25 percent in the year 2000, to 88 percent in 2011.[19] These modifications can include integrating Bt pesticide toxin directly into the corn itself. There is far too little evidence of safety to conclude genetically modified corn is harmless, and animal studies have suggested GMO corn might have negative effects.

Problems with corn are increasing in recent times, as corn is a cheap, subsidized commodity crop that is everywhere in processed foods, often in the form of high-fructose corn syrup. High-fructose corn syrup is a molecularly altered sugar, which is rapidly absorbed by your body. Scientific evidence suggests high-fructose corn syrup may contribute to diabetes and obesity even more than plain sugar.[20] Samples of it have also been found to contain mercury from the manufacturing process.[21]

The presence of high-fructose corn syrup in a product is often a good indicator that it is cheaply made, without careful regard for its wholesomeness. My advice is to stay away!

Nightshades

Many people are surprised to learn that nightshade vegetables can aggravate their autoimmune condition. The most common nightshades are tomatoes, green and red peppers (both sweet and hot), eggplant, white potatoes, and spices such as cayenne, paprika, and pepper-based sauces such as Tabasco. Fortunately, for those of us who are sensitive to nightshades, yams or sweet potatoes are not nightshades, and neither are peppercorns. There are also nightshades used medicinally, such as goji berries and ashwagandha, mandrake, belladonna, and tobacco. For healthy individuals, many of these foods can be eaten without consequence. People with autoimmune conditions need to be more cautious.

The group of substances in nightshades that can adversely affect the body are called alkaloids. Plants produce alkaloids to deter insects, and different alkaloids are found in varying degrees in all nightshades. We've all heard of the alkaloid nicotine and know that it is found in tobacco. What most people don't know is that it is present in differing amounts in all nightshades.[22] The addictive quality of nicotine may be one of the reasons it is so hard for people to eliminate nightshades from their diets. The alkaloids, certain lectins, and saponins in nightshades appear to contribute to leaky gut syndrome, which can provoke an autoimmune response.

Nightshades have only been a part of the diet in North America and

Europe for a few hundred years, which may not have given us enough evolutionary time to thrive with them. If you are going to eat nightshades, consider cooking them. Cooking nightshades reduces alkaloids by 40 to 50 percent. Another way to protect yourself is to avoid green spots and sprouts on potatoes. The green you see, usually on the outside of potatoes, is a sign that the alkaloid solanine is present. Too much solanine can cause solanine poisoning. Besides color, a bitter taste can also signify a high solanine level.

Symptoms of nightshade sensitivity are similar to those of gluten or dairy intolerance: unexplained rashes, gas, nausea, headaches, muscle tremors, GERD, moodiness, and so on. Nightshades also seem to aggravate arthritis and aching joints. Many of my clients who removed nightshades from their diet reduced their pain and symptoms dramatically.

Soy and Legumes

Soy is another food that people are often allergic or sensitive to. Sensitivity can trigger digestive problems and inflammation, while an allergic reaction can provoke worse symptoms. Soy is also at the center of the GMO controversy, as the USDA states that as of 2012, 93 percent of U.S. soy is genetically modified to be herbicide-tolerant.[23] Soy contains isoflavones, which some studies have shown to negatively affect thyroid hormones.[24] Other studies don't find a thyroid problem resulting from moderate use of soy by healthy people.[25] Soy can be an ingredient in many products and supplements, so it's easy to get more of it than you realize, even if you can tolerate it in moderation. There is reason to believe that fermented non-GMO soy products such as tempeh and miso are easier for your body to digest, as fermentation reduces the lectins, or "anti-nutrients," present in the soy as part of the plant's natural defenses.

Soy is a legume, like beans, peas, and lentils. Many people who are sensitive to one legume are often sensitive to others. Beans have a reputation for giving people gas for a reason: oligosaccharides are a carbohydrate in legumes, particularly beans, that the body has trouble breaking down, and gas is a result.

Peanuts are actually legumes, not nuts. Some people are wildly allergic to even the smallest quantity of peanuts. (You know who you are.) Peanuts are one of the leading causes of death from food allergy.[26] For the rest of us, peanuts are particularly susceptible to contamination with aflatoxins, or carcinogenic molds. There are controversies regarding whether peanut oil contributes to clogging of the arteries, and about the potentially harmful effects of peanut agglutinin (PNA), a peanut lectin, associated in studies with leaky gut syndrome and colon cancer.[27,28,29]

Not everyone needs to avoid beans, lentils or even moderate use of fermented soy. The *Sensitivity Discovery Program* outlined in Chapter 14 will help you discover if soy and legumes are a problem for you.

Nuts

Tree nuts, like macadamia nuts, Brazil nuts, almonds, walnuts, pecans, pistachios, chestnuts, beechnuts, and hazelnuts, are a common food allergy. Cashews are actually a seed that's related to mangoes, pistachios, and poison ivy, but some people are sensitive to them as well. People who are allergic to one tree nut are likely to be allergic to more than one. Peanut allergy and tree nut allergies also go together frequently. Allergy to coconut is rare. Symptoms vary, from rashes and hives, nausea, diarrhea, and swelling to heart irregularities and severe difficulty breathing.

For those without an allergy to tree nuts, you should know that tree nuts, like grains and legumes, are high in phytic acid, which interferes with our absorption of minerals. Because nuts are usually consumed in smaller quantities than staple foods like grains and beans, they are less likely to rob you of iron and zinc absorption. It helps if you snack on nuts between meals so the nuts are digested separately.

If you do want to eat a lot of nuts, please soak and sprout them, which will reduce or eliminate the enzyme inhibitors, lectins, and phytic acid content.

Food Additives and Salicylates

Many people are also unable to tolerate natural and synthetic chemicals, such as sulfites, that appear in abundance in our commercial food supply. These sulfur-containing preservatives are used in dried fruits, wines, and many other processed foods. Between 1980 and 1999, the United States Food and Drug Administration received more than 1,000 reports of adverse reactions, some fatal, to sulfites. It has been estimated that at least 1 percent of all people with asthma are sensitive to sulfites.

Synthetic food colorings, including food dyes and Color Yellow No. 5 (tartrazine), are problematic for many people as well. Monosodium Glutamate (MSG) is another example of an additive used to increase flavor, particularly in Asian foods. After eating at restaurants that use MSG, many people become bloated, experience severe headaches, or have other adverse reactions. Yeast extract, autolyzed yeast, calcium caseinate, sodium caseinate, hydrolyzed protein, and "hydrolyzed yeast" are other common ingredients that contain naturally occurring MSG.

While food colorings and additives like MSG are examples of human-created substances that many people react to, salicylates and amines are examples of naturally occurring food substances found in many vegetables, herbs, spices, fruits, and chocolate. Even though they are naturally occurring, these substances may also create adverse reactions. Salicylates and amines have been associated with a variety of symptoms including mental confusion, depression, and migraine headaches.

The following is a partial list of natural foods and prepared products that contain salicylates and amines:

Tomatoes	Broccoli
Olives	Spinach
Mushrooms	Avocado
All dried fruit	Smoked meats
Canned fish	Hard cheeses
Soy sauce	Miso
Chocolate	Cocoa
Beer	Cola drinks
Vinegars	Yeast extract

If you have an autoimmune condition, it's much more likely that there are foods that negatively affect you, and it's possible that you've been living with those harmful effects for years, thinking that's it's just normal to be bloated, gassy, overweight, tired, or any of the other symptoms created by eating foods your body can't handle.

In Chapter 14: Optimize Your Nutrition, I'll offer a *Sensitivity Discovery Program* that allows you to discover firsthand what foods make you feel bad and may be contributing to your autoimmune condition. In my time as a nutritional counselor, I've enjoyed seeing many people feel dramatically better in a short time once they stop eating the particular foods their body can't handle. I hope a careful exploration of your own diet can yield life-changing results for you, too!

Symptoms related to poor nutrition, individual sensitivities and allergic foods can show up all over the body—from minor irritations to major health conditions.

Here is a list of some of the most common ones:

- Impaired liver function
- Impaired thyroid function
- Nutritional deficiencies
- Inflammation
- Anemia
- Sinus congestion or hay-fever-like symptoms
- Dark circles or puffiness under the eyes
- Fluid retention
- Chronic skin conditions such as acne, hives, rashes, eczema, rosacea, and psoriasis
- GI symptoms—gas, bloating, constipation, diarrhea
- Gastroesophageal acid reflux (GERD)
- Fatigue
- Joint inflammation
- Mood swings and mood disorders
- Headaches and migraines
- Asthma
- Poor memory and cognition
- Anxiety and depression
- Psychiatric disorders
- ADD and ADHD
- Craving sweets and carbs
- Celiac disease
- Diabetes
- Cancer
- Heart Disease
- Autoimmune conditions

List any of the above symptoms you have here. Do you have any symptoms not on the list?

_____
_____
_____
_____
_____
_____
_____
_____

Splinter #4: Gastrointestinal (GI) Stress

In Chapter 5: Understand Your Immune System, I review the gastrointestinal tract (GI) and discuss how it functions as a barrier and is part of our "internal skin." The GI tract has the important job of screening out toxins while breaking food down into nutrients to be absorbed into the body. It's also home to as much as 60 to 80 percent of the cells of the immune system, which live in the gut-associated lymphoid tissue, or GALT for short.

The GI tract is a muscular "inner tube" that runs from our mouth to our anus and is made up of a special layer of cells, called epithelium. If laid out flat, the GI tract has a surface area equal to that of a tennis court, due to millions of finger-like projections called villi and hair-like bristles called microvilli.

The GI tract is a critical area where those of us with an autoimmune condition are especially vulnerable. A sick, tired, and toxic colon is a major part of the GI splinter in many autoimmune conditions. In fact, I have never met anyone with an autoimmune condition who had a "perfectly healthy" GI tract.

Let's review the causes of GI stress and the accompanying symptoms.

Causes of GI Stress

Eating When We're Upset, Rushed or Stressed

When we are stressed or upset, our normal digestion process slows down as the body gathers its resources to either "fight or run away." Digestion actually begins in the mouth when we chew our food well and mix it with the digestive enzymes in our saliva. That doesn't happen when we choke down food in a hurry. To make matters worse, when we're upset or stressed, we produce less stomach acid and our food may be only partially digested by the time it reaches the small intestine. This undigested food puts enormous pressure on the small intestine as it tries to break down huge food particles in order to extract their nutrients. When it can't, the food just sits there and putrefies, causing a disturbance in GI flora, malabsorption, and a host of uncomfortable symptoms.

What's worse is that large undigested food particles can seep through the gut and enter the bloodstream, triggering an immune response.

Sugar, Caffeine, Alcohol, and Carbs

Overuse of sugar, caffeine, alcohol, and refined, processed carbohydrates can irritate and erode the delicate lining of the GI tract, feed yeast, and disturb healthy bacteria. Fungi love sugar in all forms, and will overpopulate when given their food of choice. Not only does the overuse of coffee and alcohol create an acidic environment (which bad bugs love), it also puts a huge stress on the liver, pancreas, and gallbladder.

Eating Disorders

Images of emaciated women offered by the fashion industry and the media as the guidelines of "perfection" have created an unhealthy standard of beauty in our society. The attempt to be as skinny as a runway model drives many women to eating disorders. I have observed that, like me, many of my female clients have suffered from some form of eating disorder at some time in their lives.

One of the most common conditions is called anorexia, and occurs when one deeply fears gaining weight to the point that one stops eating properly, or at all. Anorexics have an unrealistic perception of their bodies, and see themselves as overweight, even if they are very thin.

Anorexia carries all the consequences of moderate to severe

malnutrition, leading to heart problems, low blood pressure, loss of bone and muscle mass, and without treatment, even death. The emotional stress is great as well, as anorexics have risk of suicide 32 times greater than that of the general population.

Nobody knows how many people suffer from anorexia, because few anorexics seek treatment until it's a full-blown crisis. The feeling of shame associated with anorexia is itself a great stress, one that also stands in the way of seeking treatment.

Bulimia is an eating disorder characterized by binge eating, followed by purging to avoid weight gain. Purging can mean self-induced vomiting, obsessive exercise and compensatory fasting. Bulimics often have relatively normal body weight and can sometimes even be overweight.

Repeated vomiting erodes the esophagus and teeth as well. Dehydration is also a common issue with bulimia. Along with dehydration can come electrolyte and chemical imbalances, loss of vitamins and nutrients, chronic GI tract irregularity, heart problems, and even death.

Overuse of Laxatives

Some people overuse laxatives as a strategy to avoid gaining weight. This may be a form of bulimia, or just overzealous dieting, but laxative abuse has additional consequences for the GI tract. Larger and larger doses of laxatives are required and the body can basically lose the ability to have a bowel moment on its own. Many electrolytes are lost and dehydration is common. Other people may use diuretics to keep their water weight at a minimum. This creates dehydration, which leads to adrenal fatigue and a chronic state of GI dysfunction.

Overuse of laxatives and diuretics puts your GI tract in a constant state of imbalance and disturbance.

There are no real statistics regarding the overuse of laxatives in our society, perhaps because people are too embarrassed to ask for help.

Your GI tract is designed to extract the essential ingredients your body needs from the food you eat. If you don't eat enough food, or you purge the food you eat, you starve yourself and disturb the function of that life-giving mechanism.

The imbalances and insults your GI tract suffers through anorexia, bulimia, and abuse of laxatives and diuretics will ultimately weaken your body and immune system, which may turn into a factor in your autoimmune condition.

Celiac Disease

The condition called "celiac disease" has gotten a lot of media attention these days, as the numbers of people who have wheat intolerance continues to rise. But just what is celiac disease? Some people equate it with simple gluten intolerance. In truth, however, it is a multi-system autoimmune condition involving changes in function of the liver, digestive tract, and other organ systems. The role of a specific enzyme called tissue transglutaminase, or tTG, appears to be especially important in celiac disease. Short strands of protein (polypeptides) found in gliadin (one family of wheat proteins) are acted on by this enzyme, resulting in many of the problems associated with this condition. For some individuals, a blood test measuring the ratio of antibodies to tTG can be an effective screening test for celiac disease.

However, wheat is still a primary cause of celiac disease. The bottom line is that there is a lot more wheat in our diet than there used to be, and it turns out that some people are extremely sensitive to it. One study showed that celiac patients have a 300 percent greater chance of having thyroid disease as well. When doctors put those celiac patients on a strict gluten-free diet for one year, most dramatically improved, and the study concluded that in certain cases, gluten withdrawal might single-handedly reverse the thyroid dysfunction.[30] Celiac disease goes hand in hand with leaky gut syndrome, which allows undigested gluten proteins into the bloodstream.

Gluten: The Big GI Splinter

Among the most common GI stressors are food allergies and sensitivities—especially to gluten.[31] I write about gluten all throughout this book, since it is my experience that it is a major issue for many people with autoimmune conditions. While many healthy people seem to be able to eat gluten with no problem, wheat, barley, rye, and other grains containing gluten can aggravate inflammation and immune responses in people with leaky gut syndrome, which allows undigested gluten proteins and other toxins past the intestinal wall and into the bloodstream.

When undigested food particles get through the tiny junctions in the GI wall into the bloodstream, the immune system identifies them as antigens and an immune response is launched. For a person with an autoimmune condition and sensitivity to gluten, this immune response is constant as long as they continue to eat food that contains these proteins.

The problems don't end when gluten proteins trigger an immune response, tagging them as antigens for destruction. If you eat gluten every day, as most Westerners do, you will likely have a large number of antibodies to gluten circulating through your bloodstream at all times. This can be a major trigger for many autoimmune conditions because of something called "molecular mimicry."[32] Scientists postulate that the immune system profile of the gluten protein is molecularly similar to many of the tissues in the human body. When our immune system tags gluten proteins as antigens, it can mistake the thyroid and other tissues for gluten and tag them as well, resulting in an autoimmune attack on the thyroid gland. We keep eating gluten, so we keep aggravating an immune response, and the result is the continual destruction of our thyroid gland.

Most of us love to eat many of the foods made with wheat, barley, rye, and the other grains containing gluten. Gluten is also hidden in many processed foods, such as soups and salad dressings. If you are sensitive to gluten, it's just not worth it to suffer the inflammation, poor digestion, and weight gain that gluten can provoke, not to mention an autoimmune response and its debilitating effects.

Antacids and NSAIDS

Overuse of antacids can neutralize stomach acid so much that food cannot be properly digested in the stomach, which puts stress on the small intestine. Over time, the abuse of antacids can cause the stomach to produce less of its own acid, leading to chronically low stomach acid and a dependence on medication.

Chronic use of over-the-counter and prescription, non-steroidal anti-inflammatory drugs (NSAIDS) such as ibuprofen (Advil, Motrin, Nuprin), naproxen (Aleve), and aspirin can damage the mucosal lining of the GI tract causing ulcers and bleeding.

Antibiotics

Antibiotics might seem like a good idea when you're sick, but they are notoriously indiscriminate killers. When you take an antibiotic for an infection, it kills healthy bacteria along with the target pathogen, making way for the overgrowth of yeast and other unfriendly flora.

Many times, doctors prescribe antibiotics for symptoms caused by fungus and viruses. This is worse than useless, as it exacerbates the situation by killing the good flora we have in our gut. To add insult to injury, the over-prescribing of antibiotics has created drug-resistant strains of bacteria that require an even stronger arsenal of antibiotics. These drug-resistant strains may evolve into "superbugs" (MRSA and Staphylococcus aureus are two examples) that are completely resistant to therapy.

Even if we don't take antibiotics, we're still exposed to them in our food and water supplies. According to a 2009 paper published in *Environmental Health Perspectives*, different antibiotics and anti-infectives have been identified in processed waste water, natural surface water, ground water, and drinking water supplies. We also get doses of antibiotics by consuming conventionally-produced (non-organic) meat and dairy products.

GI Tract Infections

GI tract infections are another major source of GI stress in many autoimmune conditions. We become more vulnerable to GI tract infections through chronic fight-or-flight states, poor food choices, food allergies and sensitivities, and toxins like alcohol and caffeine, which can damage the inner lining and disturb the delicate balance of intestinal flora. When this happens, pathogenic bacteria, parasites, and fungus can crowd out the good bacteria and disturb the GALT tissue.

Common GI pathogens include the following:
- Fungal infections such as Candida
- Pathogenic bacteria such as H. pylori, Clostridium difficile, Campylobacter sp. and E. coli
- Opportunistic bacteria such as Salmonella sp., Yersinia sp, and Klebsiella sp, and M. morganii
- Parasites, which include amoebas and worms

Chronic low-grade bacterial and fungal infections of the gut can reduce our overall immune function, leading to vulnerability to further infections and viruses. Many times, this leads to "stealth" low-grade infections in other parts of the body that can linger undetected for years. These stealth infections put an additional strain on our immune system.

Leaky Gut

Our intestinal walls function by absorbing nutrients and keeping out waste and substances that might harm the body. If the inner tubing of the GI tract becomes inflamed due to food intolerance, lectins, toxins or infections, the villi and microvilli become damaged and the surface area of the inner part of the GI tract is reduced.[33] Just a reminder that lectins are "anti-nutrient" chemicals that plants naturally use to protect themselves from insects and are particularly prominent in grains, soy, legumes and nightshades. This irritation and inflammation ultimately leads to compromised digestion, malabsorption and immune stress. Over time, the constant irritation breaks down the tight junctions of the GI tract, resulting in a condition called leaky gut. In this condition, undigested proteins and toxins escape into the bloodstream, triggering an immune response, which in turn triggers allergies and autoimmune conditions.

Even healthy guts leak substances into our bloodstream. Otherwise, how could the GI absorb nutrients? The problem arises when the gates of the gut open too wide and undigested proteins and toxins enter the bloodstream. They don't belong there, and this triggers the body to stage an immune response that can contribute to an autoimmune condition.

A study spearheaded by Alessio Fasano at the University of Maryland School of Medicine has documented increased levels of the protein zonulin in patients with celiac disease.[34] Zonulin controls the permeability of the tight junctions in the GI walls that allow substances to pass into our system. Too much zonulin and the junctions open wide enough for the gluten proteins to enter and trigger an immune reaction. Again, celiac disease is associated with increased intestinal permeability (leaky gut), and celiac patients often suffer from other autoimmune disorders.

Science has observed that for sensitive individuals, gluten actually provokes the gut to leak, but we also know that when gluten-sensitive people eliminate it from their diet, the integrity of the intestinal wall can be restored—no more leaky gut.[35,36] An imbalance in the healthy flora of the gut, due to the effects of antibiotics on our good bacteria, for instance, can also make the GI vulnerable to leakage. Besides eliminating offending foods like gluten or excess lectins, probiotics and supplements can play a strong supportive role in re-establishing the integrity of the intestinal wall.[37]

More research is needed to determine what factors account for excess zonulin. For now, if you have an autoimmune condition, there's a good chance your GI tract is irritated and allowing substances into your bloodstream that can trigger allergies, food sensitivities, and immune responses. This means you might react to foods that many others can eat with no problem. Reclaiming your health and vitality depends on discovering if certain foods aggravate you, and then healing your gut so it can protect your system.

Chronic fungal infections of the GI tract such as Candida can migrate to other parts of the body through a leaky gut and develop into "systemic" infections, which can cause inflammation and trigger autoimmune reactions. They have even been implicated in certain cancers.[38]

Symptoms of GI Stress

- Gas
- Bloating
- Constipation
- Diarrhea
- Acid reflux/GERD
- Nausea
- Vomiting
- Abdominal discomfort
- Feeling bloated after meals
- Undigested food in stool
- Impaired liver function
- Food allergies, or reactions
- Anal itching
- Inhalant allergies
- Craving sweets and carbs
- Chronic abdominal pain
- Canker sores

- Sores anywhere in the mouth
- Nausea after taking supplements
- Chronic skin conditions such as acne, hives, rashes, eczema, rosacea, and psoriasis
- ADD (Attention deficit disorder)
- IBS (Irritable bowel syndrome)
- IBD (Inflammatory bowel disease)
- Celiac disease
- Anemia

List any of the above GI symptoms you have here. Do you have any symptoms that are not on the list?

_____
_____
_____
_____
_____
_____
_____
_____

> **What You Need to Know:**
> The "heavy lifting" cells of your immune system live in your gut. If you have an autoimmune condition, your GI tract should be the first place to look for clues as to what's triggering your illness!

Splinter #5: Adrenal Exhaustion, Adrenal Fatigue and Adrenal Burnout

Our bodies are designed to handle a healthy amount of stress, and the flight-or-fight response can save our lives when we are in danger. But as you've learned, stress becomes chronic when the stressful situations don't end, and we are forced to sustain an unnatural fight-or-flight response.

Over time, our adrenals can become overworked and exhausted, which can cause us to feel fatigued, depressed, and sick. If the stress goes on for too long, we can experience a condition called "burnout," which makes our bodies begin to break down on a cellular level.

Chronic stress in all of its forms can cause chronically increased levels of the adrenal hormones adrenalin and cortisol, which have an impact on all your body's functions.

A technical discussion follows, but the bottom line is that when you are stressed-out and can feel it in your body, that stress is affecting your body. Stress out too often and you'll experience the effects of adrenal fatigue or burnout.

Effects of Elevated Stress Hormones

- Blood sugar imbalances, dysglycemia, and insulin resistance
- Redistribution of fat in the body—typically weight gain around the middle
- Decreased DNA repair
- Inhibition of pro-inflammatory interleukins[39]
- Impaired cognitive function and damage to a part of your brain called the hippocampus, which is involved in memory
- Inhibited conversion of thyroid hormones T4 into T3, suppression of TSH, and blockage of thyroid hormone receptors—a measure your body takes so that you don't just completely burn out!
- Negative effects on the cells of the immune system—elevated cortisol will reduce the amount of secretory immunoglobulin A (IgA), which is your body's first line of defense against bacteria and viruses. (This is why you get sick more easily when you are stressed.)
- Feeling wired but tired, with disrupted sleep patterns—these are the hormones that wake you up at 3 a.m.
- Inhibited skin regeneration while you are sleeping, resulting in premature wrinkles and aging
- Decreased bone density
- Elevated blood pressure
- Decreased muscle mass

Causes of Adrenal Burnout

Adrenal burnout is caused by stress in all its forms. Everything we've been discussing—emotional, psychological, infectious, toxic, allergic, and environmental factors—have an effect on the adrenal glands. All of these stresses are enough on their own, but most of us find ourselves bombarded by multiple types of stress, and over time, these accumulate and become chronic. The condition of constant, unrelenting stress leaves the adrenals working overtime, and without a rest, they eventually give out. After a while, you begin to feel like you're "beating a dead horse," and your body simply says, "No!"

Symptoms of Adrenal Burnout

- Suppressed thyroid function—poor conversion of T4 to T3
- Waking up in the middle of the night and being unable to get back to sleep
- Trouble falling and staying asleep
- Difficulty waking up in the morning
- Not feeling rested after a full night's sleep
- Needing caffeine to start the day
- Being lightheaded upon standing up
- Feeling wired but tired
- Lack of energy
- Being easily startled by loud noises
- Cold hands and cold feet
- Constipation
- Panic attacks
- Feeling shaky and weak
- Craving salt
- Craving sweets
- Mental fogginess
- Memory problems
- Needing increased time to recover from illness, injury, or trauma
- Feeling that little things put you over the edge
- Feeling depressed
- Lack of interest in the things that used to bring you joy

- Decreased libido
- Increased PMS symptoms
- "Hitting the wall" at 3-4 p.m. only to feel "up" again after 6 or 7 p.m.
- Feeling tired but resisting going to bed before 11 p.m.

Please list any of the above symptoms of adrenal burnout that you have here. Do you have any symptoms not on the list?

_____

_____

_____

_____

_____

_____

_____

_____

> **What You Need to Know:**
> Your body responds to every kind of stress in the same way; it can't tell the difference between that huge stack of unpaid bills, an argument with your spouse, an old grudge, and a saber-toothed tiger!

Splinter #6: Hormonal Stress

Our bodies are healthy and vibrant when all of our hormones are in balance. Our sex and adrenal hormones work synergistically with our thyroid hormones. In fact, if one hormone is off, it can cause stress on the body and affect all the other hormones. It's important to remember that hormonal imbalance is your body's way of trying to correct something or communicate to you that something is amiss.

Let's take a look at the main hormones:

Pregnenolone: Sometimes called "the mother of all hormones," pregnenolone is made primarily in the adrenal glands, from cholesterol. It's the precursor for all the sex hormones: testosterone, estrogen, progesterone, DHEA, and cortisol. Low levels of pregnenolone are common in people with hypothyroidism and adrenal burnout.

Estrogen is produced from cholesterol, primarily by developing follicles in the ovaries, the corpus luteum, and the placenta. A small percentage is produced in the liver, adrenal glands, fat cells, and breasts. In men, estrogen is produced in the adrenal glands and testes. There are three types of estrogen: estrone (E1), estradiol (E2), and estriol (E3). The estrogens have many functions and are important for tissue growth, sex drive, and healthy bones and, when balanced, may protect from heart disease. Too much estrogen can lead to low thyroid function in two ways: it can inhibit the conversion of thyroid hormones T4 to T3, and it can bind to thyroid proteins, blocking thyroid hormone from its own receptors.

Progesterone is primarily produced from pregnenolone in the ovaries in the second half of a woman's cycle, but small amounts are produced in the adrenal glands. Men produce small amounts of progesterone in the adrenals and testes. Progesterone is the hormone that supports a healthy pregnancy. Progesterone can enhance thyroid hormone function, but if your thyroid hormones are out of balance, it can lower your progesterone levels.

Testosterone is a male hormone, but both men and women have it. Testosterone is produced by the ovaries or testicles, and adrenal glands. Like estrogen, it plays a crucial role in the growth, maintenance, and repair of reproductive tissues.

DHEA is produced in the adrenal glands and is responsible for proper immune function, fat burning, muscle building, tissue repair, proper liver function, and energy production. DHEA will also convert into other sex hormones, such as estrogen and testosterone.

Cortisol is produced in the adrenal glands and affects every organ and tissue in the body. Cortisol has thousands of effects on the body, but its primary role is to control inflammation, help the body respond to stress, and maintain glucose levels in the blood for energy.

Human Growth Hormone (HGH) is secreted by the pituitary gland, which causes the liver to produce another hormone called IGF-1. IGF-1 affects almost every cell in the body. It's often called "the hormone of youth," because it's responsible for rejuvenating the skin and bones and regenerating the tissues of the heart, lungs, liver, and kidneys. At optimal levels, it helps build muscle mass and burn fat. It enhances sexual performance and produces increased energy levels. It lowers blood pressure and improves cholesterol profiles. It encourages hair growth, removes wrinkles, eliminates cellulite, and improves memory, mood, and sleep. Thyroid hormones regulate the release and synthesis of HGH, and many people with low thyroid levels have low IGF-1. Chronic illness, stress, hypothyroidism, liver toxicity, and aging all slow the production of IGF-1, which results in accelerated aging.

The causes of hormonal stress are everything we have been talking about!

Here are a few examples of pathways that can result in hormonal stress:

- Chronic stress causes elevated stress hormones cortisol and adrenalin, which can cause adrenal fatigue and affect all of our other hormones.
- Over consumption of sugar, alcohol and carbs leads to blood sugar imbalances, dysglycemia and insulin resistance.
- Birth control pills, hormone replacement, and exposure to xenoestrogens require the system to contend with hormonal signals introduced from outside sources.

As if these first two factors weren't confusing enough for the body's hormone production, even more of the natural balance can be lost when the third comes into play. While some stressors prod the body into producing more of its own hormones in unbalanced amounts, others simply enter the body and pretend to be those same hormones. This disrupts the endocrine cycle, because the body thinks its hormone-producing work is already done.

Exposure to Xenoestrogens and Endocrine Disrupting Compounds (EDCs)

EDCs are synthetic compounds that mimic our natural hormones when they are absorbed by the body. When these compounds mimic estrogen, they are called xenoestrogens. They can turn on, turn off, or even change normal hormonal signals. EDCs can dock in our body's hormone receptors, thus blocking natural hormones. When this happens, there can be no hormone activity, or it may become altered or mutated, resulting in unnatural hormone expression. In some cases, it's like having a key that fits in the lock but doesn't unlock the door. In other cases, it fits and opens it, but then you can't close and relock the door. Any system or bodily function controlled by hormones can also be affected, including the immune system.

Xenoestrogens and EDCs are everywhere—from lotions and sunblock to pesticides, plastics, and industrial and household chemicals. We find them in non-organic meat and dairy products as well. Cattle are injected with estrogen to create weight gain and increase milk production (more pounds and more milk = more profit). Exposure to xenoestrogens and EDCs has been directly linked with allergies, autoimmune conditions, and elevated antinuclear antibodies (ANA).[40]

We will talk in greater detail about how to identify the most common EDCs in *Splinter #8: Toxic Stress.*

Women and Autoimmunity: Elevated Estrogen and Inflammation

Many experts believe that estrogen-induced inflammation may be the reason why women account for 75 percent of all autoimmune cases.[41] After all, we make our own natural estrogen, but then we're exposed to much more in the environment. Excess levels of estrogen can cause inflammation in the body and push the immune system to make too many antibodies.[42] Excess inflammation caused by estrogen is of particular concern for women under stress, in perimenopause and menopause, or those who have high exposures to xenoestrogens.

Particularly at risk are women on hormone replacement therapy (HRT), who take synthetic estrogens and progestins such as Premarin, Prempro, Provera, and birth control pills. These "therapies" have been linked with an increased risk of developing systemic and discoid lupus, scleroderma, and Raynaud's disease, as well as certain cancers.[43]

Bad Estrogens and Impaired Liver Detoxification

The liver plays an important role in processing and metabolizing all of our hormones—not just the ones we make naturally, but also the ones we are exposed to through birth control pills, HRT, and xenoestrogens.

The liver works to clear our bodies of excess hormones and toxins using two pathways, known as Phase I and Phase II. We'll talk more specifically about these pathways in Chapter 17: Restore Your Liver.

Once your body has used the estrogen it needs, it will break down or oxidize the excess into different estrogen metabolites during Phase I through an enzyme system called cytochrome P450, in order to convert the fat-soluble estrogens into more easily excreted water-soluble forms. These leftover metabolites have varying levels of estrogenic activity; some are weak and some are strong (and more troublesome).

The bottom line is that some estrogen metabolites are good, but others can be harmful if produced in excess or out of proper balance. Good estrogen metabolites like 2-hydroxyestrone don't seem to increase inflammation or cancer risk, and may even protect us from the bad estrogen. One harmful estrogen metabolite is 16-alpha-hydroxyestrone, which causes inflammation and has been linked to breast cancer and lupus. In fact, one study found this bad estrogen to be 10 times higher in patients with rheumatoid arthritis and lupus![44]

How well your liver metabolizes estrogens depends on many factors. Your liver may have difficulty detoxifying due to stress, poor nutrition, or toxic exposures. It can also be affected by exposure to hormones originating outside your body (exogenous) such as birth control pills, synthetic hormone replacement therapy, and substances that your body mistakes for estrogens (xenoestrogens.)

In the future, health care will likely focus more on reducing disease by improving genetic expression through diet, lifestyle, and supplementation. For instance, soy isoflavones, flax lignans, exercise, fish oil, and the phytonutrients in cruciferous vegetables all stimulate the genetic expression and metabolism of estrogen into a safer form the body can handle (2-hydroylated). On the other hand, alcohol and pesticides stimulate genetic expression to create the dangerous forms of estrogen (16-hydroxylated). Many people's alcohol intake and pesticide exposure are contributing to the widespread incidence of estrogen-related cancers such as breast cancer.

Sure, some people are genetically predisposed to make more of the bad estrogens than the good ones, but as you have learned, genes are not your entire fate. By supporting your liver function you can improve your detox pathways and work around this predisposition.

We'll talk about how to improve liver function in Chapter 17: Restore Your Liver.

Symptoms of Hormonal Stress in Women

- Thyroid conditions
- Irregular cycles or heavy bleeding
- PMS
- Breast tenderness or fibrocystic breasts
- Fluid retention, swelling, or puffiness
- Hot flashes
- Loss of interest in sex
- Weight gain around the middle
- Migraines/headaches before period
- Mood swings—crying spells
- Polycystic ovarian syndrome
- Uterine fibroids
- Infertility
- Facial hair
- Poor memory
- Trouble sleeping
- Cramping at ovulation
- Acne around the time of your period
- Menopausal symptoms
- Depression

Symptoms of Hormonal Stress in Men

- Thyroid conditions
- Low libido
- Impotence
- Lack of drive or sense of purpose
- Fatigue
- Low sperm count
- Decreased muscle mass

- Losing hair in places other than your head
- Increased abdominal fat
- Bone loss
- High cholesterol
- Insulin and blood sugar imbalances
- Depression
- Memory loss
- Frequent urination and prostate problems

List any of the above hormonal stress symptoms you have here. Do you have any symptoms that are not on the list?

_____
_____
_____
_____
_____
_____
_____
_____
_____
_____

Splinter #7: Inflammatory and Infectious Stress

Inflammation is our immune system's response to an infection, irritation, or injury. It's a common occurrence: we see it whenever we twist an ankle and it swells up, or when a popcorn kernel gets stuck in our gums, making the area sore and swollen. The inflammation arises when immune cells have been called to the site through the bloodstream. These cells produce proteins called cytokines, which we learned in Chapter 5 are responsible for calling in T-cells and B-cells to fight the infection or injury. You experience this as a warm, hot, or swollen area. This is a normal reaction to a trauma, and without it, our wounds would never heal.

With chronic inflammation, there is no swelling or pain, but your immune system is producing silent inflammatory cytokines, starting little fires all over your body. The result is the destruction of healthy cells and tissues.

Chronic inflammation is present in all autoimmune conditions, from Graves' and Hashimoto's to rheumatoid arthritis, psoriasis, lupus, and others.

Causes of Inflammatory Stress

The cause of chronic inflammation often can be linked to our individual sensitivities, and to toxins, infections, chemicals, foods, and even certain emotions. Over the years, these sensitivities become more and more apparent, and as our body burdens increase, our inflammatory responses become magnified.

Over time, many of us find it difficult to tolerate the things we've been exposed to for decades. We may begin to notice symptoms such as digestive disorders, allergies, sore joints, and a host of other chronic conditions.

Chronic inflammation is epidemic in the Western world—just take a stroll down the aisles of your local drug store and count the hundreds of over-the-counter remedies designed to provide temporary relief of inflammation (i.e. ibuprofen, aspirin, cortisone creams, allergy pills, and antacids). In acute situations, these remedies are valuable. Unfortunately, many of us take these every day, masking little fires all over our bodies.

Treating chronic symptoms without addressing the underlying cause just kicks the can down the road (and adds more damage along the way). To remove the inflammation splinter, we need to identify and treat the cause(s).

Here are some of the major causes of inflammation:

Chronic Stress

Chronic emotional stress can be uncomfortable to endure, but even more concerning are the little fires that may start in the body as a result. Studies have shown that chronic stress raises the levels of pro-inflammatory cytokines such as IL-6, which are associated with cardiovascular disease, osteoporosis, arthritis, type 2 diabetes, certain cancers, periodontal disease, and accelerated aging.[45]

As you have been learning, chronic stress affects literally every cell in the body![46]

Sugar and White Flour: the Toxic Twins

Sugar and white flour are finally being recognized for what they are: highly toxic, body-burdening "foods" that cause inflammation and a deadly array of harmful effects on the body. On average, people eating the SAD (Standard American Diet) consume a staggering 160 lbs. of sugar and 200 lbs. of white flour per year. These deadly white powders spike blood sugar, which contributes to the twin epidemics of obesity and diabetes. Sugar, in all its forms—high-fructose corn syrup, and the "healthy," but just as harmful forms such as organic cane sugar, brown rice syrup and agave—is a hidden ingredient in countless processed foods such as ketchup, baked goods, and many other everyday, "healthy" foods.

Remember, just because a food is organic or from the health food store that does not mean that it's a guaranteed healthy food choice.

White flour and sugar can cause inflammation and disease by forming advanced glycation end-products, or AGEs. When certain proteins react with sugar, AGEs are produced, resulting in damaged, cross-linked proteins. When immune cells respond to these AGEs, they secrete large amounts of inflammatory chemicals. Appropriate to their acronym, AGEs accelerate aging and diseases we associate with aging. Arthritis, cataracts, memory loss, diabetes, and wrinkles are some of the sweet treats that sugar can bestow through AGEs.

> It's tempting to break off a piece of warm toasted French bread, a biscuit, or a dinner roll fresh from the oven and feel these are "real" foods, more virtuous than a dessert. But actually, from your body's point of view, eating white bread products is not much different than spooning table sugar into your mouth. White bread is particularly bad, because of its structure. The yeast in bread causes it to have a bubbly structure, like a sponge. This means that it has tremendous exposed surface area, so when it hits your digestive system, it gets turned into sugar almost as fast as cotton candy. Similarly, angel hair pasta, although it has the same ingredients as thick noodles like ziti, will spike blood sugar more quickly. But whatever form white flour comes in, it is always harmful.

High-Glycemic Carbohydrates

Besides the toxic duo above, there are other carbs that are almost as bad. The body converts many so called "healthy" foods into sugar so quickly that the result is very unhealthy. The measurement of how quickly a food is converted into sugar is called its glycemic index. The glycemic index is a scale of one to one hundred, with pure glucose sugar at the top of the scale at 100.

A more sophisticated measure of the glycemic effects of foods is called "glycemic load." Glycemic load considers the actual amount of carbohydrates present in a typical serving of a food. A glycemic load number below 10 is considered low, 11-19 medium, and 20 or above is high. For example, while watermelon has a high glycemic index number of 72, its glycemic load number is only 7.21 because of the limited amount of carbs in a serving.

Excess consumption of high-glycemic foods has not only been strongly linked to obesity and diabetes, but even to cancer and heart disease. White rice, white pasta, white flour, and white potatoes are common high-glycemic offenders. Substitute sweet potatoes or yams in any recipe calling for white potatoes. If you are sure you don't have sensitivity, substitute brown rice for white rice (many Asian restaurants offer it if you ask). Another option is quinoa, which is a seed, not a grain, and also a complete protein. Go to www.thethyroidcure.com/glycemicload to calculate the glycemic load of the foods in your diet and cut back on the ones higher on the glycemic scale.

Remember that all high-glycemic foods cause inflammation and accelerate aging!

Partially Hydrogenated Oils: Trans Fats, Bad Saturated Fats

Most of the fats and oils in the American diet, as well as most of the fats in processed foods, are inflammatory because they contain excessive amounts of the wrong kinds of fat.

Processed foods are typically loaded with oils that encourage inflammation, such as corn, soy, peanut, safflower, sunflower, and canola oils.

Partially hydrogenated oils (trans-fatty acids) are highly inflammatory, and are still found in all sorts of processed and restaurant foods. These highly toxic, factory-made fats sabotage the activity of enzymes that make anti-inflammatory compounds, but allow other enzymes to produce pro-inflammatory substances.

Unlike the wild animals we once consumed, corn-fed cattle, poultry, and farmed fish contain excessive amounts of inflammatory saturated fats.

Artificial Sweeteners

Splenda® (Sucralose)

Sucralose is a synthetic compound created by chlorinating sugar, and it causes a host of problems. It has been found to shrink thymus glands (remember, this is where your T-cells learn to protect you) and produce liver inflammation in rats and mice. Chlorine also disrupts iodine molecules in the body, causing them to be excreted. This, of course, worsens thyroid conditions.

While manufacturers claim the chlorine in sucralose is identical to that in table salt, the reality is that it has a chemical structure that more closely resembles that of the pesticide DDT.

Sucralose consumption is associated with numerous reported side effects, including liver and kidney problems, stomach cramps and diarrhea, inflammation, vertigo, bladder problems, headaches, and muscle aches.

According to a study conducted by Duke University, sucralose diminishes crucial healthy bacteria in the gut, which, as you've already learned, can cause a host of health issues![47]

Equal® and NutraSweet® (Aspartame)

Aspartame is found in more than 6,000 products, such as toothpaste, cough medicine, gum, breath mints, sports and juice drinks, and, of course, soda.

Even in low doses, aspartame has been linked to a variety of diseases and conditions, including:
- Migraines
- Asthma
- Tinnitus
- Chronic fatigue
- Diabetes
- Depression
- Multiple sclerosis
- Fibromyalgia
- Lupus
- Rheumatoid arthritis

Sweet 'N Low® (Saccharin)

Saccharin was accidentally discovered in 1878 by two chemists working on coal tar derivatives at Johns Hopkins University, when one of them noticed a sweet taste on his hands at dinner one evening.[48]

These days, saccharin is made by combining anthranilic acid with nitrous acid, sulfur dioxide, chlorine, and ammonia.

Saccharin is primarily benzoic sulfide, a sulfa-based compound. People with sulfa allergies who ingest saccharin have reported side effects such as diarrhea, nausea, and skin problems. Saccharin has also been shown to cause bladder cancer in rats.

Hidden Allergies and Sensitivities

Allergies and sensitivities are a major cause of inflammation for most people with autoimmune conditions. But why do people have allergies in the first place? Even though one out of every five Americans today suffers from allergies, and even more suffer from sensitivities such as gluten intolerance, modern medicine still can't seem to figure out why so many people are having allergic reactions to their environments. Instead, doctors are quick to prescribe medications for their patients that merely mask the symptoms. Sadly, many people rely on prescription and over-the-counter medications for years, and yet their conditions never improve.

There are many hypotheses about why we are becoming more sensitive. One is the hygiene theory, which postulates that the environments we are living in are too clean (sterile), and as a result, our immune systems don't fully mature. Another theory is that we are stressed-out, our guts are a mess, and we're exposed to too many environmental toxins, including GMOs and many types of processed foods.

Common Hidden Food Sensitivities

Gluten	Dairy
Soy	Corn
Fish	Shellfish
Nightshades	Legumes (peanuts are legumes)
Nuts	MSG and other food additives

Chronic and Low-grade Infections

Many times, low-grade chronic infections precede an autoimmune condition. In other cases, it's an acute infection or virus that turns out to be "the straw that breaks the camel's back," and a person experiences a full-blown autoimmune attack. These infections may or may not be symptomatic, and include:

- Viruses such as Epstein-Barr, herpes, hepatitis B, coxsackie B, and parvovirus B-19
- Chronic fungal infections such as Candida albicans
- Helicobacter pylori
- Yersinia enterocolitica
- Periodontal disease and/or infected root canals or dental implants
- Proteus mirabilis infection of the urinary tract
- Mycoplasma infections, which cause pneumonia and can linger for years after the initial exposure. (Many people who get "walking pneumonia" report never feeling the same afterwards.)
- Chlamydia, which can be silent and may infect the respiratory or urogenital regions (as a sexually transmitted infection.)
- Mycobacterium Tuberculosis
- Other infections, such as Brucella, Borrelia burgdorferi, Streptococcus, and Staphylococcus
- Chronic sinusitis: The Mayo Clinic did a study in 1999 that found fungus in the sinuses of 96 percent of patients with chronic sinusitis.[49] Since that time, many doctors have helped their patients reverse autoimmune symptoms by treating their sinusitis with antifungal drugs along with healthy lifestyle choices.

It's important to note that not only can some of these infections trigger an autoimmune condition, but many also interfere with normal thyroid function and the conversion of T4 to T3 in the liver and GI tract.

Environmental Toxins

We are living in a world where we are immersed in tens of thousands of man-made chemicals everyday. By the time we get to work in the morning, we are already eating, breathing, and wearing most of them. All environmental toxins are inflammatory. Even low doses of some of these toxins can derange your immune system and result in inflammatory autoimmune disease. Examples of such toxins include adhesives, cleaning products, air fresheners, synthetic fibers, plastics, perfumes, and anything that has a "new car" smell. Take a sniff under your kitchen sink. Whatever you can smell is entering your body and having an effect on your health. Indoor air pollution is often much worse than outdoor air pollution!

Being Overweight

Being overweight, particularly around the belly, is the cause of excess inflammation as well (not to mention lots of extra wear and tear on your body). The inflammatory effects of excess fat are one of the main hazards of being overweight, and are a cause of higher levels of disease and disability in people who are overweight and obese.

Injury

Inflammation was designed by nature as a response to injury, but it's supposed to subside once the injury heals. Because of all the sources of inflammation in our lives, injuries often never heal completely, and then become sources of inflammation affecting the whole body. Athletes, especially those who have played contact sports, often have disabling problems with injuries as they age.

Sedentary Lifestyles

Research indicates that being sedentary, particularly sitting for long periods of time in chairs, is associated with a variety of deleterious effects, including inflammation and insulin resistance. These effects are not canceled for people who sit for long periods and then do a rigorous workout. Research indicates that women are much more seriously affected than men.

Nutritional Deficiencies

Research indicates that nutritional deficiencies can cause inflammation. Deficiencies in omega-3 fatty acids, antioxidants, and vitamin D all contribute to chronic inflammation. Deficiency in iron can cause inflammation and anemia, which affects the conversion of T4 to T3. The good news is that correcting deficiencies by proper nutrition and supplementation is one of the simplest things you can do right away to calm the inflammatory response in your body.

Here are just a few symptoms and conditions caused by inflammation:
- Any autoimmune condition
- Suppressed thyroid function
- Impaired liver function
- Adrenal fatigue
- Allergies and sensitivities
- Asthma and bronchitis
- Anemia
- Acid reflux
- Atherosclerosis
- Chronic obstructive pulmonary disease (COPD)
- Cancer
- Cirrhosis
- Emphysema
- Dementia
- Gastroenteritis
- Sugar or alcohol dependency
- Chronic infections—fungal, bacterial, or viral
- Slow healing or recovery
- Systemic Candida
- Chronic pain
- Heart disease
- Diabetes, insulin resistance, metabolic syndrome
- Skin conditions such as dermatitis, acne, eczema psoriasis
- Chronic digestive symptoms, GERD, IBD, IBS, Crohn's
- Overweight/obesity
- Arthritis (degenerative osteoarthritis)
- Edema
- High blood pressure
- High cholesterol
- Gingivitis and periodontal disease
- Osteopenia
- Hepatitis
- Fibromyalgia
- Interstitial cystitis
- Tendonitis

Please list any of the above inflammation symptoms you have here. Do you have any symptoms not on the list?

_____
_____
_____
_____
_____
_____
_____

Splinter #8: Toxic Stress

Toxic stress can be a huge body burden and contribute to, if not cause, an autoimmune reaction. Even if you eat well and live a healthy lifestyle, you are still constantly exposed to numerous chemicals and potential antigens every day. Currently, there are over 3,000 chemicals that have been added to our food supply and more than 70,000 chemicals used for other purposes in North America alone![50]

Toxic stress includes exposure to heavy metals, petrochemicals, endocrine disrupting chemicals (EDCs), food additives, herbicides, fungicides, pesticides, volatile organic compounds (VOCs), and compounds found in most commercial cleaning products.

Here are some causes of toxic stress:

Endocrine disrupting chemicals (EDCs)

EDCs are synthetic compounds that mimic our natural hormones when absorbed by the body. They can turn on, turn off, or otherwise change normal hormonal signals. They can alter normal hormone levels, triggering excessive action, or completely block a natural response. Any other body function controlled by hormones can also be affected, including the immune system.

We find EDCs in everything these days: they make our plastic products softer and easier to handle, our lotions smoother and longer lasting, and our clothes and furnishings resistant to fire. They are used in clothing dye (especially denim), cars and computer casings, Teflon® coatings, and disinfectant bleaches. They are diffused throughout the atmosphere by the burning of industrial waste, and they leach into groundwater from landfills. What's more, some scientists are concerned because these chemicals have a tendency to biomagnify, or increase their concentration, as they pass up the food chain.

EDCs are now being found in living tissue at dramatically higher concentrations than natural hormones. A Centers for Disease Control report from July 2005 found that the bodies of Americans of all ages contain an average of 148 synthetic chemicals. These chemicals can hang out in our fat cells for years, and can even be passed from mother to child in breast milk.[51]

The Most Common EDCs

Bisphenol-A (BPA) is commonly used to make the plastics found in food and drink containers, baby bottles, toys, flame retardants, dental sealants, plastic wraps, and often comprises the linings of tin cans. Studies have linked BPA to autoimmunity, breast and prostate cancer, and infertility. In genetically susceptible mice, BPA has been shown to simulate the production of autoantibodies.[52] BPA has been shown to affect the human immune system, and is associated with cardiovascular disease, miscarriage, diabetes, childhood behavioral problems, and hormonal imbalances.[53] In a recently published study in the *Journal of Biochemical and Molecular Toxicology*, one University of Michigan team found a wide range of BPA in the livers of 50 first- and second-trimester fetuses, indicating that there is considerable exposure to the chemical during pregnancy. The team also found that the babies' livers could not eliminate the chemical over time like adult livers can. We really don't know what BPA is doing to the DNA of our babies and children, but I think it's safe to say it's not doing anything good! In recent years growing awareness of the dangers of BPA has led some manufacturers to eliminate it from their products and advertise the item is "BPA-free."

Phthalates are chemicals added to plastics for flexibility, resiliency, durability and softness. Phthalates are found in plastic bags, children's toys, IV tubing, perfumes, food packaging, vinyl flooring, pesticides, glues, nail polish, inks, shampoos, detergents, shower curtains, hair spray, and soaps. A report by the Centers for Disease Control and Prevention (CDC) and the National Toxicology Program stated that phthalate exposure is increasingly widespread, especially in women ages 20 to 40. Other studies indicate potential links with asthma, rhinitis, and eczema in children, and altered development of the sexual organs of male infants. Scientists in the Life Sciences department at Indiana State University accidentally discovered that phthalates cause lupus in genetically susceptible mice, but researchers are hesitant to say whether they affect humans in the same way. Phthalates don't have to be disclosed on the label and are often included under the generic label of "fragrance." Beware of "V," "PVC," or the "3" recycling code on an item or its packaging. The Environmental Working Group's page at www.ewg.org/skindeep is a good resource for identifying companies that don't use phthalates in their products.

Parabens are compounds used as preservatives in thousands of cosmetics, foods, and pharmaceutical products. They are used as inexpensive antifungal/antibacterial agents and can mimic the hormone estrogen, which is known to play a role in the development of breast cancers. According to the Environmental Working Group's Web site, parabens can disrupt the hormone (endocrine) system, and were found in the breast cancer tumors of 19 of 20 women studied. The CDC tested urine from 100 adults and found parabens in nearly all.[54] Check all your self-care products for parabens (also known as ethyl paraben; methyl paraben; butyl paraben; propyl paraben; benzyl paraben, etc.) and be wary, as manufacturers have come up with hundreds of ways to rename these chemicals to confuse consumers. Again, www.ewg.org/skindeep is a good resource for identifying companies using healthy ingredients in personal care products.

PBDEs (polybrominated diphenyl ethers) are common flame-retardants used on furniture, curtains, mattresses, carpets, pillows, beds, car seats, car interiors, rugs, drapes, pajamas, television and computer monitors, and a host of materials where flame resistance might be helpful. PBDEs are persistent organic pollutants, which accumulate up the food chain in animal fats, and consequently are found in fish, dairy products, meat, and even human breast milk. PBDEs have been banned in several countries. PBDEs used in foam furniture were taken off the U.S. market in 2005. PBDEs can interfere with thyroid hormones as a result of their bromine. The Environmental Working Group has helpful information at http://www.ewg.org/pbdefree on how to handle items that potentially contain PBDEs and which manufacturers have pledged to eliminate them from electronic products.

PCBs (polychlorinated biphenyls) are toxic chemical compounds on the list of Persistent Organic Pollutants (POPs). PCBs were banned in 1976, but degrade very slowly, so PCBs still pollute the environment and find their way into our bodies. They were once used for many industrial applications in electrical transformers, pipeline lubrication, and plastics, and mixed with paints, adhesives, inks, dyes, and paper.

Dioxins and dioxin-like compounds (DLCs) are a class of highly toxic chemicals that have remained in the environment long after their use was restricted. Dioxin is a byproduct of industrial processes involving chlorine in the pesticide, paper, and chemical industries. Small particles of dioxins accumulate in the food chain in fish, meat, dairy products, and even breast milk. We are mostly exposed to dioxins through contamination of our food. Dioxins and DLCs are still one of the most prevalent toxic chemicals even though levels have been decreasing due to regulations instituted in the 1990's.

Pesticides and herbicides: Organophosphates and organochlorines in pesticides and herbicides can be toxic to the nervous and reproductive systems. They play a role in autoimmune diseases such as Parkinson's, as well as childhood acute leukemia.[55] Some pesticides have recently been implicated in the serious issue of the widespread death and disappearance of honeybees. The chemicals we use to make things easier and cheaper often have unintended consequences and by the time we realize the danger, it's difficult to remove the harmful chemicals from the marketplace.

Volatile Organic Compounds (VOCs)

Volatile organic compounds (VOCs) are a class of organic chemicals that are usually gaseous at room temperature. The World Health Organization defines VOCs as organic compounds with a boiling point between 50-100 °C and 240-260 °C. Formaldehyde is often considered to be a VOC even though it does not fall within this definition. VOCs are found in such a wide variety of products, particularly home maintenance products, that it's hard to list them all, but be mindful around any substance off-gassing chemical odors. Increasing public awareness of the toxic qualities of many products has led some manufacturers to advertise "No VOCs" on their packaging.

The Most Common VOCs are:

Methyl tert-butyl ether (MTBE) is a common gasoline additive used to replace the lead formerly used in gasoline, increase octane ratings, and ironically, reduce air pollution from vehicle emissions. Unfortunately, now MTBE pollutes our water instead. Most people are exposed through inhalation of fumes while fueling their car. Another source of MTBE exposure is through drinking water as MTBE has contaminated groundwater supplies where gasoline is stored. There is a controversy over just how harmful MTBE might be to humans although it causes cancer in animal studies, and it appears some people may be more sensitive to MTBE than others.

Formaldehyde is found in tobacco smoke, certain foam insulation (UFFI), wood products like plywood, chipboard and particleboard, fabrics, household cleaners and water-based paints.

Esters are found in plastics, lacquer solvents, resins, plasticizers, perfumes and flavorings.

Ethers are found in varnishes, resins, lacquers, paints, dyes, cosmetics and soaps.

Acrylic acid esters and epichlorohydrin released from aerosols, window-cleaners, paints, paint thinner, cosmetics and adhesives like epoxy.

Ketones are found in adhesives, lacquers, nail polish removers and varnishes.

Polycyclic aromatic hydrocarbons (PAH) are released when burning hydrocarbons like gasoline, coal, diesel, or kerosene but also by incomplete burning of wood, fat, tobacco and even incense. PAHs have been found in meat cooked at high temperatures and oils, like coconut oil, that were used repeatedly at high temperatures. PAHs vary in their toxicity but some have been found to be carcinogenic and mutagenic, and to cause developmental problems.

Halogens: Chlorine, Bromine and Fluoride

Our bodies operate via chemical signals, and require certain chemicals to sustain our needs. Toxic chemicals and substances that the body mistakes for a needed constituent can disrupt the miraculous way our body sustains itself out of food, water, and air.

The body uses iodine to make thyroxine thyroid hormone. Iodine deficiency can lead to hypothyroidism and cause a goiter, which is an enlargement of the thyroid gland. When science discovered that lack of iodine caused goiters, makers of table salt began to add iodine, in the form of sodium iodide.

Iodine is a member of a group of chemically similar elements called halogens. Chlorine, bromine, and fluorine are the other common members of the halogen family, along with a very rare radioactive element, astatine. All these substances are toxic and cause particular trouble to the thyroid because of their similarity to iodine. Thyroid receptors accept them as look-alikes to iodine, but can't convert them to thyroid hormone. (If you put salt in your coffee because you thought it was sugar, you'd agree that looking alike and working alike are not the same.)

Chlorine is used to sterilize public water supplies, to sanitize pools and spas, and in the manufacture of pesticides, fungicides, plastics like PVC, and the artificial sweetener Splenda®. Chlorine is in bleach and other cleaning products. Many of chorine's uses are dependent on its toxicity; it was used as a chemical weapon in World War I. The body needs chlorine in certain forms, although too much is toxic. Ordinary table salt is sodium chloride, and the stomach uses hydrochloric acid to break down food.

Bromine is also used to sanitize hot tubs and in the manufacture of pesticides. Non-organic strawberries, tomatoes, and potatoes are often sprayed with methyl bromide. Bromine is found in the form of brominated vegetable oil in Mountain Dew® and many citrus-flavored sodas and Gatorade®. This is despite the fact that brominated vegetable oil is banned in 100 countries! Bromine is also used in flour for bread and other baked goods. In the 1990's, the United Kingdom and Canada banned the use of bromate in bread. Other places we are exposed to bromine are in plastics, flame-retardants, certain medicines, hair dyes, toothpastes, and mouthwashes. Bromine sits next to iodine on the Periodic Table of Elements. It is a culprit in taking the place of iodine in the thyroid, and is a particular danger to people who are iodine-deficient. Scientific studies have noted that polyhalogenated aromatic hydrocarbons (PHAHs), particularly polybrominated diphenyl ethers (PBDEs), resemble thyroid hormones, affect thyroid function, and could be responsible for the increase in thyroid cancer in many parts of the world, particularly the United States.[56,57] Bromine is a depressant to the central nervous system, and can cause depression, irritability, and lethargy, as well as rashes and heart problems.

Fluorine, as fluoride, is often added to municipal water supplies to prevent dental cavities in the public. Most common brands of toothpaste contain fluoride. Green and black tea, along with bottled tea drinks, contain a surprising amount of fluoride, as the tea plant (camellia sinensis) absorbs fluoride from the soil. Studies have linked heavy tea drinking with skeletal fluorosis, a bone condition, and also found that a liter of tea may contain more fluoride that previously thought.[58,59]

Sodium fluoride is a byproduct of various industries like aluminum manufacturing, and is used in rat poison, Prozac, and sarin nerve gas. Fluoride is highly toxic and even more so for people with iodine deficiencies. Fluoride has been associated with tooth discoloration (fluorosis), bone cancer, kidney problems, and impaired glucose metabolism. There is also evidence it may negatively affect the brain. In 1997 the FDA required a poison warning on all fluoride toothpastes, cautioning not to swallow toothpaste. The Teflon® in non-stick cookware contains fluorine and harmful gases can be released if the cookware is overheated.

Most European countries do not fluoridate their water; nor does China. Even the benefits of fluoridating water to prevent tooth decay are questionable, as numerous studies show that dental decay is declining worldwide, even in areas that don't fluoridate the water.[60] Fluoride occurs naturally in some drinking water, and 200,000 Americans receive greater concentrations of fluoride in their water than the FDA limit of 4 parts per million.

Organochlorines are substances that contain carbon, chlorine, and hydrogen. You may remember some of them from the section on endocrine disrupting chemicals. They are a primary component of many pesticides, many of which are now banned, but they may persist for decades in the environment anyway, since they do not break down easily. (DDT is a famous example.)

PCBs (polychlorinated biphenyls) are notorious organochlorines, and were used in electrical transformers and a variety of varnishes, inks, fire-resistant coatings, and cosmetics. Dioxins are another toxic class of organochlorines, which are also used in bleaching paper, wood treatments, and pesticides. Dioxins are also released into the air when PVC (polyvinyl chloride, another organochlorine and a very common plastic) is burned.

Besides the variety of other toxic effects that come with exposure, organochlorines are endocrine disrupters that build up in your fatty tissues. This means they interfere with your body's chemical regulating signals and aren't easily metabolized or removed from your system.

It might seem strange to be concerned over chemicals that have since been banned, but at least one scientific study has shown that even the thyroid hormones of polar bears in the remote frozen north were negatively affected by PCBs that had somehow reached habitats far from industry, or even people.[61]

The halogens chlorine, bromine, and fluorine are chemicals of particular concern for people with thyroid conditions. Be sure to read labels, as compounds of these chemicals may be found in a variety of products and even medicines.

Heavy Metals

Heavy metal toxicity can damage or reduce the function of the central nervous function, the blood, liver, kidneys and other organs. It can lower energy levels and give rise to a host of mental symptoms such as insomnia, memory loss, confusion, headaches and depression. Continued exposure can lead to gradually increasing muscular, physical, and neurological degeneration. The symptoms of chronic heavy metal poisoning can resemble muscular dystrophy, Alzheimer's, multiple sclerosis or Parkinson's disease. Heavy metals compromise the GI, leading to food allergies and sensitivities and greater vulnerability to viral, bacterial or fungal infection. In fact, heavy metals may compromise the immune system and are linked to inducing autoimmunity.[62] Some heavy metals are carcinogenic.

Aluminum

We are exposed to aluminum virtually everywhere. It is in food, water, air, soil, cookware, antacids, antiperspirants, drugs like buffered aspirin, and in tobacco and marijuana smoke.[63] Trace levels of aluminum may not be a concern for most adults, but exposure during infancy and adolescence is a different matter, because it accumulates over time. Infant formulas and cow's milk can have up to ten times higher levels of aluminum than breast milk. Aluminum is also found in vaccines where it is added specifically to intensify the immune system's response. Aluminum is a known neurotoxin and although controversial, has been implicated in Alzheimer's disease.[64] Aluminum poses particular hazards for those with kidney disease, especially those on dialysis.

Arsenic

You've probably heard of arsenic because it has been used as a poison. There are two forms of arsenic. The form of arsenic found in seafood is non-toxic and expelled from the body rapidly, while the non-organic form of arsenic found in contaminated drinking water and in industrial use like metal foundry is highly toxic. Arsenic was applied as a treatment for wood used in construction until the EPA banned that usage in 2003. Still, existing arsenic from construction will continue to contaminate water for years to come. Arsenic poisoning can also result from contaminated wine or moonshine.

Acute arsenic poisoning can kill you but long-term exposure to arsenic at lower levels can cause skin disorders and white lines (Mees' lines) in the fingernails. Arsenic can lead to sensory and motor nerve defects and compromise liver and kidney function. The EPA classifies arsenic as a carcinogen and long-term exposure can lead to cancer.

Cadmium

The most common source of cadmium exposure is through tobacco smoke and some laboratories that measure cadmium exposure expect smokers to have double the levels of non-smokers. Cadmium has generally poor GI bioavailability so it is often absorbed by the lungs and then concentrates in the liver and kidneys. Some other common sources are post-industrial waste, auto emissions, organ meats and shellfish. Cadmium can cause respiratory and kidney problems, cancer, bone loss, high blood pressure and impaired endocrine function. Rechargeable batteries made with cadmium are considered toxic waste and must be disposed of through a proper recycler. (Radio Shack also takes used rechargeable batteries.)

Lead

Lead has been around and used by humans since at least 3,000 B.C. Environmental regulations banned it from paint back in the 1970's and gasoline in the 1980's, but it persists in the soil around homes that were painted with lead-based paint, and in the soil around highways. Lead is present in lead pipes in old homes and crops grown in soil contaminated by lead. It has also been found in the breast milk of women who live in lead-contaminated areas. Exposure to lead can occur by ingestion, inhalation, or contact with the skin. Occupational exposure is a danger for those who work around lead in industry and as many as 3 million workers in the United State are exposed to lead at work. Children are at greater risk from lead exposure than adults. All your body's tissues can absorb lead.

Adult symptoms are headache, kidney failure, abdominal pain, high blood pressure, memory loss, and weakness, tingling or pain in the extremities, and male reproductive dysfunction. Early symptoms are often non-specific and include loss of appetite, nausea, malaise, fatigue, sleep disruption, depression, intermittent abdominal pain, constipation, muscle pain, diarrhea and a strange taste in the mouth.

Mercury

You've probably heard the phrase "mad as a hatter." Its origin says a lot about the effects of mercury on human health: 17th-century milliners (hat makers) used mercury in the manufacture of felt-brimmed hats. Mercury exposure can cause brain damage, and that's what happened to the milliners. Mercury is a notorious toxin, and its use in many applications is now prohibited. Paradoxically, however, there is one place where it *is* legal to put mercury and even charge people money for it…inside your mouth! According to the Centers for Disease Control and Prevention in Atlanta, mercury amalgam dental fillings may account for 75 percent of a person's mercury exposure (advanced research into human anatomy also indicates that the mouth is very close to the brain!). You don't have to be a rocket scientist or have any sort of letters after your name to realize that having a mouth full of mercury alloys is probably not a good idea.

A study conducted in 2006 took patients who had autoimmune thyroid disease and had their amalgam fillings removed.[65] Six months later, they had decreased thyroid antibodies, indicating that their thyroids were no longer responding as if they were under extreme attack. Amalgam filling removal needs to be done by a dentist competent in reducing mercury exposure during the procedure as mercury may be released in the removal process.

Mercury contamination can come from a number of other sources, too. Compact fluorescent bulbs have substantial amounts of mercury in them. These hollow glass tubes are famously easy to break, and if that happens, your home is a toxic spill site. Some fish is also contaminated with mercury. The highest amounts are found in yellow fin tuna, snapper, blue fish, and Chilean sea bass. See the section on vaccinations for information on mercury used in certain vaccines.

Mercury can trigger autoimmune disease by binding to proteins and enzymes and altering their structure, which launches an immune system response.

Vaccinations

The health consequences of vaccines have been a hotly debated topic in recent times. Vaccines have virtually eliminated certain diseases like smallpox and polio, which once killed millions of people. There is another side of the story, though, particularly for people with autoimmune sensitivity: many vaccines contain mercury and aluminum, and all vaccines are designed to provoke an immune response.

Mercury in vaccinations comes in the form of thimerosal, which is 49.6 percent ethylmercury (eHg) and is used as a vaccine preservative. Mercury is an extremely toxic heavy metal linked to all kinds of physical and behavioral conditions. A debate has raged about mercury from thimerosal contributing to autism in children.[66] While government agencies keep denying the dangers of thimerosal, in 1999 and 2000 the FDA, National Institutes of Health (NIH), Centers for Disease Control and Prevention (CDC), the Health Resources and Services Administration (HRSA), and the American Academy of Pediatrics issued two joint statements urging vaccine manufacturers to reduce or eliminate thimerosal in vaccines as soon as possible.

As a result, thimerosal use is mostly limited to multi-dose vials of seasonal flu vaccine, tetanus toxoid, and certain meningococcal vaccines. Single-dose vials of flu and meningococcal vaccines are available without thimerosal, and there are vaccines for tetanus without mercury as well. Of course, you or your loved ones might have been exposed to mercury in vaccines long before these reforms began.

Much harder to avoid is the issue of aluminum and aluminum salts as an adjuvant in vaccines. An adjuvant is a substance used to stimulate (aggravate) the immune system to make certain the vaccine is effective enough. Aluminum stirs the immune system for a reason; it is a known neurotoxin and carries a risk for autoimmunity, long-term brain inflammation, and associated neurological complications.[67,68] Evidence suggests that simultaneous administration of as little as two to three immune adjuvants can overcome genetic resistance to autoimmunity.[69] Furthermore, the very latest research demonstrates that aluminum from vaccines finds its way into the brain and spleen, where it can still be detected over a year after vaccine administration.

Not all vaccines contain aluminum or aluminum salts. Here is a list of vaccines without aluminum adjuvants: the inactivated polio virus (IPV) vaccine; the measles, mumps and rubella vaccine (MMR); the varicella vaccine; the meningococcal conjugate (MCV4) vaccine; and the influenza vaccine.[70]

The following vaccines do contain aluminum adjuvants:

- DTP (diphtheria-tetanus-pertussis)
- DTaP (diphtheria-tetanus-acellular pertussis)
- Some Hib (haemophilus influenzae type b) conjugate vaccines
- Pneumococcal conjugate vaccine
- Hepatitis B vaccines
- All combination DTaP, Tdap, Hib, or hepatitis B vaccines
- Hepatitis A vaccines
- Human papillomavirus (HPV) vaccine
- Anthrax vaccine
- Rabies vaccine

A final consideration is in order for those with autoimmune sensitivity. Vaccines work by provoking an immune response by introducing an antigen into the system so that immune cells become informed about the pathogen and mount a defense against it. Anything that provokes the immune system runs a risk of increasing autoimmune responses in susceptible individuals.

Just because there is a vaccine for something, doesn't mean it will protect you. Some vaccines like the one for whooping cough have notoriously high failure rates.[71] Many people take the flu vaccine and get the flu anyway.[72] You have to wonder about the safety and effectiveness of vaccines when even many health care professional themselves don't accept vaccinations, even though they are at particularly high risk.[73]

I'm not saying there isn't a place for vaccines. I'm saying that there are dangers and consequences associated with vaccines. We have to use them wisely when truly necessary so that the side effects of prevention don't become worse than the diseases we are trying to prevent.

Symptoms of Toxic Stress are:
- Impaired liver function
- Allergies and food sensitivities
- Suppressed thyroid function
- Constipation or difficult-to-pass bowel movements
- Low-volume, dark, strong-smelling urine
- Inability to sweat
- Chronic pain
- Being overweight or obese
- Skin conditions such as dermatitis, acne, eczema, or psoriasis
- Sensitivities to perfumes, candles, room sprays, and other chemical odors
- Headaches
- Fatigue
- Jaundice or Gilbert's syndrome
- Swollen lymph glands
- Fibromyalgia
- Chronic fatigue
- Parkinson's disease
- Alzheimer's disease
- Multiple sclerosis
- Neurodegenerative conditions

- Any autoimmune condition
- All types of cancer

Please list any of the above symptoms of toxicity you have here. Do you have any symptoms not on the list?

_____
_____
_____
_____
_____
_____
_____
_____

Review of the Top Autoimmune Triggers

Now that you have gone through the workbook, you can see that there seems to be no end to the stress and body burdens we can experience. The previous section is not designed to overwhelm you or turn you into a hypochondriac. Please don't get bogged down with the science and symptoms of disease!

I wrote this book and this section in particular so that you could become more aware of how stressed-out we have become as a society, and so that you could make the connections between any chronic, disease-causing stressors you may be experiencing and your "incurable" condition.

With this awareness you will be able to recognize how your body's autoimmune condition is actually telling you that something has to change—and soon!

I have witnessed radical change in people's health when they reduce stress, change their nutrition, heal their GI tracts, improve their liver function, and clear up infections!

Take some time to write a few notes under the areas where you may be feeling the most stress right now.

Splinter #1: Chronic Emotional Stress

_____
_____
_____
_____
_____
_____
_____

Splinter #2: Unhealthy Coping Patterns

_____
_____
_____
_____
_____
_____
_____

Splinter #3: Poor Nutrition

_____
_____
_____
_____
_____
_____
_____

Splinter #4: Gastrointestinal (GI) Stress

Splinter #5: Adrenal Burnout

Splinter #6: Hormonal Stress

Splinter # 7: Inflammatory and Infectious Stress

Splinter #8: Toxic Stress

CHAPTER 10

Perform Your Personal Assessment

"Know well what leads you forward and what holds you back, and choose the path that leads to wisdom."
– BUDDHA

If you read through Chapter 9, you have a better understanding of how many factors can be at the root of autoimmune dysfunction. Now it's time to take your personal assessments to determine the areas where you may be experiencing the most stress. These assessments will help you and your practitioner determine where to begin looking for the "splinters" that may be triggering your autoimmune condition.

This section has seven assessments to evaluate the following:
Emotional Stress • GI Stress • Adrenal Stress • Infectious Stress Inflammatory Stress • Toxic Stress • Hormonal Stress

The key to these assessments is as follows:
0 – Never/Symptoms do not apply/Disagree
1 – Occasionally/Symptoms are mild/Somewhat agree
2 – Regularly/Symptoms are moderate in intensity/Agree
3 – Frequent/Symptoms are severe and intense/Strongly Agree

Emotional Stress Assessment

Please examine your life and experience and determine to what degree each issue affects you. Pay extra attention to the questions that impact your life strongly. Look for patterns.

If you find yourself agreeing with numerous questions in this section, it's a signal that emotional stress is a big splinter for you.

0 1 2 3   I have recently lost my spouse or a loved one.
0 1 2 3   I am recently divorced.
0 1 2 3   I am in an unhappy marriage or relationship.

0 1 2 3   I do not have loving, fulfilling relationships that nurture me.
0 1 2 3   I have recently lost a pet.
0 1 2 3   I don't love my vocation or feel very stressed at work.
0 1 2 3   I work far from home and deal with traffic every day.
0 1 2 3   I have recently moved or changed careers.
0 1 2 3   I did not grow up in a happy family environment.
0 1 2 3   I worry a lot.
0 1 2 3   I have significant financial stress.
0 1 2 3   I over-commit and find it difficult to say "No."
0 1 2 3   I have a difficult time keeping my commitments.
0 1 2 3   I don't feel supported emotionally by my spouse/partner.
0 1 2 3   I feel guilty a lot.
0 1 2 3   I feel shame a lot.
0 1 2 3   I don't have a fulfilling sex life.
0 1 2 3   I don't have friends I can laugh with and confide in.
0 1 2 3   I don't get adequate sleep.
0 1 2 3   I anger easily.
0 1 2 3   I feel frustrated a lot.
0 1 2 3   I don't have a spiritual practice.
0 1 2 3   My home is cluttered and I find it difficult to manage my household duties.
0 1 2 3   I have unfinished business.
0 1 2 3   I don't have healthy relationships with my parents and/or siblings.
0 1 2 3   I have a hard time speaking my truth.
0 1 2 3   I tend to be a martyr—I have a difficult time asking for help.
0 1 2 3   I don't have a creative outlet such as painting, writing, gardening, etc.
0 1 2 3   I don't have time to play.
0 1 2 3   I rarely feel grateful.
0 1 2 3   I don't feel understood or loved.

Please list anything else you feel is relevant to this assessment and assign a number 1–3 reflecting whether this is occasional, moderate or severe.

_____

_____

_____

_____

_____

Total _____

Score   **Splinter Level**

0–6   This may be a splinter for you.

7–10   This is most likely a splinter for you.

10 +   This is very likely a splinter for you.

GI Stress Assessment

Please read the following questions and enter the appropriate response.

0 1 2 3   I have been diagnosed with IBS (Irritable Bowel Syndrome).

0 1 2 3   I have been diagnosed with GERD.

0 1 2 3   I take antacids such as Maalox, Mylanta, Gelusil, Rolaids, or Tums regularly.

0 1 2 3   I take Tagamet, Pepcid, Axid, or Zantac regularly.

0 1 2 3   I take Prevacid or Prilosec regularly.

0 1 2 3   I have taken antibiotics for two weeks or longer recently or in the past.

0 1 2 3   I have taken prednisone or other steroid drugs for two weeks or longer.

0 1 2 3   I am on the birth control pill.

0 1 2 3   I take over-the-counter painkillers regularly.

0 1 2 3   I experience food allergies, hay fever, or skin rashes.

0 1 2 3   I have often have cramps or intestinal pain.

0 1 2 3   I have a white/yellowish or dark coating on my tongue.
0 1 2 3   My gums bleed when I brush my teeth or floss.
0 1 2 3   I have incomplete bowel movements.
0 1 2 3   I often feel gassy and bloated after eating.
0 1 2 3   I experience anal itching.
0 1 2 3   I have undigested food in my stool.
0 1 2 3   I often feel nauseous after eating.
0 1 2 3   I am constipated more often than not.
0 1 2 3   I have diarrhea.
0 1 2 3   I have foul-smelling stools.
0 1 2 3   I often have a spacey feeling after eating.
0 1 2 3   I'm prone to acne or breakouts.
0 1 2 3   I crave alcohol, sugar or bread.
0 1 2 3   I drink more than 8 oz. of alcohol or coffee daily.
0 1 2 3   I tend to feel sick in moldy or damp places.
0 1 2 3   I have experienced food poisoning.
0 1 2 3   I drink more than one cup of coffee daily.
0 1 2 3   I eat sushi or undercooked meat.
0 1 2 3   I eat at restaurants regularly.

My sexual partner has one or more of these conditions. Please list:

_____
_____
_____
_____

Please list anything else you feel is relevant to this assessment and assign a number 1–3 reflecting whether this is occasional, moderate or severe.

_____
_____
_____

Total _____

Score	Splinter Level
0–6	This may be a splinter for you.
7–10	This is most likely a splinter for you.
10 +	This is very likely a splinter for you.

Adrenal Stress Assessment

Please read the following questions and enter the appropriate response.

0 1 2 3   I always feel stressed-out.
0 1 2 3   I need caffeine to start the day.
0 1 2 3   I get panic attacks.
0 1 2 3   I'm easily startled.
0 1 2 3   I frequently have cold hands and feet.
0 1 2 3   I'm frequently constipated.
0 1 2 3   I am easily frustrated and angry—the littlest things bug me.
0 1 2 3   I don't have the patience I used to.
0 1 2 3   I often feel wired but tired.
0 1 2 3   I often resist going to bed even when I'm tired.
0 1 2 3   I have trouble falling and staying asleep.
0 1 2 3   I get heart palpitations.
0 1 2 3   I'm hypoglycemic.
0 1 2 3   I retain water—my feet and hands swell.
0 1 2 3   I wake up feeling not refreshed.
0 1 2 3   I get dizzy when I stand up.
0 1 2 3   I have dark circles under my eyes.
0 1 2 3   I crave salt.
0 1 2 3   I crave sweets.
0 1 2 3   I have trouble concentrating or have brain fog.
0 1 2 3   I catch everything that goes around.
0 1 2 3   I have low blood pressure.

0 1 2 3   I've gained weight around my midsection and it won't budge.
0 1 2 3   I don't have the energy to work out.
0 1 2 3   I have weak muscles.

Please list anything else you feel is relevant to this assessment and assign a number 1–3 reflecting whether this is occasional, moderate or severe.

_____

_____

_____

_____

Total _____

Score	Splinter Level
0–6	This may be a splinter for you.
7–10	This is most likely a splinter for you.
10 +	This is very likely a splinter for you.

Infectious Stress Assessment

Please read the following questions and enter the appropriate response.

0 1 2 3   I have had pneumonia.
0 1 2 3   I have had mononucleosis.
0 1 2 3   I have had or have hepatitis.
0 1 2 3   I have had Candida or other fungal infections.
0 1 2 3   I have had chlamydia.
0 1 2 3   I have had tuberculosis.
0 1 2 3   I have had a mycoplasma infection.
0 1 2 3   I have herpes.
0 1 2 3   I have the Epstein-Barr virus.
0 1 2 3   I have HIV.
0 1 2 3   I have been diagnosed with an STD.
0 1 2 3   I have had a Staphylococcus aureus infection.

0 1 2 3   I have Lyme disease.
0 1 2 3   I have dental bone loss.
0 1 2 3   I have gum infections.
0 1 2 3   I have chronic sinusitis.
0 1 2 3   I have chronic UTI infections.
0 1 2 3   I have chronic yeast infections.
0 1 2 3   I have chronic ear infections.
0 1 2 3   I have athlete's foot, jock itch, or other fungal infections of the skin.
0 1 2 3   I have a low-grade fever.
0 1 2 3   I have swollen lymph glands.
0 1 2 3   I have experienced a period of illness that lasted two weeks or longer—the doctors did not know what I had, but I have never felt the same since then.
0 1 2 3   I have or have had Gulf War Syndrome.
0 1 2 3   I have or have had a serious infection not on this list: _____

My sexual partner has one or more of the above conditions/symptoms. Please list:

_____
_____
_____
_____

Please list anything else you feel is relevant to this assessment and assign a number 1–3 reflecting whether this is occasional, moderate or severe.

_____
_____
_____

Total _____

Score Splinter Level

0–6   This may be a splinter for you.

7–10   This is most likely a splinter for you.

10 +   This is very likely a splinter for you.

Inflammatory Stress Assessment

Please read the following questions and enter the appropriate response.

0 1 2 3 I am totally stressed-out most of the time.

0 1 2 3 I have toxic exposure at work and home (toxins, quantum toxins).

0 1 2 3 I catch everything that goes around.

0 1 2 3 I work out for less than 30 minutes, three times a week.

0 1 2 3 I never go in the sun without sunblock, and I don't take vitamin D.

0 1 2 3 I have allergies and sensitivities.

0 1 2 3 I have food allergies or sensitivities.

0 1 2 3 I am dependent on sugar and/or alcohol.

0 1 2 3 I have had a difficult time recovering from an injury or surgery.

0 1 2 3 I have chronic infections—fungal, bacterial, or viral.

0 1 2 3 I have chronic pain.

0 1 2 3 I have sore joints.

0 1 2 3 I have carpal tunnel syndrome

0 1 2 3 I have asthma or bronchitis.

0 1 2 3 I have heart disease.

0 1 2 3 I have diabetes, insulin resistance or metabolic syndrome.

0 1 2 3 I have chronic skin conditions such as dermatitis, acne, eczema, or psoriasis.

0 1 2 3 I experience chronic digestive symptoms, such as GERD, IBD, IBS, or Crohn's disease.

0 1 2 3 I am overweight/obese.
0 1 2 3 I have arthritis (osteoarthritis/degenerative arthritis).
0 1 2 3 I retain water (edema).
0 1 2 3 I have high blood pressure.
0 1 2 3 I have high cholesterol.
0 1 2 3 I have periodontal disease.
0 1 2 3 I have osteopenia.
0 1 2 3 I have hepatitis.
0 1 2 3 I have chronic fatigue or fibromyalgia.
0 1 2 3 I experience interstitial cystitis.
0 1 2 3 I have tendonitis.

Please list anything else you feel is relevant to this assessment and assign a number 1–3 reflecting whether this is occasional, moderate or severe.

_____

_____

_____

_____

Total _____

Score	Splinter Level
0–6	This may be a splinter for you.
7–10	This is most likely a splinter for you.
10 +	This is very likely a splinter for you.

Toxic Stress Assessment

Please read the following questions and enter the appropriate response.

0 1 2 3 I never or rarely sweat.
0 1 2 3 I'm frequently constipated, have hard, difficult-to-pass bowel movements, or only go every other day or so.
0 1 2 3 I produce low-volume, dark, or strong-smelling urine.

0 1 2 3   I have allergies and sensitivities.
0 1 2 3   I have frequent headaches.
0 1 2 3   I experience fatigue that is not caused by obvious reasons such as staying up late or strenuous exercise.
0 1 2 3   I am obese.
0 1 2 3   I am sensitive to MSG.
0 1 2 3   I am sensitive to sulfites (wine, dried fruit).
0 1 2 3   I am sensitive to chocolate.
0 1 2 3   I am sensitive to alcohol.
0 1 2 3   I have silver amalgam fillings.
0 1 2 3   I am sensitive to perfumes.
0 1 2 3   I am sensitive to tobacco smoke.
0 1 2 3   I am sensitive to soaps, detergents, or dryer sheets.
0 1 2 3   I am sensitive to chlorine and bromine.
0 1 2 3   I am sensitive to household cleaning products.
0 1 2 3   I am sensitive to room spray or candles.
0 1 2 3   I am sensitive to new clothes, dressing rooms, and fabric stores.
0 1 2 3   I am sensitive to other strong odors, such as: _____

0 1 2 3   I have trouble concentrating.
0 1 2 3   I drink water from or cook in plastic containers.
0 1 2 3   I drink tap water.
0 1 2 3   I drink unfiltered well water.
0 1 2 3   I have my living space treated for pests.
0 1 2 3   I use pesticides and garden chemicals.
0 1 2 3   I have my clothes dry-cleaned.
0 1 2 3   I live in a city or large urban area.
0 1 2 3   I live in a space with poor ventilation or windows that do not open.
0 1 2 3   I have mold in my home.

0 1 2 3   I regularly take over-the-counter medications, such as Tylenol, cold medications, allergy medications, etc.
Please list:_____

0 1 2 3   I take the following prescription medications:
_____

0 1 2 3   I get the flu vaccine.

0 1 2 3   I have had a liver condition.
Please list:_____

0 1 2 3   I have an autoimmune condition.
Please list:_____

0 1 2 3   I have or have had cancer.

0 1 2 3   I have gone through chemotherapy.

0 1 2 3   I have had a major chemical exposure.
Please list:_____

Please list anything else you feel is relevant to this assessment and assign a number 1–3 reflecting whether this is occasional, moderate or severe.

_____
_____
_____
_____
_____
_____
_____

Total _____

Score   **Splinter Level**

0–6   This may be a splinter for you.

7–10   This is most likely a splinter for you.

10 +   This is very likely a splinter for you.

Hormonal Stress Assessment for Women

Please read the following questions and enter the appropriate response.

0 1 2 3   I use birth control pills or HRT.
0 1 2 3   I have irregular cycles, cramping, or heavy bleeding.
0 1 2 3   I experience PMS.
0 1 2 3   I have breast tenderness or fibrocystic breasts.
0 1 2 3   I experience fluid retention, swelling, or puffiness.
0 1 2 3   I have dry skin/hair.
0 1 2 3   I have vaginal dryness.
0 1 2 3   I get hot flashes.
0 1 2 3   I have lost interest in sex.
0 1 2 3   I have gained weight around the middle and it won't budge.
0 1 2 3   I get migraines/headaches before my period.
0 1 2 3   I experience mood swings.
0 1 2 3   I feel anxious.
0 1 2 3   I feel depressed.
0 1 2 3   I have been diagnosed with polycystic ovarian syndrome.
0 1 2 3   I have uterine fibroid tumors.
0 1 2 3   I have experienced or am experiencing infertility.
0 1 2 3   I have facial hair on my upper lip and or chin.
0 1 2 3   I have hair on my breasts.
0 1 2 3   I have memory problems.
0 1 2 3   I have insomnia.
0 1 2 3   I experience cramping at ovulation.
0 1 2 3   I get acne around the time of my period.
0 1 2 3   I am experiencing perimenopausal or menopausal symptoms.
0 1 2 3   I have had a toxic or chemical exposure.
              Please list:_____

Please list anything else you feel is relevant to this assessment and assign a number 1–3 reflecting whether this is occasional, moderate or severe.

_____

_____

_____
_____
_____

Total _____

Score   **Splinter Level**

0–6   This may be a splinter for you.

7–10   This is most likely a splinter for you.

10 +   This is very likely a splinter for you.

Hormonal Stress Assessment for Men

Please read the following questions and enter the appropriate response.

0 1 2 3 I have lost interest in sex.
0 1 2 3 I have impotence or a weak erection.
0 1 2 3 I have lost my drive or sense of purpose.
0 1 2 3 I have fatigue.
0 1 2 3 I have a low sperm count.
0 1 2 3 I have decreased muscle mass.
0 1 2 3 I have "man boobs."
0 1 2 3 I am losing the hair on my arms, legs, and chest.
0 1 2 3 I have increased abdominal fat.
0 1 2 3 I have bone loss.
0 1 2 3 I have high cholesterol.
0 1 2 3 I have insulin and blood sugar imbalances.
0 1 2 3 I feel depressed.
0 1 2 3 I have trouble remembering things.
0 1 2 3 I experience frequent urination and prostate problems.
0 1 2 3 I have had a toxic or chemical exposure.
         Please list:_____

Please list anything else you feel is relevant to this assessment and assign a number 1–3 reflecting whether this is occasional, moderate or severe.

_____

_____

_____

_____

Total _____

Score   **Splinter Level**

0–6   This may be a splinter for you.

7–10   This is most likely a splinter for you.1

10 +   This is very likely a splinter for you.

What are Your Splinters?

The results of your assessments will give you an idea of where to begin looking for the underlying triggers in your autoimmune thyroid condition.

If you find that a particular area *may be* a splinter for you, then it is most likely not the first place you should address.

If you find that a particular area is *most likely* a splinter for you, then while it may not be the primary cause, there is a good chance that it is a contributing factor in your condition.

If you find that a particular area is *very likely* a splinter for you, then this is where you will want to begin looking first.

You may find that you have several areas that are tied together or overlapping, in which case I invite you to use your intuition and enlist the assistance of a qualified practitioner to help you determine where to begin.

Please make a note of which areas may be, most likely are, and very likely are splinters for you.

Emotional Stress   _____

GI Stress   _____

Adrenal Stress   _____

Infectious Stress   _____

Inflammatory Stress _____
Toxic Stress   _____
Hormonal Stress   _____

Now I want to ask you the same question Dr. Wake Up asked me back in 2004:

How do you think you got your condition?

_____

_____

_____

_____

_____

_____

_____

_____

_____

What to Do Next…

If you think you have a pretty good idea of what the underlying splinters in your condition may be, you're ready to move on to Part Two, where I will discuss the simple plan that you can use to heal any splinters you may have uncovered.

You will be happy to learn that while the ways we experience stress and illness are endlessly complicated, the path to wellness is surprisingly simple.

It's simple—but not easy. You didn't "catch" an autoimmune condition overnight, and chances are you'll have some lifestyle changes to make.

The goal of this book is to help you become aware of and then minimize the chronic stressors in your life. I'd like to see you reverse your condition, become symptom-free, and start experiencing a more fulfilling life.

PART TWO: TRANSFORMATION

The Thyroid Cure Repair Program

The knowledge of how to gain vibrant health is not reserved for the doctor or licensed healthcare practitioner. In fact, the wisdom resides in your own heart and the cells of your infinitely wise body. Listen to your heart. Listen to your body. Become whole.

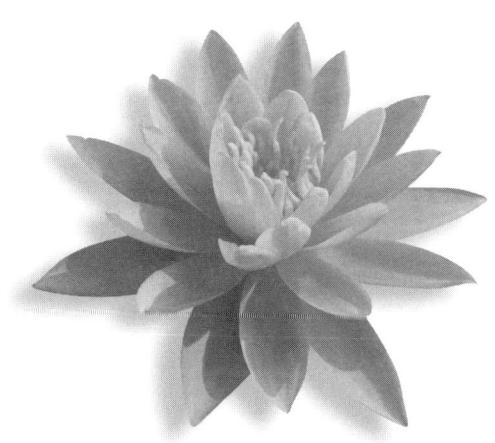

CHAPTER 11

Take the Splinters Out!

"Wisdom is knowing what to do next, skill is knowing how to do it, and virtue is doing it."
– DAVID STARR JORDAN (American ichthyologist, educator, writer b.1851)

Identify and Heal the Underlying Causes of Your Autoimmune Thyroid Condition

While each of us is unique, I have found that people with autoimmune disorders experience many of the same underlying triggers, such as chronic stress, poor coping mechanisms, poor dietary choices, food sensitivities, leaky gut, inflammation, low-grade infections or viruses, and chemical or heavy-metal toxicity. In order to reverse your condition, you will need to determine if you have any of these triggers and then work to heal them.

If you've gone through the Chapter 9 workbook and taken your personal assessments, you probably have a pretty good idea of what the splinters may be in your condition. This is great news, because awareness is the first step in healing. Now it's time to begin the process of taking the splinters out and allowing your body to heal.

You may have found that you have several "splinters," or some that overlap. Don't worry, because while the splinters may be many, the healing program is the same!

In fact, you might be surprised to learn that you can heal many splinters at the same time just by optimizing your thyroid hormones, improving your nutrition, lowering your stress, and detoxing your life. What I have noticed is that many, if not all, of the splinters will heal on their own when you make the healthy changes outlined in this section.

Part Two of this book is designed to walk you through the process of making the same healthy lifestyle changes that worked for me, and later for my clients.

Part Three, The Mind-Body Connection, is designed to be an exploration of how our emotions can affect our health. It's my opinion that chronic negative thoughts underlie many autoimmune conditions. You might ask, "Why don't I begin by exploring the emotional connection?" We start with the body instead because I have observed that once a condition has manifested in the body, it usually makes the most sense to work in the body before tackling the complexities of one's emotional life.

An autoimmune thyroid condition can affect brain chemistry. I have observed firsthand the anxiety, depression, and unstable moods that go hand in hand with unbalanced thyroid hormones. I know from my own experience, and from what I have witnessed with my clients, that once you stabilize your thyroid hormones, optimize your nutrition, and reduce inflammation, you will think and feel much clearer. After all, a healthy body houses a healthy brain, and a healthy brain is better able to process and release negative thoughts and unresolved traumas than a toxic and inflamed one.

I've worked hard to make this section simple to follow, and have included a lot of case studies to illustrate the process.

I'm going to start with the basics of thyroid testing and what to do first if you are hypothyroid or hyperthyroid.

CHAPTER 12

Test—Don't Guess!

"Risk comes from not knowing what you're doing."
— Warren Buffett

If you are reading this book, chances are you have already been diagnosed with an autoimmune thyroid condition. If you suspect that you have a thyroid condition, but have not been tested, you will need to test your thyroid hormone levels, as well as for any antibodies to your thyroid gland. This can only be accurately accomplished by laboratory blood tests.

You should be prepared to bring a letter to your practitioner requesting a full thyroid panel. You can download a request for thyroid tests from: www.thethyroidcure.com/testrequest.

If your practitioner refuses to order the tests, ask them to document that denial in writing and make it part of your permanent medical record. Many times, that will be enough to persuade your practitioner to order the tests. If not, you are most likely under the care of a practitioner who may not be open or willing to guide you through the process of healing. If that is the case, my suggestion is to begin looking for another practitioner. For a list of practitioners, check out my database at: www.thethyroidcure.com/practitioners.

Alternatively, you can order your own thyroid tests without a doctor's prescription at: www.mymedlab.com/thyroid/thyroid-complete-panel

Below are the tests you should ask your health practitioner for:

Thyroid Tests

TSH (Thyroid Stimulating Hormone): A TSH test measures the amount of thyroid stimulating hormone (TSH) in your blood. TSH is produced by the pituitary gland and signals the thyroid gland to make and release the hormones thyroxin (T4) and triiodothyronine (T3).

Free T4: This test measures the unbound form of thyroxin in the blood. This test is considered to be a more accurate reflection of thyroxin than total T4.

Free T3: This test measures the unbound "active" form of triiodothyronine (T3) in the blood. Remember, the thyroid makes large amounts of T4 and then relies mostly on the liver to convert it into the active form of the hormone T3 by an enzyme called 5'deiodoinase. If you don't have enough selenium, or if your liver is compromised by stress, infection, or toxins, you may not be converting T4 into T3.

Thyroid Antibody Tests

If you have hypothyroid symptoms, you should ask for these tests:

Anti-TPO: This tests for antithyroid peroxidase antibodies, which are commonly found with both Hashimoto's and Graves'.

TgAb or antithyroglobulin antibodies: This tests for antibodies to the protein thyroglobulin, which are also commonly found with both Graves' and Hashimoto's.

If you have hyperthyroid symptoms, you should ask for this additional test:

TSI (thyroid stimulating immunoglobulin), also called TRAb (Thyroid Receptor Antibodies): This tests for antibodies to TSH receptors. These antibodies are more commonly found in people with Graves'.

The Importance of Testing for Antibodies

It's very common for a person to be diagnosed with a "thyroid condition," but not be told why they have it. This is because most practitioners are not trained to test for antibodies right out of the gate. This is changing as more and more consumers are discovering their thyroids—thanks to the several thyroid patient advocate groups on the Internet. Still, many practitioners are not routinely testing for antibodies. If you have been diagnosed with a thyroid condition and you don't know why, you must ask that your thyroid antibodies be tested.

It's also common that once most practitioners find antibodies, they never retest for them. This is most likely because it's not commonly accepted that antibodies can be lowered or reversed by lifestyle adjustments.

It's important to explain to your practitioner that you are in the business of reversing your condition, and that you would like your antibodies monitored every six to twelve months!

The danger of not assessing the autoimmunity aspect of your condition is that every minute you have active antibodies in a part of your body, that part is being attacked by your immune system. The goal is to halt and reverse the autoimmune process as soon as possible to save your beautiful body from being harmed!

Other Important Tests for Autoimmunity

If you have other symptoms that indicate a more serious autoimmune condition, such as aching joints; chronic fatigue; vision changes; a rash over your face; sensitivity to the sun; numbness or tingling in the extremities; dizziness; tremors; low-grade fever; mouth sores/ulcers; or severe gastrointestinal symptoms, you should consult your health care practitioner and ask for further testing.

Below are some common tests for autoimmunity:

ANA (Antinuclear Antibodies): This tests for antinuclear antibodies (ANA), and is used to screen for autoimmune disorders, such as lupus, scleroderma, Sjögren's syndrome, and some types of chronic hepatitis. Many people with autoimmune thyroid conditions also have these antibodies.

Rheumatoid Factor (RA): Rheumatoid Factor may be found in the blood and joints of people with rheumatoid arthritis.

Inflammation Tests

CRP: This tests for levels of C-reactive protein in the blood. High values indicate inflammation somewhere in the body, which may be caused by insulin resistance, metabolic syndrome, food allergies, or infections.

Erythrocyte sedimentation rate (ESR or SED): This measures the speed at which red blood cells fall to the bottom of a test tube filled with blood. Your doctor may use this test to detect inflammation in the body. The faster the red blood cells fall to the bottom, the more inflammation is present. A high ESR or SED can be caused by some cancers, infections, and autoimmune conditions such as lupus, rheumatoid arthritis, etc.

Normal Versus Optimal Thyroid Lab Ranges

The "optimal" ranges for lab tests will vary from person to person. Remember that what the lab considers to be "normal" is based on 95 percent of the population who routinely go in for medical tests. Take a look around at the general population in the U.S., and you'll see that "normal" does not equal healthy! I will do my best to give you an idea of what "optimal" lab results might be, but the real gauge is how you feel. Many people who fall within the range of what the lab considers to be "normal" feel awful!

Let's take a look at the latest guidelines for thyroid lab tests.

TSH Ranges

Over ten years ago, in 2002, the National Academy of Clinical Biochemistry (NACB) issued new Laboratory Medicine Practice Guidelines for thyroid testing. Here is what they wrote:

> "In the future, it is likely that the upper limit of the serum TSH euthyroid reference range will be reduced to 2.5 mIU/L because 95 percent of rigorously screened normal euthyroid volunteers have serum TSH values between 0.4 and 2.5 mIU/L.
>
> "A serum TSH result between 0.5 and 2.0 mIU/L is generally considered the therapeutic target for a standard L-T4 replacement dose for primary hypothyroidism."[1]

In 2003, the American Association of Clinical Endocrinologists (AACE) issued a press release in support of lowering the upper limit of the reference range.

> "Until November 2002, doctors had relied on a normal TSH level ranging from 0.5 to 5.0 to diagnose and treat patients with a thyroid disorder who tested outside the boundaries of that range. Now AACE encourages doctors to consider treatment for patients who test outside the boundaries of a narrower margin based on a target TSH level of 0.3 to 3.0. AACE believes the new range will result in proper diagnosis for millions of Americans who suffer from a mild thyroid disorder, but have gone untreated until now."[2]

Unfortunately, many labs and doctors are not aware of these guidelines, and still use the old outdated reference ranges shown below. I've seen some ranges even higher, which explains why many experts believe that millions of people are walking around with undiagnosed thyroid conditions!

Old TSH Range: THS 0.5 - 5.0 mIU/L
New TSH Range: TSH 0.3 - 3.0 mIU/L
Optimal TSH Range: TSH .05 – 2.0 mIU/L

I have found that most of my clients (including me) feel great when our THS is between 1.0–2.0 mIU/L.

You will have to find your own "sweet spot" for TSH. I recommend starting by bringing this information to your practitioner's attention. You may download the full version of the NACB's official recommendations at their Web site: http://www.aacc.org/sitecollectiondocuments/nacb/lmpg/thyroid/thyroid-fullversion.pdf

The lab ranges for Free T3 and Free T4 are listed below:

Lab Range: Free T4 0.8 – 1.8 ng/dL
Lab Range: Free T3 230 – 420 pg/dL

Most integrative and functional medical practitioners like to see their patients at the higher end of what the lab considers to be normal. It's important to remember that you are not a lab result—you are a living, breathing human being with unique physiology and stress levels. Getting to the optimal thyroid levels should be based more on how you feel than how you look on paper!

Lab	Low	Optimal	High
Free T4	0.8	1.2-1.4	1.8
Free T3	230	320-340	420

If you are not taking thyroid replacement, you want to ensure that you are in the middle to the upper part of the lab range and that you feel good. The same applies if you are taking thyroid replacement. Only you can sense the best way over time to adjust your dosage until you find the optimum levels that make you feel your best.

When the results are in

Once you have received your blood results, you will know if you have antibodies to your thyroid (or other tissues, if you ran any other antibody tests).

Autoimmunity is confirmed by a positive result in ANY of the following areas:

- Anti-TPO: Antithyroid Peroxidase Antibodies
- TgAb: Antithyroglobulin antibodies
- TRAb: Thyroid Receptor Antibodies/TSI (thyroid stimulating immunoglobulin)
- ANA: Antinuclear Antibodies
- RA: Rheumatoid Factor

If there are no antibodies to your thyroid or other tissues, then your symptoms are not likely due to an autoimmune condition. Your symptoms may be caused by other factors, such as toxicity, adrenal insufficiency, nutritional deficiencies, inflammation, or in rare cases, a pituitary condition. You will need to work with your practitioner to uncover the roots of your condition, but you will definitely benefit from following the *Sensitivity Discovery Program*, optimizing your nutrition, reducing stress, healing your gut, and supporting your liver.

If your lab tests reveal antibodies to your thyroid or other tissues, the next step is to take a load off your body by starting on the *Sensitivity Discovery Program* and optimizing your nutrition. If you are diagnosed with Hashimoto's and your TSH is above the optimal range, you may benefit from starting on thyroid replacement medication to reduce inflammation in the thyroid gland itself, and to ensure you have the benefit of optimal thyroid hormones in your system so your body can begin to heal itself.

The program will follow one of two paths, depending on whether you have hypothyroid (Hashimoto's) or hyperthyroid (Graves') symptoms.

CHAPTER 13

The First Steps Toward Reversing Your Autoimmune Thyroid Condition

*"Why should I stay at the bottom of a well,
when a strong rope is in my hand?"*
– Rumi

What to Do First If You Are Hypothyroid Due to Hashimoto's

If you are diagnosed with Hashimoto's, and you have hypothyroid symptoms but are not on medication already, you will probably need to get a prescription from your doctor for thyroid hormone replacement. This will reduce the inflammation of your thyroid gland and help relieve some of your symptoms. Your symptoms will get better, because your body is getting the important thyroid hormone it needs to function well. You will need to work closely with your doctor at this stage, because prescribing the right thyroid replacement is tricky and takes expertise. It usually takes a few rounds of trial and error to find the product and dose that will work best for you.

If you are on medication but still have symptoms, and your lab tests are not optimal, it may be time to explore other medication options.

Let's look at some possible scenarios.

Early Hashimoto's with Normal Thyroid Labs and No Symptoms

If you test positive for antibodies (Anti-TPO or TgAb) to your thyroid and your thyroid levels are within the normal/optimal range, and you have mild or no symptoms, this is great news! It means you have caught the condition early, before it has done significant damage to your thyroid gland. If you follow the steps outlined in this book, you might not need to take thyroid replacement medication at all.

Sample lab results:

- Anti-TPO – mildly elevated
- TgAb – mildly elevated
- TSH: < 3.0 mIU/L
- Free T4 > 1.2 ng/dL
- Free T3 > 300 pg/dL

Remember, these are only guidelines; you will have go by how you feel, not what you look like on paper. If you have even slight symptoms of hypothyroidism, you'll probably feel better by lowering your TSH to the optimal range with thyroid replacement hormone while you are healing. I have found that many of my clients feel better when their TSH is within the optimal range.

Optimal TSH Range: TSH .05 – 2.0 mIU/L

Hashimoto's with Borderline/Low Thyroid Labs and Mild Symptoms

If you test positive for antibodies (Anti-TPO or TgAb) to your thyroid, your TSH is elevated, and your thyroid levels are below the normal/optimal range, you're probably experiencing symptoms. I doubt you would be reading this book otherwise. Some people just assume that their fatigue, weight gain, and other health issues are just a part of life, but often the thyroid is responsible. You'll likely feel better with the addition of a thyroid hormone replacement.

Sample lab results:

- Anti-TPO – elevated
- TgAb – elevated
- TSH: > 3.0 mIU/L
- Free T4 < 1.2 ng/dL
- Free T3 < 300 pg/dL

Full-Blown Hashimoto's with Low Thyroid Labs and Raging Symptoms

If the antibodies (Anti-TPO or TgAb) to your thyroid are very elevated, your TSH is very elevated, your thyroid levels are below the normal range, and you are having raging symptoms, you will very likely feel better with thyroid hormone replacement.

Sample lab results:

- Anti-TPO – very elevated
- TgAb – very elevated
- TSH: > 4.5 mIU/L
- Free T4 < 1.0 ng/dL
- Free T3 < 200 pg/dL

Note to My Readers

I was reluctant to put sample lab values in this book, because as any practitioner who works with thyroid clients will tell you, in the real world, thyroid labs are as individual as the people who have them. I'm not a doctor; I am a patient advocate, and so by the time people come to me, they have been to several practitioners and are at their wit's end. You could say that I don't get the "normal" cases, but honestly, after hundreds of clients, I just don't see much consistency in thyroid lab results, or the relationship between those results and how a person feels. For this reason, you will have to feel and experiment your way through what it will take to recover, and you have to do that work with a skilled practitioner—one who is familiar with the many nuances of autoimmune thyroid conditions. The most important "test" to consider is how you feel. The truth is that no matter what the labs say, you are the only one who can gauge how you feel. When you choose a treatment, it should be based on how you feel, not what you look like on paper. Whether you choose thyroid replacement or not, the guidelines in this book will help you to feel better…that much I do know!

Choosing a Thyroid Medication

You have a few options when choosing a thyroid hormone replacement. The most commonly prescribed treatment for Hashimoto's is a synthetic version of thyroxin (T4) called l-thyroxin or levothyroxine. The brand names are Synthroid, Levoxyl, Levothroid, and Unithroid.

In my personal experience, very few people with Hashimoto's feel better with T4 replacement alone. This is because T4 is the relatively inactive form of the hormone, and must be converted in the liver and other organs to the more active form triiodothyronine, or T3. Unfortunately, because of heavy toxic body burdens and nutritional deficiencies, most people's livers do not function optimally, and therefore cannot effectively covert T4 into T3. For this reason, I highly recommend that you add T3 to the mix while you work to find out why you're not converting effectively.

T3 comes by the brand name Cytomel, and also in prescription compounded time-released and immediate release formulas. The compounded time-released formulas are the only form worth taking though, because T3 has a relatively short half-life in the body.

Two other options are Armour Thyroid and the less allergenic Nature-Throid. These are prescription medications made from desiccated (dried) porcine (pig) thyroid, and contain both T4 and T3. They also contain T1, T2, and calcitonin, which make them closer to what your own healthy thyroid would produce. The only caveat about desiccated thyroid is that it can provoke an immune response in some people, because it's mostly not thyroid hormone but is thyroid tissue instead, which is what the antibodies are attacking in the first place. I have personally seen antibodies go up when people make the switch to a desiccated thyroid. Since the goal of this book is to reverse your autoimmune condition, it makes sense to avoid substances that are known to trigger an immune response. Many thyroid sufferers will swear by Armour. They will tell you that nothing makes them feel as good. My personal opinion is that if you feel better and your antibodies disappear while you are on a desiccated thyroid, then you are on the right track. However, if you're taking desiccated thyroid, you've removed all the other possible splinters, and your antibodies are still elevated, it may be time to try another type of hormone replacement.

Finally, there are prescription synthetic compounded T4/T3 combinations in sustained-release form that are made by a compounding pharmacist. Personally, I feel these are superior preparations, but they are rarely covered by insurance companies, and can cost significantly more than the other options. I always recommend calling the compounding pharmacy first to inquire about the costs. I list the names of some reputable compounding pharmacies in the resources section.

Like I have said before, I have noticed that everyone is different when it comes to thyroid hormone replacement. There is no one-size-fits-all medication. You and your practitioner must be willing to try different options until you find the right one for you.

Beware of Sensitivity to Fillers

I have observed that quite a few of my clients have not felt as well on Synthroid, Armour, or Cytomel. It's likely that many people with autoimmune conditions have sensitivities to the fillers used in these preparations. Synthroid has both cornstarch and lactose. Cytomel has a modified food starch that contains gluten and Armour has dextrose. It's hard to believe that a person can react to such tiny amounts of these substances, but they definitely do.

Finding the Correct Dose

With all hormone therapy, it's always best to start low and go slow. Your doctor will be able to find a starting dose that is appropriate for you. I agree with Dr. Alexander Haskell's approach of raising the dose incrementally until your TSH is 1.0 or lower. This gives your thyroid a break, and reduces inflammation in the gland itself.

Don't Stop Here!

Taking thyroid medication alone will not reverse your condition. Even if you feel better and some of your symptoms improve, you must start to reduce your body toxicity and look for the splinters aggravating your condition if you want to completely heal. This requires further investigation, and in most cases, some lifestyle changes.

The next step is to follow the *Sensitivity Discovery Program* to discover what foods may contribute to your condition.

Why You May Need Thyroid Replacement Hormones to Get Better

"The thyroid prescription is very, very important. I have not known of a single person that has been able to recover from Hashimoto's who didn't have to initially use this medication."

— Dr. Alexander Haskell

I have found that lowering TSH is essential for recovery from Hashimoto's in many cases. This is probably because lowering TSH reduces inflammation in the thyroid gland. Dr. Alexander Haskell in his book, *Hope for Hashimoto's*, explains that elevated TSH increases the production of hydrogen peroxide in the thyroid gland, and is likely one of the mechanisms involved in the development of autoimmune thyroiditis. As you know, the thyroid needs iodine to make thyroid hormones. But the thyroid gland can only absorb iodide, which has to be converted into iodine in the body using a process that requires hydrogen peroxide (H_2O_2) and thyroid peroxidase (TPO).

It's a bit like the chicken-and-the-egg story, but try to follow along. If there is not enough iodide/iodine in the body, the thyroid can't make thyroid hormones. If there are not enough circulating thyroid hormones, your TSH will go up. When TSH goes up, it triggers the thyroid cells to produce hydrogen peroxide in anticipation of converting iodide to iodine. If there is not enough iodide (or any other necessary nutrient), TSH will remain elevated, and so will hydrogen peroxide. Extra hydrogen peroxide causes oxidative damage and inflammation, because the white blood cells release hydrogen peroxide as part of the inflammatory process, and all of this extra oxidative stress can lead to thyroid cell destruction. When thyroid cells destruct, they leak H_2O_2 into the surrounding areas, further exacerbating an immune response. The immune cells are there to clean up the H_2O_2 and the dead cells, but as you have learned, a stressed-out immune system can sometimes begin to attack healthy tissue, and, *voila*, you have a raging autoimmune situation!

I've had some full-blown Hashimoto's clients try to work this program "naturally" and insist on no thyroid replacement. I can say from experience that this is not a good idea, because all of our body's systems depend on optimal thyroid hormones. This means that if you have Hashimoto's and your thyroid levels are low, healing the roots of your condition will be almost impossible. It's like trying to drive a car without gas—you won't get anywhere.

It's important to remember that bio-identical hormones are substances that are recognized by the body as "self," and should not be feared or thought of as drugs or foreign chemicals.

Low T3 Can Be Due to Poor Conversion of T4 to T3, or Due to Stress and Reverse T3

The conversion of T4 to T3 happens in the liver, the GI tract, and other organs, and the conversion is affected by stress, deficiencies in nutrients such as selenium and zinc, liver dysfunction, infections, inflammation, and other toxicities.

In times of acute and prolonged stress, the body will naturally slow the process of converting T4 to T3 in the liver and other tissues. In its wisdom, the body will render the thyroid hormones to an inactive form called reverse T3, or rT3. The job of rT3 is to block the active hormone T3 so that you don't totally burn out. The production of rT3 is not a disease, but rather a survival mechanism. The body knows that under times of extreme stress, processing more thyroid hormones will be like kicking a sick, worn-out horse…and if you're not careful, it could drop dead!

If your T4 is normal/optimal but your T3 is low, it could be that either you are not converting T4 to T3 due to some deficiency or liver toxicity, or you are stressed-out and fatigued and the body is making more reverse T3 (rT3). If you are not converting T4 to T3, you may feel better with the addition of T3 hormone replacement. However, if you are super-stressed, the addition of T3 may make you feel worse.

If You Have Symptoms of Adrenal Fatigue

If you scored high on the adrenal questionnaire and you feel that your adrenals are stressed, you will need to treat them at the same time you treat your thyroid. As you have learned, the adrenals are the glands that control the fight-or-flight response. If you are very stressed and your adrenal glands are exhausted, you may feel worse with the addition of thyroid replacement. This is because extra thyroid hormones will boost your metabolism, but if your adrenals are exhausted, they won't be able to handle the extra energy.

Taking too much thyroid hormone when your adrenals are exhausted is like beating a dead horse!

If adrenal stress is one of your splinters, and you want to add thyroid hormones, it's always best to start very low and go very slow. At the same time, you will need to reduce your stress levels and get adequate rest. I have found that many of my clients with exhausted adrenals bounce back quite fast if they take the time to slow down and rest.

Don't add more pressure on yourself by attempting to heal yourself overnight. I have outlined ways to reduce stress and heal your adrenals in Chapter 15: Reduce Stress. It may be best for you to start there, even before you do anything else or make any major lifestyle or nutrition changes.

Should You Take High-Potency Iodine?

It is argued that one of the underlying causes of Hashimoto's is a deficiency of iodine. That may be true for some people, but if that's the case, why not just take high doses of iodine? The reason you don't want to do that is because iodide/iodine stimulates TSH, and as we have discovered, TSH stimulates the production of hydrogen peroxide (H_2O_2), which causes more inflammation. For a person with autoimmune thyroiditis, more inflammation is not a good idea.

So if you're deficient in iodine and that causes inflammation, but you can't take iodine because it causes more inflammation, what can you do?

First, you must realize that single deficiencies rarely exist. If you are deficient in iodine, you are most likely deficient in other important minerals and antioxidants, such as selenium. Selenium is the mineral found most abundantly in Brazil nuts, seafood and organ meats and it's needed to make glutathione peroxidase. One of the roles of glutathione peroxidase is to detoxify hydrogen peroxide. If you have inflammation in the thyroid gland and you're low on selenium, you don't have the right tools to clean up the inflammation. Selenium is also a cofactor for the deiodinase enzyme, which converts T4 to the more powerful T3.

Other compounds that detoxify hydrogen peroxide are phenolic acids—better known as the antioxidants found abundantly in plant-based foods, such as seeds, berries, leafy greens, green tea, and even red wine.

It makes sense, then, that people who don't have a diet high in selenium or other antioxidants would have a difficult time detoxifying free radicals like hydrogen peroxide. Over time, that can to lead to chronic inflammation, and a stressed-out immune system—perhaps triggering an autoimmune condition.

Let's say you are eating foods rich in iodine, selenium, and antioxidants, but you still have the symptoms of deficiency. As you have learned, if you're stressed-out and have a leaky gut, you could be malnourished because you're not absorbing all the nutrients from your food.

Even if you're eating all the right foods and your gut is healthy, you could have toxic halogens such as chlorine, bromine, and fluorine, blocking your thyroid receptors and taking the place of iodine.

Your body is a complex interplay of integrated systems that work together in harmony under ideal circumstances. But as you have seen, there are many ways that stress can disrupt that harmony. The situation is different for each individual. What you need to know is that taking high doses of iodine while you have inflammation can cause more inflammation and make you feel worse.

I have observed that it's better to reduce inflammation with thyroid replacement, along with a diet rich in selenium and other important antioxidants, while you look for the underlying causes of your autoimmune condition.

If you find that you are grossly iodine-deficient, you and your practitioner can work to uncover the reason, and then add it back in safe amounts. Many times, simply eating sea vegetables like nori a few times a week is enough to get your levels back up. Many excellent multivitamin formulas contain a small amount of iodine (150 mcg or less), which is a safe amount for many people with autoimmune thyroiditis. In more extreme cases of deficiency, it may be appropriate to take a high-potency supplement like Iodoral, but please only do this under the care of a knowledgeable practitioner, and always take selenium and other antioxidants along with it!

I do recommend taking additional bioavailable selenium during the Phase One of the healing protocol. I have found it to be very effective in reducing inflammation, and when that happens, people start feeling much better!

A Case for Lowering TSH: Julie's Story

Julie came to me after three years of struggling with Hashimoto's. As a Doctor of Oriental Medicine, she had been working to reverse her condition naturally, without any thyroid hormone replacement. She admitted that she was skeptical about my approach, but she had seen the labs of a mutual client who was able to reverse her antibodies and wanted to know how she did it. On her first visit, she brought an arsenal of herbs and remedies with her, each designed to support particular deficiencies in her body. She was also taking 12.5 mg of Iodoral, a high-potency iodide/iodide supplement. I could tell she was frustrated that all her efforts had not produced the results she had hoped for. Her biggest worry was that she was 36, and she and her husband had been trying to conceive. She tearfully explained that they had suffered three miscarriages, and that the stress was taking a toll on the marriage. Because of her excellent diet and self-care, she had been relatively symptom-free, but now, symptoms had started appearing, and that was adding to her anxiety. She had a gut feeling that the year she had spent in China had exposed her to heavy metals, and she was considering a heavy metal detox. She brought in all her labs from the previous years, and this is what they looked like:

First lab test:
- TSH: 4.7 mIU/L
- Free T4 .08 ng/dL
- Free T3 203 pg/dL

Nine months later:
- Anti-TPO – 154
- TSH: 5.3 mIU/L
- Free T4 .08 ng/dL
- Free T3 190 pg/dL

Two years after diagnosis and taking 12.5 mg of Iodoral per day:
- Anti-TPO – 437
- TSH: 5.7 mIU/L
- Free T4 .06 ng/dL
- Free T3 174 pg/dL

Her lab tests revealed that in spite of a healthy diet and adding iodine/iodide, her thyroid levels were going down, and her TSH and antibodies were going up!

I suggested she try lowering her TSH with a compounded T3/T4 combination, stop taking the Iodoral, and add 400 mcg of selenium and a good multivitamin. I also suggested she add 3000 mg of an omega-3,

3000 mg of GLA, and some extra vitamins C and D3. She was on a dairy/gluten-free vegetarian diet, and since she had an excellent understanding of nutrition, she was getting an adequate amount of protein. The only dietary suggestion I made was to take out the corn, soy, and nightshades to see if that made a difference.

She elected to wait on heavy metal testing and wanted to try far-infrared sauna therapy and Epsom salt baths first.

She followed up seven months later with a new set of labs, and this is what they looked like:

- Anti-TPO – 54
- TSH: .08 mIU/L
- Free T4 1.5 ng/dL
- Free T3 330 pg/dL

What a difference in antibodies in just seven months! They had reduced from 437 to 54! With renewed enthusiasm, she decided to test for heavy metals. She was slightly high in mercury and cadmium, so she decided to do an herbal heavy metal detox in addition to the far-infrared sauna treatments. At her six-month checkup, her antibodies were gone. She slowly weaned herself off the thyroid medication, and was feeling great. She and her husband now have a bouncy baby girl!

Will You Need Thyroid Hormones for Life?

The short answer is: I don't know. Everyone is different. If antibodies have been attacking your thyroid for many years, it may be so damaged that it's unable to produce adequate thyroid hormones. I have been free of antibodies for over four years, and I am on half the dose of thyroid replacement that I used to take. I'm now at the point where I can gauge how I feel, and I take the amount I feel is right for me. Personally, I feel better with a little extra thyroid hormone. It's hard to say how long I was brewing antibodies before I was diagnosed, so I'm not sure how much of my thyroid was damaged, or if it will ever produce optimal thyroid hormones. I continue to remain hopeful!

I have some clients who have weaned themselves off their medication, their labs are optimal, and they feel great. I think it's important to remember that thyroid hormone replacement is simply replacing a natural hormone your body needs to function optimally. I understand some people's aversion to taking a pill every day, but this is not the same as taking a drug to mask symptoms.

Studies have shown that the thyroid has the ability to regenerate after the autoimmune response is reversed, and that 20% of Hashimoto's patients may recover satisfactory thyroid function so that replacement hormones are unnecessary.[1] I believe that percentage will be markedly higher for those following the recommendations in this book as the ones studied were not necessarily removing the splinters aggravating their condition.

Checking for antibodies can test whether the autoimmune response has stopped. Checking to see if the thyroid itself is recovering is another issue. Some people gradually reduce their hormone dose while testing TSH to ensure it stays low. The thyroid can be visualized by ultrasound but a clearer indication of thyroid regeneration comes from administering Thyroid Releasing Hormone (TRH). If the thyroid has recovered, TRH will cause an increase in T3 and T4 released from the thyroid.[2]

Remember that even if your thyroid has sustained extensive damage requiring you to take ongoing thyroid hormone replacement, it is still worthwhile, even critical, to reverse the autoimmune process in your system. Autoimmune thyroid conditions are an indication that the immune system is being triggered and is overreacting, which can affect other aspects of your health. It is common to find other autoimmune conditions existing side by side with thyroid conditions.

The most important things to focus on are reducing/eliminating the antibodies to your thyroid and feeling better!

My Personal Program

Everyone always asks what thyroid medication I take. If you read my story, you know that I tried Synthroid when I was first diagnosed. I felt terrible on this medication, and my night sweats and rashes got much worse. Then my doctor switched me to Levoxyl, and I felt a little better. He suggested I try adding T3 in the form of Cytomel, but I reacted very badly to that—I had rashes, night sweats, and my hair started falling out again. One year later, another doctor recommended that I add a compounded time-released T3 to the Levoxyl, and for the first time in years, I felt better.

I've stayed on this combination for over seven years with optimal results. I've tried switching to Nature-Throid a couple of times, but I've never felt as good as I do on this combination. I now take less than half the dose of thyroid medication I did four years ago, and I feel amazing!

But remember, I healed my gut, I had my silver fillings replaced, and I detoxed from mercury. I've found the nutrition program that works best for me, which is a modified Paleo diet with plenty of healing fats; organic, non-starchy veggies; berries; soaked and sprouted nuts and seeds; fermented foods like kimchi; and live green juices. I never eat gluten, or any grain for that matter, and I completely avoid sugar, nightshades, legumes, and all conventional meat and produce. I take my own super nutrient complex, "The Women's Empowerment Formula," along with digestive enzymes and a good probiotic. I live in a green home, with no harmful chemicals in my cleaning or personal products. I've addressed the emotional patterns that were at the root of my chronic stress, and I have a spiritual practice that includes daily doses of love and joy.

I make much healthier choices than I did when I was sick, and have found the balance that works for me. But there is no one single path to wellness—there are many. I'm not asking you to do what I do; I'm asking you to find the balance that works best for you and then thrive with me!

What to Do First If You Are Hyperthyroid Due to Graves' or Hashimoto's

If you have been diagnosed as hyperthyroid due to Graves' or are in a hyperthyroid stage of Hashimoto's, your next step will depend on the severity of your symptoms. I have found that working with hyperthyroid clients can be difficult due to the high anxiety and increased emotionality they experience. If you are very anxious and emotional and have severe symptoms, your doctor may recommend a beta blocker, an antithyroid medication, or an anti-anxiety medication. This is perfectly acceptable, and may be necessary to help you to feel better right away.

If your symptoms are mild, you may decide to try some calming botanical preparations, such as bugleweed, valerian root, and lemon balm. Some of my clients have also found relief from eating a lot of the foods known to suppress thyroid activity, such as broccoli, kale, and Brussels sprouts, etc. You can read more about these foods in Chapter 14: Optimize Your Nutrition.

Please keep in mind that taking medication and herbal treatments to reduce your symptoms will not reverse your condition. In order to heal, you will still need to find out why you have antibodies to your thyroid or other tissues in the first place.

Once you and your doctor have decided how to manage your hyperthyroid symptoms, your next step is to begin the *Sensitivity Discovery Program*, and then address any splinters you may have uncovered.

Graves' and the Stress Connection

I have found that reducing stress is a big factor in recovery from Graves' and the related symptoms. I'm not being trite; I realize that what you are going through is very difficult, and the symptoms can be awful. The hyperthyroid symptoms that accompany Graves' and sometimes Hashimoto's can make you feel like you are running from a pack of saber-toothed tigers! The last thing you probably want to hear is that you "should reduce your stress." But what I have found is that in order to feel better, you must take your health into your own hands, and that includes your emotional health. You will benefit greatly from reading Chapter 15 and beginning a stress reduction program while you work on positive lifestyle changes.

Things You Can Do to Start Feeling Better Fast!

Healing involves restoring balance to the core systems of the body. While you work to get the proper thyroid tests to balance your thyroid hormones, you can begin to support your healing process by strengthening your body with good nutrition, supplementing deficiencies, and reducing your stress.

The following chapters discuss just how to do that. Remember, the body knows how to be healthy and will naturally move toward vibrant health if given what it needs: positive thoughts; sufficient rest; stress relief; vibrant food and proper nutrients; healthy GI and eliminatory systems; good detoxification pathways; and healthy environments!

Thyroid Repair Program at a Glance

Phase I: 30 to 90 Day Overview

People always ask me what is the quickest, most effective way to reverse an autoimmune condition. I have outlined the path that works the fastest most of the time. It's important to stay on Phase I until your symptoms have resolved. This can take anywhere from 30 to 90 days if you follow it 100 percent. It will take longer if you are unable to make all the healthy changes required to heal.

You can take as long as you like to work the program. Some people can't or don't want to make lifestyle changes that quickly. It's okay. Just do the best you can. I always tell people that reversing their condition is like taking a trip from California to New York. You can hop on a plane and get it over with quickly, or you can walk across country. It's totally up to you how fast you want to get well. If you follow the program 100 percent for a full 90 days, I guarantee you will see a marked improvement in your health; in many cases, you may see a complete reversal. Remember, you are doing this for yourself, so do it at the pace that feels comfortable.

Start with a full panel of blood tests so that you have a starting line for your journey to better health. If your most recent labs are from within the last 90 days, it's okay to use those. You will be retesting in 90 days or when your symptoms have resolved, whichever comes first.

Baseline lab tests and their codes:
- 85025 CBC with differential
- 80053 Comp metabolic panel with Glucose
- 86141 CRP
- 80061 Lipid Panel
- 83036 Homocysteine
- 83525 Insulin
- 82627 DHEA-Sulfate
- 84305 IGF-I
- 83519 IGFBP-3
- 84481 Free T3

- 84439 Free T4
- 84443 TSH

To check for anemia:
- 82728, 83540, 83550   Iron, TIBC and Ferritin Panel

Thyroid antibodies:
- 84442 TPO

If you have hyperthyroid symptoms:
- 83520 TRAb

If you have other symptoms of autoimmunity, such as sore joints, rashes, fever, etc:
- ANA (Antinuclear Antibodies)
- Rheumatoid Factor (RA)
- Erythrocyte Sedimentation Rate (ESR or SED)

Hashimoto's: Balance thyroid hormone levels with the addition of thyroid replacement medication if necessary. Ideally you should aim to reduce thyroid inflammation by lowering TSH to 1.0 or lower by using thyroid hormone supplementation, selenium, zinc, essential fatty acids and antioxidants. Compounded T3/T4 is optimum if you can afford it. This treatment may only be short term—3 to 6 months—after which you can reassess your condition and medication needs. This recommendation is only if you are hypothyroid. Hyperthyroid patients do not need thyroid hormone replacement.

Graves': Control hyperthyroid symptoms with medication (beta blockers, antithyroid) or botanicals (bugleweed, valerian root, and lemon balm).

Chapter 14: Follow Phase I—*Eating for Your Good Genes,* and for 30 to 90 days stop eating gluten, dairy, eggs, sugar, nightshades, grains, legumes, nuts, and processed foods. Start eating fresh organic berries, tons of certified organic veggies, fermented foods, healing fats, and small amounts of lean organic fish, meat, or poultry. If you are adverse to animal protein you can try hypoallergenic rice protein powder. Cook with anti-inflammatory herbs and spices: turmeric, cumin, fennel, parsley, cinnamon, cardamom, ginger, garlic, sea salt, etc.

Chapter 15: Reduce stress by becoming aware of stress and your unique Mind-Body type. Heal your adrenals with mindfulness practice, exercise, laughter, and 8 to 10 hours of sleep every night. Try a media fast. Adrenal supplementation if indicated.

Chapter 16: Heal your GI tract if necessary and reduce inflammation by removing foods and substances that cause leaky gut (staying on Phase I). Test for and treat dysbiosis (imbalance among the colonies of microorganisms within your body), parasites, fungus, and other GI pathogens if indicated. Support GI tract with medical foods, HCl, digestive enzymes, and probiotics.

Chapter 17: Restore your liver by staying on Phase I of the nutrition program and steering clear of harmful substances such as alcohol, sugar, caffeine, and drugs. Improve methylation and boost glutathione with supplementation if necessary.

Chapter 19: Detox your home, garden, and office. Look for hidden sources of toxic stress. Replace toxic chemicals with clean and green alternatives. Try some detox treatments:
- 3- or 10-day detox
- Far-infrared sauna
- Epsom salt bath.

Phase II: Sensitivity Discovery Phase

Once your symptoms have completely resolved, you can begin the process of reintroducing foods and tracking how you feel.

Theoretically, if you've healed your GI tract, you may be able to reintroduce many of your favorite foods and find that you can now "tolerate" them fairly well. The universal exceptions are gluten, junk, and processed foods. Many people report feeling better by staying off all grains, dairy, nightshades, and legumes long-term.

If you're still not feeling well...

If you've followed the program 100 percent for a full 90 days and you still don't feel well, you most likely have some other splinters that need to be addressed, such as a stealth infection or a toxin like mercury. In that case, you will want to move on to the next step:

Chapter 17: Test for toxic splinters such as heavy metals and work with a practitioner to improve detoxification naturally.

Chapter 18: Look for sources of hidden inflammation, such as infections. Treat any systemic infections, sinusitis, dental infections, mycoplasma, Candida, etc.

Phase III: Vibrant for Life!

The lifestyle program is the custom mind-body program you create for yourself after following the guidelines in this book. Once you feel well, you'll want to stay well. Most people find that they love the healthy changes they've made and want to stick with them for life.

At 3–6 months into the program or after your symptoms have resolved, you'll want to retest antibodies and thyroid hormones. It's very likely that if you feel good, your labs will have improved too. In this phase, you will work with your practitioner to adjust your thyroid hormone dosage if necessary.

Many people are able to keep up with the lifestyle changes long-term by using the 80/20 rule, which means sticking to a healthy program 80 percent of the time. You will have to find the ratio that works best for you!

CHAPTER 14

Optimize Your Nutrition

"The very fact that we are having a national conversation about what we should eat, that we are struggling with the question about what the best diet is, is symptomatic of how far we have strayed from the natural conditions that gave rise to our species, from the simple act of eating real, whole, fresh food."
– MARK HYMAN

"Leave your drugs in the chemist's pot if you can cure the patient with food. Our medicine should be food and food should be our medicine."
– HIPPOCRATES, 420 B.C.

The Thyroid Cure Mind-Body Nutrition Program

Autoimmune conditions develop when the immune system becomes confused and overwhelmed by multiple aggravating factors, which I call "splinters." One of the biggest splinters is poor nutrition, which eventually leads to other splinters, such as disrupted digestion; malabsorption of nutrients; malnutrition; allergies; blood sugar imbalance; weight gain; hormonal imbalance; inflammation; and toxicity.

Poor nutrition sets off a cascade of problems, from lack of essential vitamins, minerals and nutrients to imbalanced gut flora, depleted enzymes, and the eventual breakdown of the mucosal layer of the intestines—the condition called "leaky gut."

I have never met anyone with an autoimmune condition who has optimal nutrition and a healthy digestive tract. Hmmm… Are you starting to connect the dots?

Remember that the GI tract is home to almost 80 percent of the cells of our immune system. Although our stress levels and emotions have an influence, our gut health is determined first and foremost by what we put into our mouths every day! I'll discuss the functional tests available to determine intestinal health in Chapter 16: Heal Your Gut, but you can create huge shifts in your GI health by simply making an effort to clean up your diet.

Optimizing your nutrition will help by:

- Providing your body with the essential nutrients needed to heal
- Healing your GI tract
- Reducing inflammation, which is itself an immune response
- Balancing your blood sugar
- Supporting your liver and detoxification pathways
- Regulating your hormones

Good nutrition will make you feel better every single day once the healing process is underway. You will be amazed at how fast you can bounce back from a chronic condition when you begin eating the foods your body was designed to eat.

You may have been told that you are genetically predisposed to autoimmune disease, and that there is nothing you can do to reverse it. In Chapter 6, you learned that nothing could be further from the truth. In fact, you have a lot of control over the health of your body and how your genes express themselves—much more than most people think. I've seen hundreds of people reverse their autoimmune conditions. It's more than possible. In fact, it's nearly certain that if you do what it takes to remove the splinters, you will reverse your condition. It's time to discover which foods may be turning on your bad genes and contributing to your symptoms, and which foods turn on your good genes and make you feel vibrant!

> **What You Need to Know:**
> Your genes are NOT your destiny! You can heal many of your "splinters" at once, simply by optimizing your nutrition!

Eat for Your Unique Mind-Body Type

In this section, I will walk you through the basic principles of a nutrition discovery program that has helped hundreds of people regain their health and vitality. This is not a one-size-fits-all "diet"—it's a nutrition program that helps you determine what works for your unique physiology.

The ancient healing practice of Ayurveda recognized that humans come in different mind-body types, or constitutions, called prakriti, which simply means "nature." In other words, your prakriti is your unique biological and psychological nature. Since we are unique in body and mind, it makes sense for each of us to tailor our nutrition according to that unique nature. One of the simplest ways to discover what foods are best for your particular mind-body type is to eat only from the foods known to be healthy for all human beings for a period of 30 to 90 days, or until your symptoms disappear, and then follow it with a *Sensitivity Discovery Program.*

This section is designed to give you the basic tools to discover which foods create an imbalance in your body, and which foods restore you to balance.

Food is Information

The science of nutrigenomics reveals that all food carries information directly to our genes, influencing every aspect of our health. Food speaks to your body and controls how your genes express themselves. In fact, as Nora T. Gedgaudas, CNS, CNT, says in her book, *Primal Body, Primal Mind*, "…(T)here is no drug anywhere that can regulate genetic expression better or more powerfully than your diet can." Every cell and system of your body is affected by the foods you eat. The quality of your food choices is of utmost importance. This is not about counting calories—it's about prioritizing the quality of the foods you eat.

Have you ever considered eating ONLY the foods that turn on your good genes and contribute to vibrant health? I can guarantee that if you do, you WILL look and feel amazing. Many times, changing your diet alone can completely reverse your autoimmune condition!

Think About What You Eat!

Every time you reach to put something in your mouth, ask yourself the following questions:

"Is this the highest quality food available at this time?"

"How will this food make me feel emotionally and physically?"

"Is there an emotional reason I want to eat this?"

"Is there something more nutritious that I can eat instead right now?" "How will this food speak to my genes?"

You will be surprised how effective this little mindfulness exercise is, and how it can help you make healthy choices for the rest of your life.

A Calorie is Just a Calorie, Right?

Wrong! For years, we were told that maintaining a healthy weight was a matter of "calories in and calories out." Science has now proven that this theory is flawed. If you eat 1,500 calories in the form of chips, burgers, and beer, you're going to have a very different body and genetic expression than if you ate the same amount of calories in the form of lean proteins, organic fruit, veggies, and healing fats!

Trade Inflammation for Inspiration

All autoimmune disorders have something in common, inflammation, which you'll remember can be caused by stress, poor nutrition, food allergies, and sensitivities and infections. Inflammation is a sign that your immune system is fired up and on high alert.

Our goal will be to remove foods known to cause inflammation while adding foods that help calm and heal the body.

If this sounds simplistic, that's because it is. It's simple, but it's not easy. The first phase of the program can be challenging, because you will eat ONLY healthy, vibrant foods. You will have to stay away from all foods that might be responsible for inflammation, irritation, and indigestion. The only way to discover which foods are really giving you trouble is to stay away from all the likely culprits in the beginning for a period of time that will allow your body to calm down and then add them back slowly, one by one, after all your symptoms have resolved, observing the effects of each food on your body as they are reintroduced.

As I write this, I can feel my heart sink, because I realize that words like "eliminate" and "avoid" sound depriving. No one likes to feel deprived: I know I don't! We are creatures of habit, but sometimes we have to break our habits to see their effects.

I want you to feel inspired as you embark on this journey, and I want you to reverse your autoimmune condition, just like I did! Give yourself some credit. You can do this!

If you read my story in the prologue, you know that I felt so sick that I was willing to do ANYTHING to feel better. I was motivated more by pain than inspiration in the beginning. It wasn't until I started feeling better that I became really inspired.

If you are reading this, you probably have an autoimmune condition, and you're regularly suffering uncomfortable symptoms. I assure you from my experience that embracing this nutrition program will improve your symptoms, and in some cases it will eliminate them entirely!

If you are feeling really lousy, you may not be inspired yet, but I guarantee that if you follow the program, you will feel better soon, and the inspiration will follow.

I'll tell you what I tell all my clients: give me 90 days, and I promise you WILL see and feel results!

> **What You Need to Know:**
> The most effective way to heal your autoimmune condition is to eat only foods that calm and heal the body, and to remove foods known to provoke inflammation and chronic illness.

Our goal will be to determine what foods cause an inflammatory response in your body and then replace them with awesome-tasting alternatives for vibrant health!

You are worth it! Love yourself enough to embrace the Sensitivity Discovery process; your immune system will feel the love, and the healing can begin! While I was healing, I put notes all over my home, including the refrigerator and the pantry, to remind me to love myself and make healthy choices. This is what the notes said:

- *"Love yourself with every choice!"*
- *"What is your most beautiful vision of yourself? Make that vision a reality today!"*
- *"I love myself. My immune system accepts my thyroid gland and my whole body."*
- *"My thyroid is completely healed!"*

Go to my Web site—www.thethyroidcure.com/inspiration—and download some beautiful affirmations to put around your kitchen, your bathroom mirror, or wherever you'd like to be reminded to love yourself.

Discover Your Unique Mind-Body Type: Sensitivity Discovery Program

The *Sensitivity Discovery Program* enables you get to know your body and how it responds to the foods you eat. There is nothing new or extreme about this program. Dr. Albert Rowe first introduced the concept of an elimination diet in 1926, and since then, medical doctors, allergists, and nutritionists have been using similar programs to help patients discover how food affects their health and emotions.

During the first phase, I ask you to remove inflammation-provoking foods from your diet for 30 to 90 days, or until your symptoms disappear. In the second phase, you can add them back (one at a time) so you can carefully monitor how each one makes you feel emotionally and physically.

I guarantee that if you follow the program 100 percent, you WILL know within as few as 90 days which foods truly nourish your body, mind, and spirit, and which foods cause inflammation and discomfort. Perhaps you've felt sick for so long that you've forgotten what it feels like to be healthy and vibrant. Once you remember what it's like to feel good again, the effort will seem like a small price to pay!

Prepare Your Mind

Before you begin the *Sensitivity Discovery Program*, it's a good idea to prepare your mind for the journey ahead. For some people, the program is a breeze. For others, it requires making some drastic changes. Change isn't easy, but it is possible. One way I found the motivation to make positive, healthy changes is by reviewing my reasons for seeking change in the first place. You might find it helpful to take another look at your answers in The Empowerment Exercise from Chapter 1. With your compelling reasons for healing fresh in mind, reaffirm your intention to reverse your condition.

I have created a *Sensitivity Discovery Program* Journal to help you stay on track. You can download the full version at my Web site: www.thethyroidcure.com/Sensitivityjournal.

Set an intention to nourish yourself with wholesome foods and plenty of rest. The reward will be a new level of health you may not have thought was possible!

Phase I:

Wellness Goal: How do I want to feel every day?

_____
_____
_____
_____
_____
_____
_____
_____

I will accomplish my wellness goal by the following actions:

_____
_____
_____
_____
_____
_____
_____
_____

My reward for achieving these goals:

_____
_____
_____
_____
_____
_____
_____

I will schedule at least 30 minutes each day for these enjoyable physical activities:

_____

_____

_____

_____

Timing is Everything

Plan to start the *Sensitivity Discovery Program* at a time when you know you won't be overly stressed or busy. For instance, if you're going on vacation or have houseguests, it's probably best to wait until your schedule is clear. You can always focus on eating better in the meantime, but wait until circumstances are on your side before embarking on the disciplined approach.

But don't put it off for too long! If you wait for the "perfect time" to begin the program, you may never get around to it.

I find it's best to begin on a weekend or when you have a couple of days off in a row. This allows you to ease into the program gently and gives you time to plan your meals for the workweek.

Get Support from Family and Friends

Since most social engagements revolve around food, you might wonder how you'll survive a nutrition program that limits certain foods. If you have a family, you might worry about eating different food than everybody else. I know firsthand that one of the biggest hurdles to overcome is dealing with family meals and social events. I've found it's critical to ask for support during your healing process. You will find that the people who love you will respond positively when you express a true desire to heal your life. Ask your spouse, parents, children, friends, and work associates to support you in the process and it will be much easier. They may even help keep you on track.

Make it a family affair to get healthy! Remember, this program is not just for "sick" people—it's for any human being who wants vibrant health! Many of my clients have asked their spouses to join them in the *Sensitivity*

Discovery Program, and the results have been amazing. I've seen the husbands of many of my clients recover from their own chronic symptoms by following the program. Many are now enthusiastic ambassadors of health!

Prepare Your Kitchen

The plan for the next 30 to 90 days is to eat only foods that heal. You'll want to prepare your kitchen and stock up on the ingredients in advance. I have provided you with a grocery list of all the items you will need in this chapter. At the same time, you'll want to get rid of all unhealthy foods. I recommend throwing junk and processed foods away and putting potentially allergic foods up and out of view. Remember, out of sight, out of mind. You don't want to be tempted during Phase I of the program.

What to Expect During Phase I

How you feel during Phase I depends on how healthy your current diet and lifestyle is. The cleaner you are, the easier it will be. If your current diet includes a lot of inflammatory substances, such as wheat, dairy, fast food, canned and packaged foods, sugar, alcohol, caffeine, and over-the-counter drugs, you may have symptoms of withdrawal as your body works to eliminate toxins and find balance. These symptoms are sometimes referred to as a "healing crisis."

This is not an ordinary detox program, but some people do have annoying symptoms of withdrawal when they remove addictive foods and substances. This is a normal response, but it can be challenging for some people. Not everyone with a lousy diet suffers withdrawals—many feel great—but understand that if you experience withdrawal symptoms when you remove caffeine, sugar, alcohol, gluten, or other addictive substances from your diet, it doesn't mean you are doing something wrong.

Common withdrawal symptoms include:
- Headache
- Fever
- Lethargy
- Mood swings
- Constipation
- Diarrhea
- Skin eruptions

It's important to remember that these symptoms won't last forever. Most people feel better after a couple of days of eating healthy, and even those who suffer a temporary reaction are soon feeling better than ever.

Again, this is NOT a "detox diet" or fast. It's not calorie-restrictive. You simply choose to eat ONLY healing foods for 30 to 90 days!

If you suspect your diet is super-toxic, you may want to ease into the program by simply eliminating gluten and cutting back on grains, junk foods, sugar, caffeine, and alcohol for a couple of weeks. Then you can plan a time to follow the program 100 percent.

If your diet is pretty clean already, you may feel a surge of energy and lightness, which is the goal!

Phase I: Eating for Your Good Genes

"Eat the way your body was designed to eat and a lot takes care of itself."
— Nora T. Gedgaudas, *Primal Body, Primal Mind*

When we cut out the foods known to cause inflammation, such as processed and junk foods, sugar, modern grains (especially gluten), dairy, eggs, legumes, and nightshades, what do we have left? We have a diet that's closer to what our hunter-gatherer ancestors ate. While we each have a unique mind-body type, our genes are 99.9 percent the same, and they're also identical to those of our ancestors. Sadly, most of the foods we eat today, especially the junk and processed stuff that hardly qualifies as food, haven't been around long enough for our genes to adapt to them.

In order to eat for your good genes, you'll want to go back to the foods your body recognizes as food. If you give it 100 percent, you'll be amazed at how well your body remembers how to be healthy!

The first phase of the program involves eating vibrant foods that we know reduce inflammation and have the ability to turn on your good genes!

You'll be choosing from an abundant variety of:
- Healing fats
- Healing carbohydrates
- Healing lean proteins

I've even included delicious recipes for breakfast, lunch, and dinner.

Special note: The only two foods on the "avoid list" that I consider safe to eat as long as you know you don't react to them are:

- Omega-3 enriched organic eggs
- Organic brown or wild rice

If you are absolutely certain that you do not react to these foods you may include them in Phase One. If you are unsure, then please wait until Phase Two to bring them back in!

Healing Fats

Healing fats such as essential fatty acids (EFAs) are essential to health and critical for recovery from any autoimmune condition. Fats have been maligned in the popular press for many years, but we now know that healthy fats are nurturing and support healing. Let me share the technicalities of essential fats, and then I'll suggest a few beneficial ones for your diet and to take as supplements.

EFAs are not manufactured in the body, and must be obtained through diet. There are four categories of EFAs: omega-3, omega-6, omega-9, and omega-12. I'm going to focus on the anti-inflammatory omega-3 and omega-6 EFAs.

The three most nutritionally important omega-3 fatty acids are alpha-linolenic acid (ALA), eicosapentaenoic acid (EPA), and docosahexaenoic acid (DHA). Food sources of ALA include flax seeds, walnuts, hemp seeds, rapeseed, and certain dark leafy green veggies.

Under ideal conditions, the body partially converts ALA from the foods we eat into EPA and DHA. However, chronic illness and other deficiencies can inhibit the conversion. EPA and DHA can also be found in certain fish, and are the most desirable of the omega-3 family. DHA is converted in the body to a group of anti-inflammatory prostaglandins, which are hormone-like substances used throughout the body. This conversion to prostaglandins is what's responsible for omega-3's therapeutic effects. DHA has been shown to reduce inflammation and aid in treating many autoimmune conditions. For this reason, I suggest that you start taking 1,000 mg of an omega-3 fatty acid complex three times a day.

Healing omega-6 fatty acids include cis-linoleic acid, linoleic acid, and gamma-linolenic acid (GLA), and are found in certain plants and vegetable oils. These fats contain critical antioxidant properties and help to inhibit and destroy free radicals and fight inflammation. GLA is the most therapeutic member of the omega-6 family. A healthy body will convert some cis-linoleic acid into GLA, but age and certain deficiencies can disrupt the conversion. GLA is also found in certain plants, such as evening primrose, black currant, and borage oil. The body then converts GLA into another group of anti-inflammatory prostaglandins, which are responsible for its therapeutic effect. I suggest you start taking 400–600 mg of GLA in the form of borage oil three times per day.

Coconut oil was once demonized along with other saturated fats, but research increasingly reveals it to be an elixir of health. Coconut oil appears to help prevent cancer, stimulate thyroid function, and even lowers cholesterol by converting it to the anti-aging hormones, pregnenolone, progesterone, and DHEA. It may help keep excess weight in check to boot. There are many reports on coconut oil benefiting dementia and Alzheimer's patients as well. Coconut oil can be stored at room temperature for over a year without becoming rancid, probably owing to its antioxidant properties.[1-4]

Coconut oil also turns out to have antimicrobial properties, as it contains lauric and capric acids, which are antibacterial, antiviral and antifungal. These medium-chain triglycerides are fuel for your cells and support immune function in the GI tract.[5]

I suggest that you start taking 2 tablespoons of this healing oil—once in the morning and once in the evening before bed. Coconut oil is also great for cooking and baking. If the taste doesn't quite fit what you're cooking, you can combine it with ghee or olive oil to balance the flavor.

Note: Because of the potential thyroid stimulating properties of coconut oil, persons with Graves' might consider avoiding coconut oil until their symptoms resolve.

Ghee is pure clarified butter that is high in butyrate, a short-chain fatty acid that is anti-inflammatory and immune boosting. In Ayurvedic medicine, ghee is believed to enhance one's "life energy." It is recognized as a healing food that balances the mind and the body. Since ghee has the milk protein removed, it's safe for Phase I, and for those with dairy sensitivities. Ghee can be used in place of butter. It has the added advantage of not burning at higher temperatures like butter does, and can be stored at room temperature for extended periods. Ghee is often available in natural markets and the ethnic foods section of some markets, but you can make your own ghee from butter by melting it gently in a small pot and skimming off the milk solids that rise to the top, until only clear milk fat (ghee) remains.

Other sources of healing fats include olive oil, avocado oil, and the fat from grass-fed, organic animals.

I have provided you with a list of the approved healing fats in the shopping list in this chapter.

> **What You Need to Know:**
> Healing fats are your friends, and are vital for healing your autoimmune condition. You particularly need anti-inflammatory omega-3 and omega-6 essential fatty acids. Take both 1,000 mg of an omega-3 fatty acid complex and 400–600 mg of GLA in the form of borage oil three times per day. Use ghee, coconut, olive, and avocado oil for cooking and get healthy fats from certain fish, grass-fed organic animals, and later, in Phase II, nuts and seeds.

Healing, Non-Starchy, Low-Glycemic Carbohydrates

The most healing foods on the planet are colorful, low-glycemic fruits and non-starchy vegetables. These foods are rich in powerful antioxidants called phytonutrients, and they contain important vitamins, minerals, and fiber.

The foundation of the *Eating for Your Good Genes* phase is eating tons of non-starchy, low-glycemic vegetables and fruits. You'll be choosing from a wide variety of these gene-loving, anti-inflammatory foods. You'll be eating red and purple berries; dark, leafy green vegetables like kale and rainbow chard; and orange and yellow vegetables like squash, sweet potatoes, and yams. Make sure you get 5–9 servings of these foods per day.

To protect yourself from unnecessary toxic stress, try to buy organic when possible. If you're on a budget, try shopping at your local farmer's market or co-op. Many times, the prices are much lower than at the natural grocery store. Purchasing foods that are available locally and seasonally is healthy for your body and easier on the planet, as they have a lighter footprint!

While it's still best to buy organic, I have included a list of conventionally grown fruits and veggies that are safe to eat online at www.thethyroidcure.com/safeconventionalfoods

Healing Complete Proteins

You can survive without carbohydrates, but you can't survive without protein! Protein contains amino acids, which are the building blocks of life, and are essential for vibrant health. Out of the 20 different amino acids you need to be healthy, your body only makes 11 of them. That's why the remaining nine are called essential amino acids, and must come from the foods we eat. We need protein for the regeneration and repair of our tissues, and for detoxification. The body detoxifies in two phases. In phase one, toxins are mobilized from fat and internal organs. In phase two, they are excreted via the skin, hair, sweat, urine, and stool. Amino acids are needed for the second phase, since they bind with the mobilized toxins and carry them out of the body.

All foods have some protein, but some are more complete than others. Certain foods contain all the essential amino acids we need to be healthy. The best source of complete protein is all-natural animal protein, free of antibiotics, hormones, and other chemicals. Other sources are quinoa, soy, buckwheat, and the combination of rice and legumes. Unfortunately, many of the plant foods that contain complete proteins are highly aggravating to people with autoimmune conditions, and in some cases, they comprise a huge dietary splinter. This is due to the high content of anti-nutrients and lectins that are part of the plant's natural defenses. For this reason, these foods are not allowed during Phase I of the program. You can experiment with properly preparing (more on this later) and reintroducing these foods in Phase II and see how you feel. Most people I have worked with can't tolerate them, but I haven't worked with everyone. You will have to find out for yourself if these foods are aggravating to your unique physiology.

While you need complete protein to be healthy, you don't need that much. Depending on your body weight, you only need between 45 to 60 grams per day, which translates to 6–8 oz., or about the size of the palm of your hand. Some people need even less.

The QUALITY of the protein you choose is vitally important. Make sure you choose from ONLY the choices I've provided on the shopping list. This list contains only natural, grass-fed red meat like beef, buffalo, and game; organic, all-natural, free-range poultry; safe fish; and approved, hypoallergenic protein powders.

If you can't find all-natural, antibiotic, hormone- and chemical-free animal protein, don't settle for the alternative. Some of the worst foods on the planet are conventionally-farmed animal products. If you can't find all-natural, go without!

In Phase II, you will be reintroducing organic sprouted nuts and seeds, organic brown or wild rice, and omega-3-enriched eggs.

If you are a vegetarian or vegan, I suggest a high-quality, hypoallergenic protein powder to ensure you are getting enough of the essential amino acids that you need to heal. Check the Resources section for suggestions.

I have found that some people do well with more protein than others. You will have to find your own sweet spot, but please, don't overdo it—too much protein is hard to digest and accelerates the aging process!

Drink Clean Water!

Proper hydration is a great aid to detoxification and helps the kidneys eliminate toxins. Make a point of drinking at least 64 ounces of clean, pure filtered water daily. Add a squeeze of lemon or cucumber and mint to make it a refreshing and detoxifying treat!

Can I Follow the Program If I'm a Vegetarian?

There is no argument that certain people can flourish on vegetarian and vegan diets. I'm not one of them, but you might be. While I have found that most people with autoimmune conditions do need some animal protein to heal, it may be possible to reverse your condition without it. The trick is to make sure you are getting enough complete protein with all of the essential amino acids that you need to heal. This may be accomplished by using a high-quality, hypoallergenic protein powder. It's equally important to make sure you're getting enough of the healing fats every day. Personally, I have only worked with one client who was able to completely reverse their autoimmune condition on a vegan/vegetarian diet, but I would be thrilled to hear about it if there are more of you out there! If you follow this program as a vegan/vegetarian and you completely reverse your condition, come share your story and tell us how you did it at www.thethyroidcure.com/veganhealing

What about Hashimoto's and Goitrogenic foods?

The cruciferous family of vegetables, also called brassicas, have been demonized for years as a cause of hypothyroidism. These foods are sometimes classified as goitrogens because over-consumption of these foods appears to block thyroid peroxidase (TPO), causing the thyroid to grow more thyroid tissue resulting in a goiter.

These foods contain sulfur-containing compounds called glucosinolates and when chewed are broken down (through hydrolysis) into biologically active, cancer-fighting antioxidants. Two of these compounds classified as goitrogenic are isothiocyanates and thiocyanates.

However, there is little evidence that it's the consumption of these otherwise healing compounds alone that cause the problem. It appears that they only interfere with TPO when there is a deficiency in iodine or selenium and other antioxidants.[6]

The truth is that foods from the brassica family are rich in antioxidants and eating them along with adequate iodine and selenium has been proven to reduce inflammation and reduce the risk of cancer—even thyroid cancer.[7] Consumption of isothiocyanates along with selenium has been shown to boost glutathione peroxidase[8] (a powerful antioxidant), which I'll talk about in Chapter 17: Restore Your Liver.

As long as you correct any nutritional deficiencies you may have, you should have no reason to worry about these foods affecting your thyroid. If you are taking thyroid hormone replacement, these foods will not interfere with the action of these hormones. Remember that cooking and steaming reduces the goitrogenic (along with some of the antioxidant) properties of these foods.

However, if you feel these foods exacerbate your symptoms then please listen to your body. After all you are the one who knows your body the best. Ideally, when your antibodies are gone and you begin to wean off your medication, you will no longer be deficient in selenium, iodine or zinc and you may eat abundantly from this family of foods!

Special Note If You Are Hyperthyroid

If you have hyperthyroid symptoms and you are worried about losing weight, make sure you are getting enough of the healing proteins and healing fats each day. Some of my hyperthyroid clients report feeling "grounded" by eating yams and sweet potatoes, which also helps to relieve symptoms and keep weight on.

Supplement for Thyroid Support

In addition to eating for your good genes, you'll want to make sure you're getting all the nutrients you need to heal. This can be accomplished by taking a high quality multivitamin that includes B vitamins, vitamin D3, healing fats, zinc, selenium digestive enzymes and probiotics.

Suggested Supplement Schedule (See my resources section in the back of the book for recommended brands.)

- High-quality multivitamin with minerals and vitamin B complex taken with meals
- Vitamin D3: 2,000–5,000 IU per day, based on lab results
- Omega-3 EPA/DHA: 3,000 mg per day in divided doses
- GLA Borage Oil: 3,000 mg per day in divided doses
- Selenium methionine: 200 mcg per day to start
- Zinc 30 mg per day
- N-acetyl-l-cysteine: 600 mg twice daily to increase glutathione production. Best if taken with 1,000 mg buffered vitamin C.
- Digestive enzymes with each meal
- Probiotics taken between meals with a light snack

You may also choose a hypoallergenic protein powder or medical food to add to smoothies. (See Resources section for recommendations.)

Why we need vitamins

Our food is no longer the nutrient-dense food that our grandparents and ancestors ate. Our soil is depleted due to modern farming practices, environmental toxins, and pesticide use. Our current food supply doesn't have the nutrients that we need to support our health leaving us to rely on supplementation for what we are missing. Ideally, we would have unadulterated foods grown from nutrient rich soils, and would not need supplements.

Studies have shown that most people have nutrient deficiencies. In my practice and personal life, I have used comprehensive nutritional testing. This testing shows specific vitamin deficiencies by analyzing serum and urine. I have yet to see a test come back that wasn't lacking several nutrients. In the case of autoimmune conditions, B vitamin and folate deficiencies along with essential amino acid deficiencies are common. If you have an autoimmune condition, you probably need additional support for detoxification and healing.

Just like the foods we eat, not all supplements are created the same, and some are actually detrimental to your health. I believe that it's important to supplement with a high quality multivitamin formula that will give your body the nutrients you need to support your healing and continued wellness. As I began my own healing process, I wanted quality supplements that would help me heal. However, I came to realize that this was difficult to find.

When I started Vibrant Way I looked closely at the supplement industry and became concerned by the lack of reliable assurances about the quality of the vitamins on the market or if they even contained what's on the label. For instance a Consumer Labs report once surveyed different brands of DHEA supplements on the market, and found disturbing variability in the actual doses compared to the amount on the label; one brand supplied only 10% of the stated amount.

Moreover, I was shocked by the addition of fillers, preservatives and colorings that do nothing to support wellness. What I found was an unnecessary amount of potentially harmful ingredients including additives such as sugar, aspartame, corn, soy, lactose; preservatives like palm oil and sodium benzoate, and a long list of food colorings. These ingredients do nothing to make your vitamins more effective, and actually aggravate autoimmune conditions and any chronic condition.

The one-a-day multi-vitamin you buy from the drug store or supermarket simply cannot contain optimal values of vital nutrients in one tablet. In order to create a nutrient dense vitamin complex that contains all of the ingredients I wanted for my family, my clients and myself, I found I needed 10 capsules in each pack. My *Women's Empowerment Formula* packs in the ingredients needed to support internal vibrancy. My raw ingredients cost over ten times more than what goes into the vitamins you find on the shelves in the supermarket.

The bottom line is that you get what you pay for. Cheap vitamins give you little more than expensive urine.

There is a way you can be assured that you're getting quality ingredients in your vitamins. Look for supplements that are made in a NSF certified, GMP registered facility. See http://www.nsf.org. NSF/GMP stands for "NSF International/Good Manufacturing Practices" and is an independent testing and certification body for the dietary supplement industry. They not only test to make sure you're getting the ingredients listed on the label but they audit facilities twice a year for every aspect of production including procedures, personnel, documentation and more. Surprisingly, less than 10% of supplement labs are NSF/GMP certified and registered.

Taking a high quality nutritional supplement each day is a habit worth acquiring in our increasingly toxic world.

Phase I Review:

Remove gluten, dairy, eggs, sugar, nightshades, grains, legumes, nuts and processed foods. Add green tea, fresh organic berries, tons of certified organic veggies, healthy fats and small amounts of lean organic fish, meat, or poultry, or hypoallergenic rice protein powder. Cook with anti-inflammatory herbs and spices: turmeric, cumin, fennel, parsley, cinnamon, cardamom, ginger, garlic, sea salt, etc. Supplement with a good multivitamin, selenium, and healing omega-3 and omega-6 fatty acids, or the Thyroid Emergency Repair Pack available at www.thethyroidcure.com.

I have included Phase I: *Eating for Your Good Genes* Shopping List and a few basic recipes in this section. For a complete 30-day meal plan and amazing Phase I recipes, please visit www.thyroidcure.com/phase1recipes. You can also check the resources section of this book for amazing paleo cookbooks!

Phase I: "Eating for Your Good Genes" Shopping List

Choose Healing, Organic, Low-Glycemic Fruits:

Apples
Blackberries
Cherries
Lemons
Peaches
Plums
Raspberries

Avocados
Blueberries
Coconuts
Nectarines
Pears
Pomegranates

Choose Healing, Organic Vegetables:

Artichokes
Asparagus
Broccoli
Cabbage
Celery
Collard greens
Fennel
Leeks
Rhubarb
Squash

Arugula
Bok choy
Brussels sprouts
Cauliflower
Chard
Cucumbers
Kale
Lettuce
Spinach
Watercress

Choose Healing Roots:

Beets
Celeriac
Onions
Turnips
Rutabagas
Sweet potatoes

Carrots
Jicama
Parsnips
Radishes
Shallots
Yams

Choose Organic, Healing Proteins:

Organic, lean meats, such as beef, lamb, and buffalo
Organic poultry: turkey, chicken, game hen, pheasant
Wild-caught fish: salmon or trout
Hypoallergenic rice protein powder or medical food

Choose Healing Fats:

Coconut oil   Ghee
Olive oil   Avocado
GLA—Borage oil
EPA/DHA—Omega-3 complex

Choose Healing Dairy Substitutes:

Coconut milk
Coconut yogurt or kefir

Choose Healing Herbs:

Basil   Bay leaves
Chamomile   Chives
Cilantro   Dill
Lavender   Lemongrass
Lemon balm   Marjoram
Mint   Oregano leaves
Parsley   Peppermint
Rosemary   Saffron
Sage   Spearmint
Tarragon   Thyme

Choose Healing Spices and Sweeteners:

Cinnamon   Cloves
Garlic   Ginger
Onion powder   Saffron
Sea salt   Shallots
Stevia   Turmeric
A small amount of organic honey*

Choose Healing Pantry Items:

Organic apple-cider vinegar
Coconut flour
Coconut flakes
Olives
Canned salmon

Choose Healing Fermented Foods:

Coconut kefir and yogurt
Fermented vegetables
Kimchi (without nightshades)
Kombucha
Sauerkraut

Choose Healing Drinks:

Water: at least 64 oz. of pure, filtered water each day
Organic green tea
Organic, diluted, unsweetened cranberry juice
Organic herbal tea
Teeccino coffee substitute
Dandy Blend

*This phase does not include added sugar, but a small amount of organic honey is acceptable in teas and salad dressings, as long as you are sure you don't react to it. Please keep it to no more than 1 teaspoon per day.

Exclude the Following

Excluded Protein:

Pork
Canned meats
Uncooked meats
Sushi
Cured or processed meats
(i.e. cold cuts, sausage, hot dogs)
Shellfish and crustaceans
Eggs*

*If you know you don't react to eggs, you may have them on Phase I.

Excluded Dairy:

All animal milk, including cow, goat, and sheep
Cheese
Yogurt and kefir

Cottage cheese
Butter
Ice cream

Excluded Grains:

All grains and products made from grains must be eliminated during this stage; the exception is organic brown rice if you know you don't react to it. So are all refined white flour products, such as macaroni and cheese, cookies, cakes, pizza dough, pasta, tortillas, pancake/waffle mixes, and cookies, as well as the carbs secretly lurking in the ingredients of many "low-carb" products. Read labels, and you'll be surprised how many foods, such as salad dressings and soups, have grains, particularly wheat, added. When dining out, make sure to ask your server if the soups, sauces, and dressings are gluten-free.

Excluded grains include:

Amaranth	Barley
Buckwheat	Bulgur
Corn	Farro
Kamut	Millet
Oats	Rye
Rice*	Sorghum
Spelt	Teff
Wheat	

Quinoa *(not technically a grain, but excluded in Phase I)*

If you know you don't react to rice, you may have it on Phase I.

Excluded Nuts and Seeds:

Walnuts	Almonds
Brazil nuts	Coffee
Cocoa	Hazelnuts
Pecans	Macadamias
Anise	Hemp
Canola	Caraway
Chia	Coriander
Cumin	Fennel seeds

Fenugreek	Mustard
Nutmeg	Poppy
Pumpkin	Sesame
Sunflower	

Excluded Grasses:

Wheatgrass	Barley grass
Oat grass	Alfalfa

Excluded Fruits:

Tropical fruit	Oranges and orange juice
Grapefruit	Strawberries
Grapes	Melons

Excluded Beans and Legumes:

Adzuki beans	Black beans
Black-eyed peas	Chickpeas
Fava beans	Lentils
Lima beans	Peanuts
Kidney beans	Soybeans

Excluded Nightshades:

Cayenne	Chili peppers
Eggplant	Goji berries
Ground cherries	Habaneros
Jalapenos	Paprika
Poblanos	Tomatillos
Potato—all forms (especially chips)	
Sweet peppers (green, red, yellow peppers)	
Tobacco	Tomatoes

Excluded Sweeteners:

Sugar in all forms—brown, white, or in the raw
Honey*

Sugar alcohols—xylitol
Artificial sweeteners: Equal®, Splenda®, Sweet'N Low®
Fructose, glucose, sucrose
High-fructose corn syrup
Maple syrup
Evaporated cane juice
Agave

*A small amount of organic honey is acceptable as long as you are sure you don't react to it.

Excluded Condiments and Dressings:

Regular table salt
Soy sauces, distilled vinegars, ketchup, mayonnaise, conventionally pickled (not fermented) foods
Bottled salad dressings
Ketchup
Relish
Mayonnaise
BBQ sauce
Teriyaki

If it comes in a bottle and contains salt, sugar, thickening agents, or any other potentially compromising additives, it's not part of a successful Phase I.

Excluded Drinks:

Alcohol
Caffeinated drinks—coffee, energy drinks
Concentrated fruit juices
Soft drinks

Excluded Fats:

Butter and butter substitutes
Margarine
Canola oil
Processed oils
Excess dietary fats, especially trans-fats

Miscellaneous:

ANYTHING YOU ALREADY KNOW THAT YOU REACT TO!

All over-the-counter drugs (allergy medications, Tylenol, Advil, etc.) unless prescribed by your doctor

Performance bars, drinks, gels, and protein shakes unless listed in the Resource section

Hold the Green Powder!

Green powders typically contain grasses, such as barley and wheatgrass, alfalfa, and other potentially allergic substances. I have found that many people with autoimmune conditions are especially sensitive to these powders. Also, many green powders contain multiple substances, which makes it impossible to pinpoint which substance triggers a reaction.

A Final Word on Artificial Sweeteners…

As you have learned, artificial sweeteners such as aspartame and NutraSweet® are not good for anyone, but are especially bad for people with autoimmune thyroid disease. These are highly toxic to the liver and contribute to inflammation. Splenda,® or sucralose (which is chlorinated sugar), can worsen iodine deficiency problems, which can worsen autoimmune thyroid problems. Please stay away from these terrible fake sweets!

A Typical Day

Upon rising, drink 1 cup of hot water with lemon. This helps to stimulate bile and aid in detoxification. Take thyroid medication. Eat within 90 minutes of waking up. Aim for a balance of 50 percent healing carbohydrates (low-glycemic fruits and non-starchy vegetables), 25 percent lean protein (fish, turkey, lean beef), and 25 percent healthy fats (olive oil, avocado, coconut oil) with each meal.

For a downloadable sample day and a complete 30-day meal plan with amazing Phase I recipes, please visit www.thyroidcure.com/phase1recipes or check the resources section of this book for recommended paleo cookbooks and websites!

Phase I Recipe Suggestions

Very Berry Green Smoothie

1 cup organic unsweetened coconut milk
1–2 scoops vanilla hypoallergenic protein powder or medical food
1 cup mixed blackberries, blueberries, and raspberries
1 cup chopped dandelion greens or spinach
1 tablespoon coconut oil
Stevia to sweeten if necessary
Place all ingredients in blender and blend until smooth.

Creamy Peachy Smoothie

1 cup unsweetened coconut water
1–2 scoops hypoallergenic vanilla protein powder or medical food
1 cup frozen peaches
1 tablespoon coconut oil
Stevia to sweeten if necessary
Place all ingredients in blender and blend until smooth.

Healing Bone Broth

4 quarts of filtered water
1 medium onion, chopped medium
3 carrots, chopped medium
3 celery stalks, chopped medium
2 bay leaves
3 garlic cloves, chopped finely
2–3 lbs. natural beef or chicken bones
2 tablespoons apple cider vinegar
Sea salt to taste
Stovetop:
Fill a large stockpot with all the ingredients, pour in water and bring to a boil. Cover and reduce heat to a simmer. Cook for a minimum of 8 hours and as long as 24 hours.

Pressure cooker:

I like to make all my soups and broths this way, because it saves so much time. Place ingredients in pressure cooker and cover with water. It's okay if the bones are frozen. Do not exceed the fill line. Lock the lid and place over high heat until the gauge reads high or 15 psi. Immediately decrease the temperature to the lowest possible setting to maintain high pressure. Cook for a minimum of 1 hour and up to 3 hours. Remove the pot from the heat and let the pressure release naturally. Let the broth cool, strain, and you've got a tasty, healing broth that can be drunk alone or used as a base for other soups.

Healing Vinaigrette

1 cup organic olive oil
1 cup organic apple cider vinegar
½ teaspoon organic honey*
¼ teaspoon sea salt

Whisk ingredients together in a small stainless steel bowl until emulsified and then flash freeze for 5–8 minutes. *Omit honey if you know you react to it.

Killer Kale Salad

6 cups chopped kale
2 large carrots, grated
1 cup red cabbage, finely sliced
¼ cup organic dried cranberries or cherries

Wash kale and strip the leaves off the stalks. Discard the stalks and chop the kale into bite-sized pieces. Toss in carrots and cabbage. Sprinkle with cranberries/cherries and serve with healing vinaigrette. (In Phase II, you can add goat feta and sprouted sunflower seeds.)

Coconut Salmon Chowder

1 pound lightly poached salmon filet—skin and bones removed
1 medium onion, finely chopped, or 1 ½ cups leeks, sliced
2 cups carrots, diced into small pieces
1 tablespoon of fresh dill, chopped

2 tablespoons olive or coconut oil
1 bay leaf
2 cups of chopped cauliflower florets
3 cups of chicken stock or organic chicken broth
1 can of organic unsweetened, full-fat coconut milk
Sea salt to taste
Fresh dill to garnish

In a large stockpot, add olive oil, onions/leeks, and carrots and sauté 5 minutes, or until tender. Add the chicken broth, coconut milk, cauliflower, bay leaf, and dill and bring to a simmer. Add poached salmon filets and simmer until filets break apart easily. Stir well to break apart the salmon and cook until tender.

To poach salmon: Sprinkle salmon fillets with a dash of sea salt. Place salmon fillets skin-side down in a sauté pan. Cover with 1 cup chicken or fish stock and bring to a simmer on medium heat. Cook 5 to 10 minutes, depending on the thickness of the fillet.

Phase II: Sensitivity Discovery

If you've been eating for your good genes for the last 30 to 90 days, you probably feel dramatically better. You may have noticed that many of your symptoms have improved, or even disappeared. Now you realize just how powerfully food impacts your health! If you're feeling great, you can begin to add certain foods back to your diet and track how you feel.

If you're still very symptomatic, please continue with Phase I until your symptoms improve or disappear. Remember, the goal is a complete reversal of symptoms and antibodies. You didn't catch an autoimmune condition overnight, and reversing it may take some time. Most people notice significant results in the first 30 to 90 days. If it's been that long and you still don't feel well, it's time to start looking for other possible triggers or "splinters" in your condition. You may need to do more to heal your GI, or to support your liver. You may have an infection that needs to be treated, or you may have high levels of heavy metals in your body that need to be removed before your health can flourish. It's helpful to revisit the

Chapter 9 workbook as well as your answers to your personal assessments in Chapter 10. While there is a lot you can do on your own, you may want to enlist the help of a functional medical practitioner who can help you uncover any core imbalance that's preventing you from healing.

How Long Does the Sensitivity Discovery Phase Last?

The sensitivity phase can last anywhere from 30 to 60 days, depending on how many foods you plan to reintroduce. I suggest you start with ONLY the foods on the reintroduction list and continue to avoid inflammatory foods.

In this phase, you will begin with reintroducing omega-3 enriched eggs, organic goat or sheep yogurt and kefir, organic cultured butter, organic brown or wild rice, quinoa, rice milk, and organic, sprouted nuts and seeds. I have chosen these foods because they seem to be "well tolerated" by many people. That simply means that some people can get away with eating these foods and not get sick again. For instance, I can eat eggs, sprouted nuts and seeds, and the occasional tiny bit of goat or sheep dairy and quinoa. These foods do not trigger an autoimmune response in my body. However, if I eat dairy and quinoa more than once a week I notice that I start to retain water and get puffy.

Please resist the urge to reintroduce multiple foods at once! The whole point of this discovery phase is to discover which of your favorite foods may be contributing to your symptoms and your autoimmune condition. Reintroducing multiple foods at once defeats the purpose of the program. If you have a reaction, you won't be able to determine which food you are reacting to and you will have to go back to Phase I for a couple of weeks and start over.

In order to be able to tell most clearly what contributes to your symptoms and what doesn't, it's best to add one food group at a time and eat it every day for a minimum of four days. Use your diet journal to track the foods you eat and your symptoms. If you have a reaction to a food, it's best to stop eating it and then wait until the reaction clears and you're feeling good before reintroducing another food. Otherwise, it may not be clear if you're reacting to the new food or still hung over from the last one.

It's time to get out your healing journal or download some pages at www.thethyroidcure.com/journal. When you add a food or food group back, be mindful of how you feel—and this includes your emotions and state of mind. Keep track of your energy levels, your moods, and your digestion.

Watch for symptoms such as:

- Brain fog
- Headache
- Flushing
- Gas and bloating
- Constipation
- Diarrhea
- Congestion—clearing your throat or sniffles
- Sinus pressure or pain
- Rashes or breakouts
- Fatigue
- Insomnia
- Irritability
- Moodiness
- Increased pulse

Since you'll be reintroducing foods one at a time, you will have the opportunity to really observe how that particular food makes you feel. Any reaction is a clue that the food is troublesome for you.

To minimize your symptoms and maximize the health benefits of a vibrant, natural diet for the long haul, you will continue to avoid some of the most autoimmune aggravating foods, such as sugar, all processed and junk foods, GLUTEN, grains (except organic wild or brown rice and quinoa), corn, nightshades, legumes and grasses.

Will You Ever be Able to Have Regular Bread Again?

Good question. I don't know. There may be people out there who completely heal their GI tracts and are able to have gluten every once in a while without it triggering a full-blown immune response. Who knows? There aren't many, but there might be a few, and you might be one of them. The bigger question is: why would you want to take a chance? Gluten is such a big trigger for autoimmune conditions that I recommend eliminating it for life. Believe it or not, you can live a very long and happy life without gluten. Most people who cheat and eat gluten after healing from an autoimmune condition regret it, because their symptoms and antibodies return. If you plan on staying healthy, I suggest you leave gluten behind.

A Word About Beans

Let me start by saying that beans used to be one of my favorite foods in the world. I love the taste of beans, but they don't love me (and they seem to feel this way about many people). I have had to completely eliminate all legumes to stay healthy. You may have a different experience. You can experiment with reintroducing legumes, but watch closely for symptoms such as gas, bloating, fluid retention, inflammation, and weight gain. In my experience, there are some legumes that appear to be less problematic than others, such as peas and chickpeas (hummus), but that doesn't mean I recommend them. You will have to find out for yourself how they make you feel. Remember, this is about you discovering what works for your unique physiology.

What About Nightshades?

Tomatoes, potatoes, peppers and eggplant—yum! Who doesn't love French fries with ketchup and salsa on everything? I know I used to, but I had to give all them up for better health. You will have to see how you feel with reintroducing these foods. If you notice brain fog, "spaciness," GI disturbances, rashes, or sore joints, you've got a problem. In my experience, some people can add these foods back very occasionally, and only after they have healed their GI tract.

Corn

Corn comes in many forms: corn chips, corn on the cob, popcorn, canned or frozen corn, corn syrup, cornstarch, corn flour, and high-fructose corn syrup. If you have a sensitivity to corn, you will know it—because you will feel better without it. As you read in the Splinters section, corn is problematic for many people with autoimmune conditions, and it's mostly genetically modified these days, too. It's the same as with nightshades: if you notice GI disturbances, headaches, rashes, or sore joints, stay away from this food for life!

Soy

Soy is another food that people are often allergic or sensitive to because of its high lectin content. Sensitivity can trigger digestive problems and inflammation. Also, most of the soy available in the U.S. is genetically modified. Some people are able to reintroduce fermented, non-GMO soy products, such as tempeh and miso. You will have to see for yourself how you feel with the reintroduction of soy. If you do decide to bring it back in, make sure you choose organic, fermented soy products such as tempeh and miso.

Sugar and Alcohol

People often ask me when it's safe to drink alcohol or have their favorite dessert. Let me start by saying that there isn't a healing diet on the planet that includes sugar or alcohol. Still, for many people it's just not realistic to stay away from these substances for life. My suggestion is that you wait until you are completely symptom-free and your GI is healed before imbibing. These substances are inflammatory, and will slow—perhaps even halt—your healing process. Once you feel better, you can experiment with how you feel adding them back. After a 30- to 90-day break, your cravings will be totally gone, and you might be surprised to find that if you do try reintroducing them, they don't make you feel as good you remember. Start with small amounts of organic dark chocolate. Wine and spirits can be tricky because the vast majority of them contain so many contaminants. I suggest going with organic, biodynamic wines and grain-free spirits, as they tend to be tolerated better by most people.

In addition to the healing foods you've been eating in Phase I, here is the list of foods to reintroduce:

Protein:
- Omega-3 enriched eggs

Carbohydrates:
- Organic brown or wild rice
- Organic quinoa

Dairy:
- Goat or sheep yogurt and kefir
- Organic cultured butter

Dairy Substitutes:
- Organic rice milk

Soaked and Sprouted Nuts and Seeds

Properly prepared nuts, nut butters, and seeds are good sources of both protein and fat. If you don't have time to soak and sprout them, I have included a list of companies that sprout and package them for you. Go Raw and Lydia's Organics are both great brands. Better Than Roasted also has a line of soaked organic nuts and seeds and butters made from those nuts and seeds. What you can't find in local stores can be ordered via the Internet. Check the Resources section for a list of companies that sell properly prepared nuts and seeds.

- Almonds
- Walnuts
- Pumpkin seeds
- Sunflower seeds

Why Soak Nuts and Seeds?

Nut and seeds are packed with nutrition, but come with natural defenses that need to be neutralized so your body doesn't have to fight for that nutrition! Nuts contain phytic acid, lectins, and enzyme inhibitors that help the plant fulfill its life cycle. Nuts are designed to breed more nuts, not just become food. These chemicals protect the nut from insects and allow the nut to pass through the digestive system of an animal in order to be transported, deposited, and fertilized, which also keeps the nut from germinating until water is available. These same substances interfere with your body's ability to easily digest and assimilate these otherwise highly nutritious tidbits. Your body has to work overtime to digest nuts and seeds as they are. The enzyme inhibitors in nuts can deplete the enzyme stores in your body, and thus defeat some of the nutritious purpose of nuts in your diet.

How to Neutralize Enzyme Inhibitors

Fortunately there are ways to neutralize the enzyme inhibitors in nuts and seeds. One method is soaking them in salt water and then dehydrating them. The other technique is roasting them. Soaking has the advantage of also reducing phytic acid and retaining valuable enzymes that are destroyed by roasting. Soaking also enhances the availability of certain vitamins, unlocking the life force energy of the nut or seed as it begins to germinate.

Still, if you face limited choices, a roasted nut is better than a raw one. Beware of roasted nuts that are coated with excessive salt, sugar, or flavorings that can turn a nutritious food into another form of junk food (and avoid nuts coated with sugar or coatings that could contain grains or dairy, as you detox and discover what your system can handle). Nuts are best in moderation to begin with, and even more so if they haven't been prepared ideally.

The good news is that properly soaked and dehydrated nuts and seeds are delicious and satisfying. The basic technique is to soak them in salt water, using a couple of teaspoons of salt for each pound of nuts, in enough water to cover them. Use clean, filtered water, as the nuts will soak it up. Almonds and walnuts should be soaked for at least 8 hours, and some people soak them for 24 hours. Sunflower seeds and pumpkins seeds may require as few as 2 hours, although research seems to indicate that more is better.

It's very important to thoroughly dry them after soaking, or they may be vulnerable to mold. You should drain them in a colander and then spread them out (not touching each other) on a stainless cooking sheet and dry in the oven at 120 degrees or the lowest setting. Some people leave their oven doors slightly open if their oven settings don't allow such low temperatures. The best solution is to use a food dehydrator instead. Some models are very economical to buy and cheaper to run than your oven, which then remains free for other uses. Dry the nuts until they are crunchy and crisp. It's okay to add a modest quantity of salt or seasonings while drying. You may also find that you have to make extra because your friends and family can't resist the yummy treats you've created!

Seeds Used as Spices—You Don't Have to Soak These!

Anise Caraway
Coriander Cumin
Fennel seeds Fenugreek
Mustard Nutmeg

Phase II Recipes

Here are some basic Phase II recipe suggestions. You can find more delicious recipes by visiting my Web site: www.thethyroidcure.com/phase2recipes

The Power of Green Salad

4 cups chopped spinach
3 cups chopped green chard
1 avocado
4 cups baby greens or mache
2 cups steamed broccoli
2 cups steamed asparagus, cut into bite sized pieces
½ cup organic dried cranberries
¼ cup goat feta cheese
¼ cup soaked and sprouted sunflower seeds

Lightly steam broccoli and asparagus (about 6 minutes). Remove and put in freezer to cool (about 5 minutes). Mix spinach, chard, and baby greens together. Add cooled steamed veggies, avocado, and goat feta and sprinkle with sunflower seeds and cranberries. Serve with healing vinaigrette.

Classic Turkey Burgers

1 pound lean organic ground turkey breast
1 medium onion, chopped finely
1 omega-3-enriched egg
2 garlic cloves, minced
½ teaspoon sea salt
1 teaspoon garlic powder
Organic, extra-virgin olive oil

Using your hands, mix turkey with egg, onions, garlic, garlic powder, and salt. Divide into fourths and shape into patties. Heat grill or broiler to medium high. Grilling time is roughly 6 minutes on each side. You can also use a stovetop skillet or grilling pan. Use ghee if cooking on the stovetop so the burgers don't stick. Cook at medium-high heat for about 5 minutes on each side or until cooked through.

Phase III: Vibrant for Life!

The *Vibrant for Life* phase is the custom mind-body program you create for yourself after following the guidelines in this book. Once you feel well, you'll want to stay well. Most people find that they love the healthy changes they've made and want to stick with them for life.

If you've followed the *Sensitivity Discovery Program*, you have very likely found the nutritional triggers in your diet. By now, you know what foods are contributing to your symptoms. This is the most empowered place to be, in my opinion. From this point forward, you will no longer be mystified by what foods are causing uncomfortable symptoms.

At 3–6 months into the program, or after your symptoms have resolved, you'll want to retest your antibodies, thyroid hormones, and any other markers that were suboptimal before you started the program. It's very likely that if you feel good, your labs will have improved too. In this phase, you will work with your practitioner to adjust your thyroid hormone dose if necessary.

Many people are able to follow their new lifestyle using the 80/20 rule, which means sticking to a healthy program for 80 percent of the time. You will have to find the ratio that works best for you.

A Word on Allergy Testing

People often ask me how I feel about food allergy testing. Personally, I find an elimination diet like my *Sensitivity Discovery Program* to be the most empowering way to find out if you react to a particular food. As you learned in Chapter 9 there is a big difference between food allergies (also called hypersensitivities), and food sensitivities and intolerances. While food *allergy* testing can find out if you have a true food allergy, food *sensitivity* and food *intolerance* testing can be somewhat unreliable and in my experience, rarely finds every food you are sensitive to as accurately as a food elimination program can.

I've also seen some people rely on test results instead of paying attention to how their body feels. Let me share Kathy's story with you. At 30 years old, she was 25 pounds overweight and diagnosed with Hashimoto's. She had all the classic Hashimoto's symptoms; hair loss, chronic yeast and bladder infections, felt cold all the time, the outer thirds of her eyebrows were gone and she couldn't lose a pound despite taking 200 mcg of Synthroid every day. She was under the care of a medical doctor, an acupuncturist, a chiropractor and a psychologist. On her first appointment, she brought in a shopping bag full of supplements and herbal products. She heard about me from a clerk at our local health food store and wondered if I could help.

She came from an Italian family and her health history revealed that her daily diet included a ton of gluten and nightshade vegetables. When I began to explain the connection between gluten sensitivity, gluten allergy and Hashimoto's, she pulled some papers from a folder and waved them wildly in the air. "I'm not allergic to gluten! Look! It says so right here!" I looked at her food allergy tests and sure enough, she had no antibodies to wheat or the gliadin protein.

I explained the difference between food allergies and sensitivities and how a person may not have an immune response towards a particular food, but could still be sensitive to it. I suggested that she try Phase I of the *Sensitivity Discovery Program* to find out if something she was eating aggravated her Hashimoto's and added to her unwanted weight. Thankfully, she agreed to follow the program. Two weeks later on her follow-up appointment, she had lost 13 pounds and felt amazing. She was literally in shock, and exclaimed that she had tried many different nutrition programs but none had produced these kinds of results. Of course I was thrilled and suggested that she remain on the program until her antibodies completely disappeared.

After 6 months on the program, she had lost all the weight and her antibodies were gone. Another success story!

Two years later, I saw her in the grocery store. She had regained all of the weight plus more, and her Hashimoto's was back with a vengeance. I worried that we had missed a big splinter. When I asked what happened, she said, "Well my doctors don't think I'm allergic to gluten and since I don't test positive, I went back to my old diet." I was dumbfounded! I said, "But you felt so much better, and you lost all the weight and the antibodies by removing gluten, diary and nightshades!" "Yeah, I know but I just can't believe that I'm allergic to those foods. My allergy tests say no allergies so it must be genetic with me."

I almost fell over in disbelief. She had healed her condition by changing her diet but because the testing didn't back it up, she couldn't believe it (or perhaps didn't want to believe it).

Food allergy testing has its place and can help you identify if you have a true food allergy, for instance to wheat, dairy, nuts, soy, shellfish or eggs etc., but it cannot tell you whether you have a food intolerance or sensitivity. Experts still don't agree on whether food sensitivity/intolerance testing is accurate enough to pick up more subtle reactions to foods.

Still, I understand why many practitioners utilize food sensitivity testing. After all, most people aren't willing to give-up their favorite foods for an elimination program, and the testing can seem like a short-cut around that problem.

If you follow the *Sensitivity Discovery Program* but still have trouble identifying all of your food splinters, it may be a good idea to work with a practitioner who can help you find out if you have a true food allergy. If he or she feels that testing for food sensitivities will help, there's no harm in giving it a try.

The bottom line is this: Food allergy/sensitivity testing can be helpful in certain situations, but it should never replace your body's innate wisdom.

When You May Need a Health Practitioner

Improving your nutrition is not rocket science, but some people feel overwhelmed by making the major lifestyle changes I suggest in this book. If you feel overwhelmed or struggle with how to integrate healing foods into your diet, you may want to enlist the support of an integrative or functional nutritionist. These practitioners can help you with customizing your program, show you how to shop for healing foods, provide you with recipes and planning tools, and help keep you accountable.

There may be some of you who still don't feel well after making the recommended healthy changes outlined in this chapter. You may need extra support from a qualified health practitioner who can help you uncover any "splinters" that have not resolved by improving your nutrition. You may need extra support to heal your GI tract, or you may have a heavy metal such as mercury or an infection triggering your condition. I give more information on the functional tests available to uncover these "splinters" in the following chapters.

You may also want to consider nutritional testing to get a comprehensive view of your overall health. My favorite test right now is the ***NutrEval* Plasma by Genova Diagnostics.** This blood-and-urine combo test evaluates your need for antioxidants, B vitamins, amino acids, essential fatty acids, and minerals. You'll also find out if you have imbalances in the GI tract or problems with detoxification. The most exciting aspect of this test is if you have insurance (except some, including Aetna, Kaiser, Humana, Principal, and Tufts) the $1,500 test price is vastly reduced. With the new "Pay Assured" program, you pay a fraction of the full price up front and Genova bills your insurance for the rest. Even if your insurance doesn't cover the test, you never pay another dime.

You can learn more about this test by visiting my Web site: www.thethyroidcure.com or at www.gdx.net.

CHAPTER 15

Reduce Stress

*"When we are no longer able to change a situation,
we are challenged to change ourselves."*
— Viktor E. Frankl

These days there seems to be no end to the stress in our lives. As I've discussed throughout this book, chronic stress makes us sick. While stress is unavoidable and a natural consequence of living, some of us have experienced so much stress that we feel powerless over our circumstances. This feeling of powerlessness can intensify when we get sick, and our lives may feel out of control.

I have learned that we have a lot more control over our lives and our stress that we think. Regardless of our circumstances, we can choose how we respond to life. Even if things seem out of control, we can cultivate an inner knowing and calm. We can learn more about our unique nature, or Mind-Body type, and make choices that reduce chaos and restore balance in our lives. The more self-aware we become, the better we can take care of ourselves.

The trick to reducing stress is to consciously choose to do something — *anything*—about it.

When you restore your body's core systems by *Eating for Your Good Genes*, you take the first step by replacing junk foods and stimulants with nutrient rich foods. When you follow the *Sensitivity Discovery Program*, you take the process one step further by uncovering any food sensitivities.

Now let's discuss some of the other ways you can reduce the stress in your life.

Support Your Adrenals

Have you ever witnessed the meltdown of an overtired child? It starts out as hyperactivity and then progresses to erratic behavior and inattentiveness. She may become clingy, and if her needs aren't met, she'll start whining, and then inconsolably crying. If this goes on for long enough, she'll eventually cry herself to sleep. Now imagine handing this exhausted child a donut and a triple espresso and telling her to get a grip and get back to work! Then, when she's so totally cracked out on sugar and caffeine that she can't sleep at all, imagine handing her a double Martini or a sleeping pill to knock her out so that she can get up and do it all over again in 4 to 6 hours! "No way!" You'd protest, "That's child abuse!"

Sadly, that's what many of us do to ourselves on a daily basis, and then we wonder why we're sick. We shouldn't be mystified by the epidemics of stress-related chronic illness in Western society. We live on borrowed energy, never pay it back with rest, and wind up depleted and sick.

I call adrenal fatigue a "splinter" because I feel that it's a major underlying trigger in *all* chronic illness. Adrenal fatigue is similar to an autoimmune condition because it is the symptom and consequence of a life out of balance.

Adrenal Exhaustion, Adrenal Fatigue and Adrenal Burnout are All Names for the Same Condition: Too Much Stress in All its Forms!

Most Western medical doctors do not recognize adrenal fatigue or adrenal exhaustion. They believe that either your adrenals work fine, or they don't work at all. Unless you have a diagnosis of Cushing's or Addison's disease, they will chalk up your symptoms to depression, anxiety or some other ill-defined mechanism and then prescribe a pharmaceutical drug to mask your symptoms. This is like closing the windows and turning up the radio when your car starts smoking and making a banging sound.

Practitioners who work with patients who have adrenal fatigue will tell you it's a real condition all right. They will also tell you that it's difficult to correct, but not because the body can't heal, but because the sick, toxic, stressed out and exhausted person can't or won't *slow down for long enough and make the necessary lifestyle changes to heal.* Plus, as you read in Chapter 9: Uncover the "Splinters" in Your Autoimmunity, there are so many potential triggers to consider!

Adrenal Fatigue is Not:

- It's not "just being tired." Many times a person is told to simply "rest." While that may help, it doesn't correct the underlying functional imbalances. What is making that person tired and stressed-out? A toxin? An infection? A crazy lifestyle? All of the above? Because each of us is unique, we each have different issues; it can be challenging to find all the causes of stress.

- It's not a hormone deficiency. A person with adrenal fatigue may be deficient in adrenal hormones, but it's important to correct why that person is deficient, instead of just giving them more adrenal hormones. Imagine your car has an oil leak and uses up a quart of oil per day. Do you just add a quart of oil everyday and keep driving, or do you add the quart of oil and then try to find the leak? If you don't fix the leak, there will come a time when adding oil won't help anymore.

- It's not an herbal deficiency. There are wonderful herbs that can support your adrenals and help you feel more comfortable while you heal, but if you don't take out the splinters and reduce your stress, you're not correcting the core issue.

This chapter is about slowing down and learning to nurture your body and soul. Have the same compassion for yourself as you would have for the tired little child who needs rest. Believe me, there is no supplement, herbal formula or hormone available that will make you immune to running yourself into the ground. I encourage you to develop this kind of self-love because your body is crying out for help.

Take this time to listen. Take this time to heal.

A Word on Adrenal Testing...

There are tests available that assess adrenal function, some may be paid for by your insurance, others may not. There are blood tests that measure the adrenal hormone DHEA, and saliva tests that measure your cortisol levels over a 24-hour period. DHEA-sulfate is included in the baseline lab test suggestions in Chapter 12. Most insurance companies will pay for this test.

Saliva testing for adrenal function measures your diurnal (24-hour) cortisol levels. Cortisol is integral to your body's stress response. Some saliva tests include other hormones such as DHEA, testosterone, progesterone, estradiol and estriol. This testing may or may not be covered by your insurance. Many integrative and functional practitioners feel that cortisol is the only one of these hormones that can be measured accurately in the saliva. Only you and your practitioner can determine which testing is right for you.

I feel there is a place for cortisol saliva testing, as it can help you and your practitioner assess your stage of adrenal fatigue and where you need the most support. **If you scored high on the *Adrenal Stress Assessment*,** this test may be worthwhile, and will help your practitioner design a healing program for you.

If you did not score high on the *Adrenal Stress Assessment*, you may not really need an adrenal function test.

Before considering adrenal saliva testing, ask yourself the following questions:

- Do I really need a test to tell me that I'm too stressed out?
- If a medical test confirms that I am too stressed out, will I be **more** willing to make the lifestyle changes necessary to heal?

If you answered yes to both of the above questions, then go ahead and spend your money on an adrenal function test!

Now let's say the test comes back and it shows that your adrenals are "ok," but you know deep down inside that you're too stressed. What then?

The whole point of an adrenal stress profile is to find out if your adrenals are stressed, and to determine your stage of adrenal fatigue. The results can help your practitioner prescribe the right support, as well as inspire you to make the necessary lifestyle changes to heal.

What You can Do on Your Own to Heal Your Adrenals

- Try *Eating for Your Good Genes!* Replace junk foods and stimulants with nutrient rich foods. Eat healing proteins and healing fats with every meal.
- Follow the *Sensitivity Discovery Program* to uncover food sensitivities.
- Don't skip meals—Try to eat within 90 minutes of waking.

- Take a good multivitamin and B complex supplement as outlined in Chapter 14.
- Slow down and get some rest.
- Try adaptogenic herbs. An adaptogen is a compound that increases one's ability to adapt to environmental factors, including physical and emotional stress.
- Cut unnecessary stress from your life!

Herbs for Adrenal Support

There are herbal formulas that have been used for centuries to help support the body during times of stress.

- **Ashwaganda**—This is a powerful herb from the Ayurvedic tradition that is particularly helpful with sleep problems. It has been shown to improve DHEA-S and testosterone levels. It is available in tablet, liquid and capsule form. Standard dose is 500 mg per day or as directed by your healthcare provider. **A note of caution is in order:** Ashwaganda is a nightshade and some people are sensitive to it. If you take it and you notice symptoms such as sore joints, rash etc., discontinue use.
- **Rhodiola**—This herb also has a long tradition of use for the management of fatigue, reducing mild depression, and facilitating mental clarity. Look for formulas that contain 2-3% rosavin and 0.8-1% salidroside. Standard beginning dose is 100 mg per day and can be increased by 100 mg per week up to 400 mg.
- **Siberian ginseng *(Eleutherococcus senticosus)*** —This herb is famous in traditional Chinese medicine for increasing vitality and longevity. Western herbalists favor it to treat stress, fatigue and exhaustion, and to restore immune function. This herb is available as liquid extracts, solid extracts, powders, capsules and tablets; and as dried or cut root for tea. Because it is energizing, it's better to take earlier in the day so it doesn't interfere with sleep. Look for formulas standardized to contain 0.8% eleutheroside E & B. Standard dose is 100 to 500 mg per day. **Warning**: Siberian ginseng may boost the immune system and may interact with immunosuppressive drugs commonly prescribed

for autoimmune conditions. Please consult your healthcare provider before taking this herb.

Note: It's important to remember that just because something is natural, doesn't necessarily mean it's safe or right for you. Herbs can be powerful medicines and have side effects and interactions with pharmaceutical drugs. If you take medication, please talk to your health care provider before self-prescribing these herbs. At the very least, do your own research on the side effects and interactions.

When You May Need a Practitioner

The suggestions in this book are designed to help you reduce stress and bring the core systems of your body into balance. **If you scored high on the** *Adrenal Stress Assessment,* or if you have chronic fatigue syndrome (CFS) or a more serious autoimmune condition, you will very likely need to support your adrenals in order to heal. You may benefit from working directly with a qualified functional or integrative practitioner in addition to following the steps outlined in this chapter. A practitioner can help you uncover the splinters underlying your adrenal fatigue and help you feel better while you heal.

If you don't already have a functional or integrative medical doctor, you can find one by visiting the Institute for Functional Medicine's website at www.functionalmedicine.org. Click on the tab "Functional Medicine Resources" and choose "Find a Functional Medicine Practitioner" to find someone in your area. We have also compiled a list of practitioners on *The Thyroid Cure* Web site at www.thethyroidcure.com/practitioners.

If you find a practitioner in your area, be sure to ask if they have experience with advanced functional medical testing and adrenal fatigue. Many chiropractors, doctors of oriental medicine and certified nutritionists are also skilled in evaluating and uncovering the roots of adrenal fatigue.

Functional Testing for Adrenal Stress

I feel it's best to consult with an integrative or functional practitioner to obtain an adrenal saliva test because self-diagnosing can be complicated and the results are not always easy to interpret. Working with a qualified practitioner can save you time and money by removing the guesswork and thus avoiding unneeded treatments or supplements.

There are several labs that offer saliva testing for adrenal hormones. Here are two tests that I have used with my clients:

- **Adrenal Stress Profile** by Metametrix and Genova (two labs that have recently merged)
- **Diurnal Cortisol (Saliva) - 4x** ZRT Laboratory

You can learn more about these tests by visiting the laboratory websites listed in the Resources section or www.thethyroidcure.com/adrenaltesting

Just Breathe!

Breathing is something we often take for granted. Believe it or not, just remembering how to breathe is one of the quickest and easiest ways to reduce stress. By breathing properly, you can shut down your body's fight or flight response and activate your relaxation response. This might sound funny, but the truth is that many of us have forgotten how we're supposed to breathe.

Have you ever watched a baby breathe? You'll notice that the baby's torso rises and falls with each breath. When you take a closer look, you notice that it's not the baby's chest that rises and falls, it's actually her diaphragm, the muscle between the chest and abdominal cavity.

Now take a few moments to focus on your own breathing. If you're like most people, you may notice that your shoulders rise up slightly toward your ears and that your chest expands as you inhale, and contracts as you exhale. You may discover that your belly doesn't move at all, or that you're holding your stomach in. Perhaps you realize that you're holding your breath. This is called chest breathing. This is not your natural state of breathing; it is a conditioned response to stress. We get in the habit of breathing this way and this habit alone can keep our fight or flight response activated.

My first introduction to abdominal or diaphragmatic breathing was in Dr. Joan Borysenko's classic book on mind-body awareness entitled, *Minding the Body, Mending the Mind*. In her book, Dr. Borysenko explains how important it is to learn how to breathe correctly to initiate the relaxation response.

Abdominal/belly breathing is nothing new. In fact, many healing traditions teach that the key to calming the mind is through the breath.

The breath is the one body function that happens automatically, but that we can also consciously control. When you begin to pay attention to your breath, you discover that your breath and your mind are deeply linked.

Remembering How to Breathe:

Get into a comfortable position, sit upright in a chair or lay flat on your back. Make sure your clothes are comfortable and not restricting your belly. Try to keep your back as straight as possible. If you're sitting, make sure your shoulders are down and relaxed.

Relax your jaw.

Began by breathing in slowly and evenly through your nostrils. You might want to place your fingertips lightly on your abdomen. Take a deep breath in through your nostrils, and then release it through your mouth, making the sound "Ahh." Gently contract your abdomen to expel the last bit of stale air. You will naturally inhale a full belly breath

Feel your abdomen rise and fall with each breath. If you're having trouble, imagine that you're blowing up your belly like a balloon with each inhalation.

Dr. Borysenko suggests that you only need to breathe out deeply once or twice per session for it to be effective.

Keep practicing these slow deep breaths for a few minutes.

Don't strain or try to force air into your lungs, just breathe easily and rhythmically.

Just two or three minutes of this type of breathing activates the relaxation response, lowers your blood pressure and heart rate, and increases the production of endorphins -your body's natural painkillers.[1] Try to practice this breathing exercise two or three times daily if you can. It's absolutely free and you can do it anywhere.

Restorative Sleep

Just like breathing, sleeping is something we often take for granted. If you suffer from insomnia or other sleep disturbances, you're not alone. According to the 2011 *Sleep in America*® poll, 43% of Americans say they rarely or never get a good night's sleep on weeknights. More than half (60%) say that they experience a sleep problem every night or almost every night (i.e., snoring, waking in the night, waking up too early, or feeling unrefreshed when they get up in the morning), and about two-thirds (63%) of Americans say they don't get enough sleep during the week. [2]

Chronic stress, blood sugar imbalances, fluctuations in hormones including thyroid hormones, the use of caffeine, sugar, alcohol and other stimulants; along with "staying connected" all the time, can set us up for a cascade of metabolic imbalances. Sleep disturbance is just one of the side effects.

Unfortunately, our modern lifestyles leave very little room for normal sleeping patterns. Many of us have organized our lives so that it's impossible to get a good night's rest. We each have different sleep requirements, but generally we need between 7 ½ and 9 ½ hours per night.[3] Some people may require more sleep while healing, especially if they have adrenal fatigue.

Of all of the lifestyle changes I ask you to make in this book, sleep may be one of the most difficult, yet also one of the most important. You might be thinking,

"Yeah right, do you know how much I have to do?" Believe me, I totally understand. This is one of those areas where you're going to have to get serious. An autoimmune condition is literally your body saying "No!" You're going to have to listen to your body if you want to get well.

There are hundreds of scholarly articles on the relationship between disturbed sleep and autoimmune conditions.[4] One very recent study showed that disturbed circadian rhythm affects a protein that controls proinflammatory Th17 cells.[5] These are cells that live in the GI tract and help fight fungal and bacterial infection in mucosal tissues but have a tendency to get out of control under certain conditions and attack healthy tissue.[6]

Other new research shows that sleeping actually helps flush toxins out of your brain![7] Using mice, scientists discovered that the space between brain cells increases during sleep, which allows the glymphatic (yes with a G) system to flush out toxins from the brain. The leader of the study, Maiken Nedergaard, M.D., D.M.Sc, co-director of the Center for Translational Neuromedicine at the University of Rochester Medical Center in New York explained, "Sleep changes the cellular structure of the brain. It appears to be a completely different state. We need sleep. It cleans up the brain."

Restoring your sleep cycle isn't always easy and it may not happen overnight, but resolve to get more sleep and I guarantee that you will see an improvement in your health.

Here are a few tips to get you started:

- **Avoid caffeine:** If you drink coffee or other caffeinated beverages, make sure you don't drink them after 3 PM. It's even better if you avoid caffeine altogether.

- **Limit alcohol:** You may feel that alcohol helps you sleep, but it can actually do the opposite. Too much alcohol disrupts REM sleep and affects your hormones and neurotransmitters.[8] It can cause unstable blood sugar and you're likely to wake up between 2 and 3 AM with a blood sugar crash.[9] Alcohol is also a diuretic so you'll lose more sleep if you have to get up to pee several times during the night.

- **Plan your meals:** Try to finish eating at least 2 or 3 hours before bedtime. Don't eat a heavy meal or drink too many fluids. Heavy meals can cause indigestion, restless sleep and even nightmares. Again, if you drink excess fluids before bed, you might find yourself getting up to pee all night long.

- **Avoid sedatives:** Try to avoid sedative medications. Sleeping pills might knock you out cold, but these chemicals can disturb your natural brain chemistry and often lead to a dependency.

- **Avoid OTC medications:** Avoid over-the-counter medications such as cold, allergy, cough and pain medications. Many of these contain substances such as caffeine, pseudoephedrine, alcohol and other substances that can disturb your brain chemistry.

- **Wind down:** Try to wind down before bedtime. It can help to dim the lights around your home after 8 PM. Bright light actually tricks your brain into thinking that it's daytime, which disrupts your circadian rhythm or "body clock."

- **Update your technology:** Computers screens, smartphones and tablets emit light in the blue part of the spectrum. This doesn't cause any issues in the daytime, but at night, this blue light may limit your production of melatonin. Install free F.lux software on your computer.

There is also an app for jailbroken iPhones and iPads, and an Android version is in the works. F.lux works discreetly in the background, automatically adjusting the color temperature of your screen. It adapts your computer's display to the current time, *"warm at night and like sunlight during the day."* In effect it tries to match the light from your computer to the light in your natural environment.

- **Stick to a schedule:** Try to get to bed at the same time every night—even on the weekends—and wake up at the same time. This will help set your circadian rhythm.

- **Just do it!**: Move your body for at least 30 minutes per day. Your body was built to move. Vigorous exercise is best, but anything is better than nothing. Most people with autoimmune thyroid conditions can exercise. However, if you have adrenal fatigue, chronic fatigue or are very ill, please listen to your body and don't over do it!

- **Kill your television:** Ok, that's radical, but if you're accustomed to going to sleep in front of the television, I suggest you break the habit. For starters, take the television out of the bedroom; then gently wean yourself off late night television. Never watch the news or violent movies before bed. Believe it or not, these can activate your fight or flight response. Action movies are supposed to be exciting! Don't take my word for it, take note of your breathing and heart rate the next time you're watching a terrible news story or a scary movie.

- **Unplug:** Disconnect from your cell phone, computer, video game and iPad at a reasonable hour!

- **Make a cozy nest:** Create a peaceful environment in your bedroom. Keep the room quiet, or get used to earplugs or ambient sound recordings if you live where noise is inescapable. Make your room as dark as possible; even the glow from electronic gadgets like cell phones and alarm clocks can disrupt your sleep. Invest in a good mattress, and only use your bed for sleeping and making love. Keep the room at a comfortable temperature; not too cold, not too hot. Clean and simplify your environment for a restful sleep. It's difficult to sleep in a room that's cluttered or messy. Put a night light in your bathroom and avoid turning on the light if you get up for the restroom. For more great tips on creating a cozy bedroom, check out the National Sleep Foundation's website http://bedroom.sleepfoundation.org

- **Warm up and relax:** If you have a bathtub, take a bath before bed. Try an Epsom salt bath, which has magnesium that will help you to sleep better. I love to light a (non-toxic beeswax) candle, and slip into a bath with a few drops of essential oils such as lavender, or ylang ylang, neroli and clary sage.
- **Breathe:** If you worry and have anxious thoughts when you're trying to sleep, use the belly breathing outlined above. It takes practice but you'll be surprised at the results you can get in just a week.
- **Ask for help:** It's hard to change your sleep schedule when everyone else in the house is bustling around at night. One of my clients, a busy dental hygienist and mother of three, sat her husband and three children down and very calmly and deliberately asked them to help her to get enough sleep. She was surprised when everyone paid full attention. Now her children remind her, "Mommy, stop working! It's time for you to turn off the lights and go to bed so that you can get better!"

Supplement for Better Sleep

Finally, there are supplements that can help you sleep. Some people respond well to neurotransmitter precursors such as GABA, 5HTP and melatonin. It's beyond the scope of this book to enter into a discussion about whether these supplements might benefit you. Please consult with your integrative or functional medical practitioner before using these supplements.

Magnesium can help you sleep and just about anyone can use it. Here are two of my favorite sources:

- Natural Vitality®, Natural Calm - Two rounded teaspoons yields 235 mg of ionic magnesium citrate. Take as directed on the label.
- Pure Encapsulations® Magnesium (citrate), take as directed on the label.

Essential Oils for Better Sleep

- Lavender
- Vetiver
- Sandalwood
- Vetiver
- Roman Chamomile
- Marjoram

If You have Sleep Apnea

If you have sleep apnea (periods of breathlessness, often followed by brief gasping for air), it's a good idea to seek medical advice. While sleep apnea can be a big splinter in many chronic conditions, including autoimmunity, I have found it to be a symptom of other imbalances such as insulin resistance, metabolic syndrome and obesity.[10,11,12,13] There are exceptions, but losing weight is often the most effective treatment, and that beats having surgery.[14] Additionally, breathing exercises and surprisingly, playing the didgeridoo, can strengthen the muscles in the back of the throat that collapse to allow snoring and apnea.[15]

For more information on getting a good night's rest, check out the National Sleep Foundation's website: http://www.sleepfoundation.org.

Honoring Your Unique Mind-Body Type

"Today you are You, that is truer than true.
There is no one alive who is Youer than You." – Dr. Seuss

While most of us recognize the great stress that can accompany the death of a loved one, divorce, moving or financial struggles, we don't all experience these events in the same way or with the same intensity. What constitutes stress is not universal. In fact, one person's stress might be invigorating to another. To further complicate things, some of us were taught as kids to strive for things that we didn't want and that weren't natural for us. For instance, you might have been a naturally sensitive and creative child that needed more quiet time alone or in nature. If your parents didn't notice or honor that sensitivity, they might have pressured you into sports, academic goals and careers that ultimately didn't suit your personality. This kind of stress can ultimately wear you down.

Take Leslie, an attorney, who confessed that she had always wanted to be an artist. Her parents, who had grown up poor and uneducated, valued financial security and pressured her to go to law school. She finally graduated from law school and then endured 15 years in a law practice. Her firm asked to become a partner the same year she was diagnosed with lupus. "Every fiber of my body is revolting," she confessed. "I don't enjoy practicing law. I've never been cut out for this work. I've been sick to my stomach for over 15 years!"

I'm not suggesting that being an attorney will make you sick (or that her parents were to blame). For some people, it's a challenging and rewarding vocation. It just wasn't right for Leslie. While she had other "splinters" underlying her autoimmune condition, her career turned out to be a big factor.

Career is not the only area where you can be misfit. You might be fighting your own nature in other parts of your life. Geri came to me after "hitting the wall" with a lupus flare up. An escrow officer by day, she was a partying rock-n-roller on the weekends. She was always off to a different festival or show. "I'm totally burnt every Sunday night but somehow I get up on Monday and make it to work. My husband and friends all rock it. I guess they can just hang better than I can. I got a prescription for Adderall from my gynecologist, and I just take that so I can keep up with everyone." When I asked her if she was tired, she began to weep and said, "I've been tired my whole life."

Believe it or not, a "rock-n-roll" lifestyle doesn't trigger an autoimmune condition in everyone either. While there were other factors in her condition, Geri was often over stimulated and she pushed herself beyond what her constitution could handle. Her body was screaming for her to slow down and rest.

These are two dramatic examples but there are many subtle ways that we get out of sync with our nature. We may find ourselves attracted to people, places, foods and substances that don't support who we really are.

The trick is to listen to your heart and honor your unique nature. Find the place where you are balanced, calm, and centered. This is your natural state. If you have a hard time finding yourself at first, it's okay to start by letting go of the parts of your life that you know aren't nourishing and supporting you.

The bottom line is that we're all different. Learn to recognize your nature, your unique Mind–Body type, and then you can design a life that suits you better.

You might find that the life your body longs for is quite different than the one you have created.

If you realize you have been living "against the grain," slow down and pay attention to how your body feels in each moment. This is the practice of mindfulness, or simply "presence."

Mindfulness; Being Present in the Moment
"Being present makes you whole and empowers everything you do."
— Karl Baba

I got sick because I was unaware of my body's needs and ignored how my diet and lifestyle stressed me out. I got caught in a vicious cycle of worrying about the future, regretting the past and checking out of the present. My lack of self-awareness and self-love caused much of the suffering in my life—and in the lives of my loved ones.

I was forced to make a shift when my body finally said, "NO!" I became conscious (at least partially) of my how my own misguided thoughts and actions caused disharmony in my life. I made peace with my past, and began the journey of living more authentically. Mindful self-inquiry allowed me to discover, appreciate and even adore, my own unique nature. When I no longer had to cling to the image of who I "should" be, or who others wanted me to be, I was free to just be me—Michelle without the mask.

Healing from any chronic illness is complex. It demands deep passion and asks you to take responsibility for getting well. This response-ability is empowered by getting to know yourself, and then by honoring yourself enough to make essential positive lifestyle changes.

This shift to conscious awareness is a lifetime journey, but every step counts. I know because I'm still working on it, and things get better all the time. Mindfulness practice will help you become more in tune with who you are. Mindfulness simply means being present in the moment; it means "Being Here Now." If you think about it, the only real time is the present. The past is gone, and the future is just an idea.

Don't Worry, Be Happy!
In every life we have some trouble, when you worry you make it double don't worry, be happy… —Bob Marley

I think Bob was on to something. The University of Cincinnati did a study that discovered that 85% of what we worry about never happens. Researchers Wells and Matthews also noted that even when things actually do go wrong, we deal with the problem much better than we expected. Recognize that your resistance to life and your fear of getting hurt can be more painful than the inevitable losses and setbacks that we all face. Things often work out. Don't suffer in advance!

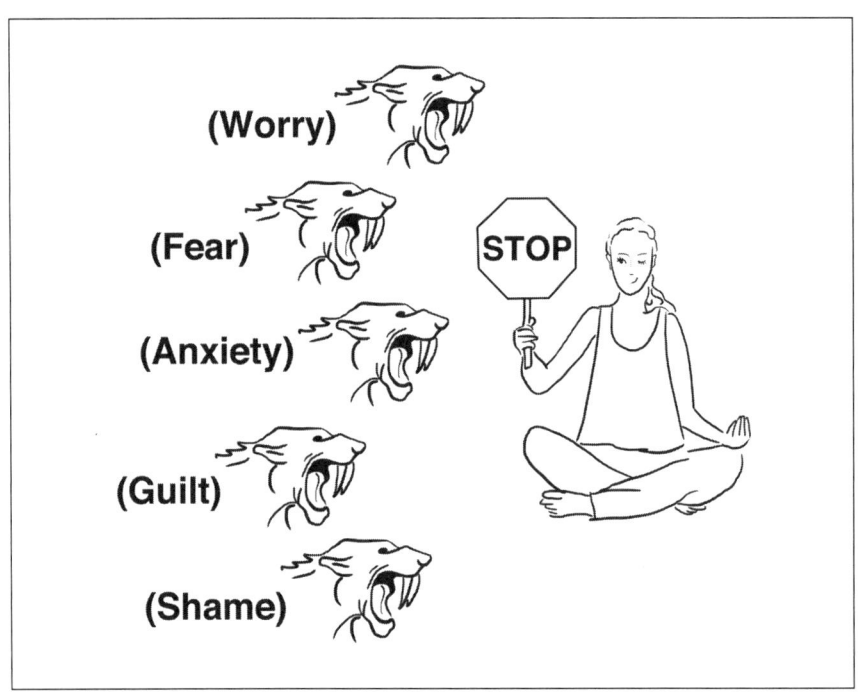

What is Mindfulness?

"Mindfulness" is the translation of a Buddhist concept that has been the subject of many techniques and meditations. Our state of "Presence" in the here and now is a universal expression of mindfulness that transcends any religion or philosophy. It is basic to our existence." – KARL BABA

Mindfulness is the non-judgmental observation of your thoughts, feelings and bodily sensations. A wonderful definition of mindfulness comes from Jon Kabat-Zinn PhD, founder of Mindfulness-Based Stress Reduction, and author of the timeless classic, *Wherever You Go, There You Are*. Dr. Kabat-Zinn explains that mindfulness is, "paying attention on purpose, in the present moment, and nonjudgmentally, to the unfolding of experience moment to moment."

If you're wondering what that means, you're not alone. As Dr. Michael Baime, creator of the Penn Program for Mindfulness says, "Trying to understand mindfulness by its definition is like trying to understand what it is like to fall in love by reading a textbook. You might get a general idea, but you'd be missing out on the best part: what it actually feels like.

Mindfulness is all about experience, about the actual aliveness, of each moment. You learn to pay attention on purpose, in the present moment, not because someone said that it would be a good thing to do, but because that is where you find your life."

How to Practice Mindfulness

Mindfulness practice asks you to keep your awareness in the here and now, to devote your full attention to the current experience. It's the opposite of multitasking. Instead of drowning in a frazzled attempt to juggle several thoughts or tasks at once, the goal is to be completely immersed and aware in whatever it is you are doing in the *moment*.

You can develop mindfulness by simply devoting your undivided attention to your everyday experiences. Simply remain focused on whatever it is you're doing - breathing, eating, washing the dishes or making love. The whole point is to be totally present with whatever you are engaged in.

You might begin practicing mindfulness for stress reduction, pain management or even weight control. After a while you will find that the effects extend to other areas of your life. You will naturally make better choices and be more compassionate. Mindfulness may transform your entire life.

Mindfulness is simple even if mastering it isn't. This kind of focused attention is like a muscle; at first it's weak, you get distracted and then have to remind yourself to return to awareness. Eventually, your attention will get into shape and you'll discover that you are happiest when centered in the present moment.

For more information on mindfulness and mindfulness-based practices, check the Resource section of this book.

Exercise

Disease is inertia. Healing is movement.
If you put the body in motion, you will change.
– Gabriele Roth

Exercise is a wonderful stress reducer and has many positive benefits for everyone, even people with autoimmune conditions. Moving your body improves every aspect of your mind, body, and spirit!

Most people with autoimmune conditions can exercise. In fact, the American College of Rheumatology recommends that people with autoimmune conditions engage in regular exercise. However, if you are in an advanced stage of illness, have chronic fatigue or **if you scored high on the *Adrenal Stress Assessment,*** it's a good idea to approach exercise with common sense. Honor your body and don't overdo it. Talk to your healthcare provider before starting a new exercise program.

Four types of exercise and what they offer:

- **Flexibility exercises:** Stretching and range-of-motion (ROM) movements can reduce stiffness and make you more flexible.
- **Strengthening exercises:** Weight lifting and bodyweight (think push-ups and burpees) workouts are examples of strengthening exercises. These build muscle and strengthen your bones.
- **Aerobic exercise:** Cardio activities such as running, swimming, cycling, walking or dancing use your body's large muscle groups and improve cardiovascular function.
- **Body awareness:** Activities that combine movement with mindful awareness like Tai chi, yoga, Chi-gung, dance and Pilates can improve your balance, coordination and posture. They get you out of your head and into your body.

Exercise and Your Mind-Body Type

We often choose the type of exercise that our body needs the least. This is one area where knowing your unique Mind-Body type can be the key to restoring balance in your life. Before I got sick, I was a "cardio queen," spending hours on the Stairmaster in the gym. I also did Bikram (hot) yoga almost 7 days a week. I was literally burning up and running myself into the ground. My body never changed. I didn't lose any weight and often felt depleted or anxious after my workouts. Eventually, I got too sick to do either activity. I had to slow down and find a routine that allowed my body to come back to balance.

Moving your body can help move emotions. If you feel overwhelmed, sad, angry or irritated, go for a walk or even dance around your living room. For me, dance is a very powerful healing practice and stress reducer.

Humans have been healing through dance for centuries. Dance wisdom is rooted in the awareness that the body and mind are inseparable. When I'm dancing, my mind stops and I'm able to just *be* in my body. My dear friend and 5 Rhythms dance instructor, Visudha De Los Santos, told me the first time we danced together, "Good, you're like me. You can dance faster then you can think!" Dance movement has helped me heal childhood emotional trauma and reclaim parts of my lost and abandoned self. In many ways, it's saved my life.

I can't prescribe a "right" type of exercise that suits everyone—it's beyond the scope of this book and we're all different. The point is, no matter who you are, you are meant to move your body. Choose an activity that you enjoy so you don't burn out or become tempted to quit. Be gentle with yourself, but make a little time to move your body every day. If you do, you'll find that your energy levels rise and so do your spirits!

Reconnect with Nature

"The earth does not belong to man, man belongs to the earth. All things are connected like the blood that unites us all. Man did not weave the web of life, he is merely a strand in it. Whatever he does to the web, he does to himself."
– Chief Seattle

Spending time in nature is restorative and grounding. In fact, new research proves what many of us already knew; nature is healing and revitalizing![16] Connecting with nature enhances your well-being and nurtures mindfulness.[17] Receive the blessings of our beautiful planet, even if it's just through a walk in your local park or time in your garden. Nature nourishes my soul and reminds me that I am interconnected with all life. You belong to mother earth…reconnect with her and she will heal you.

Manage Your Life

As you read through the suggestions in this book, you might easily think, "But… I don't have enough time for all of this!"

Get creative. Let go of activities that you don't really *want* to do or that don't really serve you. Make a list of everything you do. How do you spend your time at work, at home and everywhere else? What can you stop doing now so that you'll have the time to get enough rest and take care of yourself?

Make a list of the people, places and things that invigorate you, and then another list of the people, places and things that deplete you or stress you out. When you discover where your time and energy are going, you'll soon recognize what no longer serves you.

Cultivate Joy!

"Through humor, you can soften some of the worst blows that life delivers. And once you find laughter, no matter how painful your situation might be, you can survive it."
– BILL COSBY

Many times when we are sick, we take ourselves too seriously. One lupus client of mine confessed that she went five years without smiling or laughing! Norman Cousins illustrated the healing power of laughter and creativity in his classic book *Anatomy of an Illness*. After a stressful trip to Cold War Russia in 1964, Cousins was diagnosed with ankylosing spondylitis, a chronic, debilitating and "incurable" skeletal condition. In his famous autobiographical case history, he explains how he laughed himself back to health, defying a gloomy prognosis.

Evidence reveals that laughter triggers the brain to release catecholamine hormones, which can activate the release of endorphins, the body's natural painkillers.[18] Joy and laughter ease the anxiety and depression that often come with chronic illness. The truth is, laughter releases tension and breaks negative thought patterns. Laughter is even good for our genes! Research shows that positive emotions can downregulate (turn off) bad genes and upregulate (turn on) the good ones![19]

Focus on the bright side and find the humor in everything and you'll experience more joy. Another attitude that brings joy is gratitude. When you are thankful for the blessings that you do have, they seem to multiply.

Michelle's Laughter Rx

When was the last time you had a real belly laugh? I'm talking about the kind of laugh that makes you fall off your chair and your face hurts afterward. If it's been a while, try breaking up your day with a laughter meditation. It goes like this: For five or ten minutes each day, stop whatever it is you're doing and think about something really hilarious. If you can't think of anything funny, read a funny joke, or watch a funny video on YouTube. Make this a daily habit and you'll soon become hooked!

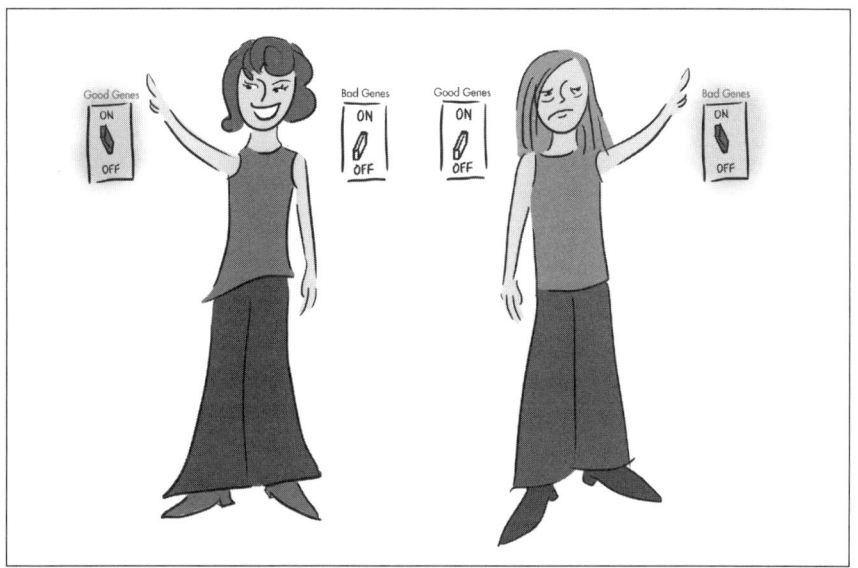

When Nothing Seems to Help

Nobody is an island. We all need help from time to time. It's essential to recognize when it's time to reach out to friends, family or a professional. It might be challenging to find the right practitioner for the issues I've explored in this chapter. Chronic stress, adrenal fatigue, anxiety, sleep disorders and depression are complex conditions that often involve many factors. **If you scored high on the *Adrenal Stress Assessment* or *the Emotional Stress Assessment,*** or if you follow the suggestions in this chapter and still don't feel well, you may need to consult with a qualified functional or integrative medical practitioner who has experience treating these conditions. It's important to remember that antidepressants, anti-anxiety medications and sleep aids have a place, but these medications are not meant to be permanent solutions. Make sure to choose a practitioner who will address the root cause and not just treat the symptoms.

Conclusion

The art of reducing stress is the art of life itself. Develop mindfulness in order to discover yourself and your own unique nature. Have an adventure creating a life that sustains and nourishes your mind, body and spirit.

CHAPTER 16

Heal Your Gut

"The road to health is paved with good intestines!"
– Sherry A. Rogers

The Gut is Your Immune System's Neighborhood

Made of a layer of epithelial (skin) cells and mucus, your GI tract is the inner tubing that regulates what enters your system and what passes through as waste. The intestinal walls have tiny gateways called "tight junctions" that allow the nutrients from food into your bloodstream, but keep undigested proteins, bacteria and toxins out, so they can be eliminated via the feces.

It may be surprising to find out that the strength of your immune system is intricately tied to the health of your GI tract. In fact, your GI tract is the "neighborhood" where up to 80 percent of your immune cells live. It also houses over 100 trillion bacteria, yeasts and other microbes. The healthy balance of these organisms is important for the cells of your immune system and your overall health.

If your GI microbes are out of balance, you have a condition called dysbiosis. If the tight junctions of your intestinal wall become loose enough to allow undigested proteins and bacterial toxins from your GI tract into your bloodstream (where they don't belong), you are suffering from a condition called leaky gut. As you have learned, this can trigger an immune response and keep your immune system on high alert. New research shows a clear connection between intestinal dysbiosis, leaky gut and autoimmune conditions.[1,2]

The following "splinters" can alter your delicate microbial balance and damage the intestinal lining, causing inflammation, dysbiosis and leaky gut: chronic stress, alcohol, antibiotics, acid blockers, NSAIDs (non-steroidal anti-inflammatory drugs such as Advil and Tylenol), steroids and infections, high-sugar diets, advanced glycosylation end products (AGEs), trans fats, food allergies, gluten and processed foods.

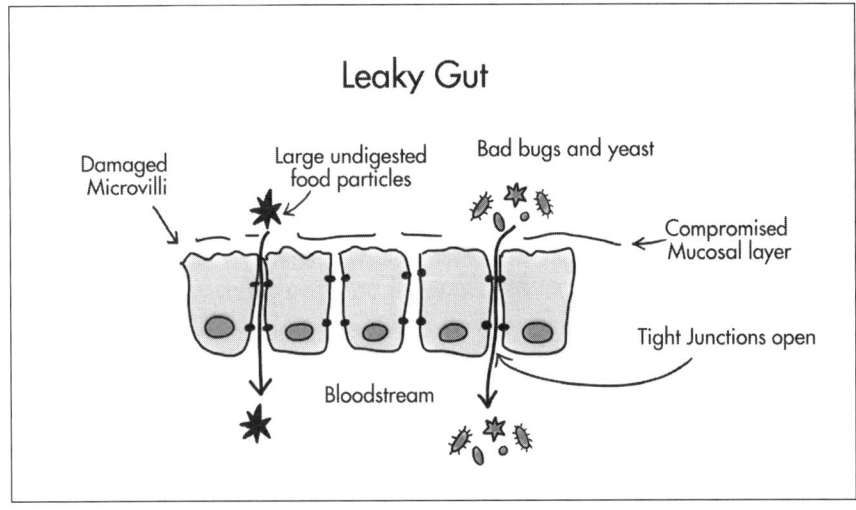

Healing your gut is not rocket science. It's simply a matter of consistently eating healing foods and avoiding unhealthy foods and substances. Of course, this is easier said than done in our modern society, where most of the food we eat is so far from its natural state that it barely qualifies as food. Sadly, many of us are not mindful of what we eat or how food affects our health. Even when we have a reaction to something, we are conditioned to take a pill to cover up our symptoms instead of listing to our body and avoiding the offending substance.

> **What You Need to Know:**
> There is no drug or supplement that will heal your GI system faster than consistently eating the right foods for your body and removing the "splinters" that cause the irritation.

The good news that you can clean up your GI and make it a safe neighborhood for your immune system. The quickest and easiest way to do that is by improving your nutrition. When you begin *Eating for Your Good Genes* and follow the *Sensitivity Discovery* program, you take the first steps by removing the foods and substances that contribute to your GI inflammation. In many cases, just following a healing diet for 30 to 90 days is enough to allow things to get back into balance.

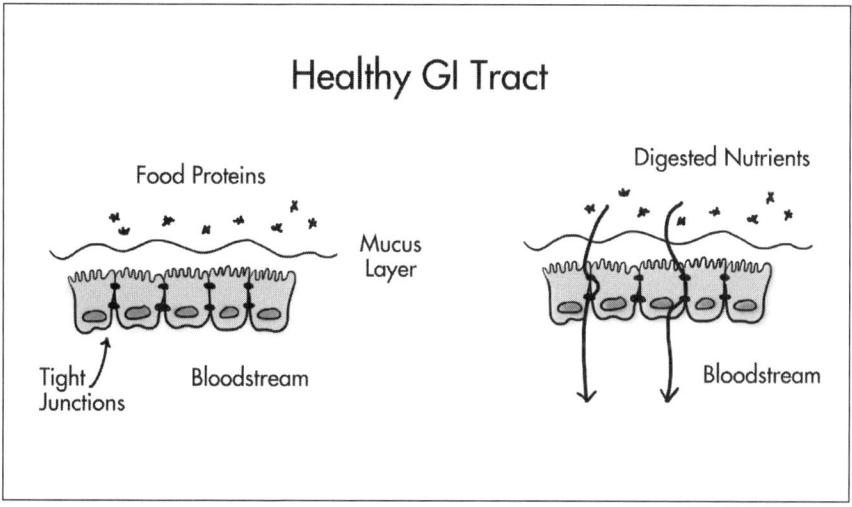

If you scored high on the *GI Stress Assessment*, have a serious GI condition, or if you begin *Eating for Your Good Genes* and follow the *Sensitivity Discovery Program,* and you still have symptoms, you may have to dig a little deeper to uncover the cause. This is where the "Function" comes into the *Functional Mind-Body Approach*! Who knows, you may have an overgrowth of yeast, or an infection such as a parasite or bacteria. Without testing you're just guessing and you can spend a lot of time and money trying different approaches. Functional medical GI testing cuts the guesswork out and saves your precious time and money. If had done this testing in the beginning I could have saved thousands of dollars! I suggest you get a comprehensive GI test (see my recommendations below) to find out exactly what is "bugging" you. Many times these conditions can be cleared up with over-the-counter botanical preparations within a few weeks. You may even need a prescription antifungal or anti-parasitic medication from your doctor.

> **What You Need to Know:**
> Your GI tract is a sensitive tube that absorbs the nutrients from your food and keeps unwanted proteins, bacteria and toxins out

> of your bloodstream and eliminates them via the feces. It's home to up to 80 percent of your immune cells. Everything you eat and drink comes into contact with this inner tubing and affects your immune system. Think of stress, bad food and toxic substances as sandpaper that wears holes in your GI tract and disrupts the delicate microbial balance (dysbiosis), leading to a condition called leaky gut. A leaky gut allows undigested food proteins and toxins into your bloodstream. When this happens, your immune system gets fired up to clean up what shouldn't be in your bloodstream. Over time, a fired up immune response can result in an autoimmune condition.

Next I'll explain what you can do on your own to heal your GI, and when you may need to see a practitioner.

What You can Do on Your Own to Heal Your GI

Remove Your GI Splinters!

Stress, bad foods, toxins and infections are like festering splinters that cause inflammation, intestinal dysbiosis and leaky gut. These splinters have to come out for your GI to heal!

- **Remove Bad Foods:** Steer clear of gluten, dairy, sugar, alcohol, nightshades, grains*, legumes*, nuts*, artificial sweeteners and processed foods. Eat fresh organic *Eating for Your Good Genes* approved fruits and veggies; fermented foods such as kimchi; healing fats such as borage oil, EPA/DHA fish oil, ghee and coconut oil; and small amounts of lean organic fish, meat or poultry (or hypoallergenic protein powder). Cook with anti-inflammatory herbs and spices: turmeric, cumin, fennel, parsley, cinnamon, cardamom, ginger, garlic and sea salt. Eating this way will starve out bad bugs and yeast that feed on sugars and calm the inflammation caused by food sensitivities, lectins, phytic acid and other antinutrients.

---

* Not everyone reacts to grains, legumes, or nuts! Certain Mind-Body types thrive on rice, quinoa (technically a seed), millet and other non-gluten grains as well as legumes and nuts. Follow the *Sensitivity Discovery Program* to find what's best for you!

- **Remove Stressful Eating Habits:** Eating when you're stressed-out lowers stomach acid and contributes to GI distress. Your body wasn't designed to digest food while running from a Saber-Toothed Tiger! Practice mindful eating. Work to create a peaceful eating environment. Think about, and take time to prepare, a healthy meal for yourself and your loved ones. Sit down, give thanks for the food and chew your food slowly. This practice helps you enjoy your meal and improves and supports digestion.

- **Remove Bad Bugs:** Kill unfriendly bacteria, yeast and parasites with over-the-counter herbal formulas that contain sweet wormwood (artemesia), caprylic acid, grapefruit seed extract, berberine and garlic. See below for my recommendations. NOTE: I recommend having GI testing done before beginning this step because it can save you a lot of time and money down the road. Different bugs require different treatments. With the functional GI testing now available, it just makes sense to identify the bug and get the right treatment. See below under *Test Don't Guess!*

- **Remove Bad Drugs:** Wean yourself off of acid blockers, proton pump inhibitors, NSAIDs and steroids. NOTE: If you have gastroesophageal reflux (GERD), heartburn or are taking proton pump inhibitors, see below for a special healing program. If you are taking NSAIDs or steroids, please talk to your functional/integrative healthcare provider about how to safely transition to natural anti-inflammatory compounds. I have found that following a healing diet greatly reduces inflammation and the need for anti-inflammatory drugs.

Replace What's Missing!

Years of stress, poor eating habits, malnutrition, infections and irritating substances can lower stomach acid and deplete pancreatic enzymes. It's important to replace these essential GI ingredients for faster healing.

- **Replace stomach acid:** Healthy digestion requires adequate stomach acid. Low stomach acid can interfere with the absorption of important nutrients such as B6, B12, folate, calcium and iron. Malabsorption of B vitamins and folate can lead to impaired methylation (a topic I will discuss later), and can affect everything from your mood, to your capability to detoxify, and even your ability to repair your DNA. Low stomach acid can be a cause of vitamin B12 deficiency related anemia, which is common in people taking antacids.[3] Low stomach acid can also cause anemia due to malabsorption of iron. People with low stomach acid are also at a greater risk for GI infections. To make sure you have enough stomach acid take betaine HCL with protein meals to help digest and break down your food. **See below** for my recommendations. **NOTE:** If you have gastroesophageal reflux (GERD), heartburn or are taking proton pump inhibitors, skip this step and **read below** for a special healing program.

- **Replace enzymes:** Enzymes assist in the breakdown of proteins, fats, complex carbohydrates, sugars and fibers. This is especially important for people with leaky gut, allergies or any kind of autoimmune condition, because enzymes break down the large proteins in food that may otherwise cross the intestinal lining and fire up the immune system.[4] I recommend supplementing with a broad-spectrum formula that contains a blend of carbohydrate, sugar, vegetable fiber, protein and fat specific enzymes. **See below** for my recommendations.

Reinoculate with "Good Bugs"

The healthy bacteria that live in your GI tract can be disrupted or killed off by stress, poor nutrition, alcohol, drugs and bad bugs. It's important to bring the good bugs back and reestablish microbial balance in your gut!

- **Reinoculate your GI tract with healthy bacteria "Good Bugs":** Numerous studies have shown that re-introducing good bugs in the form of probiotics into the intestines helps to reestablish the microbial balance, and suppress immune disorders.[5] In fact, supplementing with probiotics has been shown to bring excessive Th1 and Th2 responses back into balance and reduce allergic symptoms.[6,7] Probiotics help with the production and absorption of nutrients, especially vitamin B12, vitamin D and folate.[8] Take a broad-spectrum probiotic that contains a combination of several strains of lactobacilli and bifidobacteria. Take saccharomyces (a beneficial yeast) and eat fermented foods such as kimchi and coconut kefir to help repopulate the good bacteria in your gut. **See below** for my recommendations.

- **Reinoculate with prebiotics:** Good bacteria love fiber so eat plenty of non-starchy veggies, berries and apples. You can include soaked and sprouted nuts and seeds if you know that you don't react to them. These contain non-digestible fibrous plant compounds that ferment in the GI tract and feed your good bacteria. Aim for 30 – 50 grams of fiber per day. You can also try fiber supplements such as acacia or larch arabinogalactans. Avoid bran fiber (wheat) and fiber supplements that contain sugar or artificial sweeteners. Psyllium can be good to bulk up your stool, keep you regular and help eliminate toxins. Be cautious of fiber supplements that contain multiple ingredients because if you have a reaction, it will be impossible to know which of those ingredients is bothering you. **See below** for my recommendations.

Repair Your Inner Tube!

After you have removed your GI splinters, replaced digestive enzymes and reintroduced healthy bacteria, the final step is to heal the mucosal lining of your inner tube. Your individual need for repair will depend on how severe your GI symptoms are, and if you have leaky gut.

- *Repair your GI with healing fats:* Eating plenty of the healing fats outlined in Chapter 14 will help reduce inflammation and heal the mucosal lining of your GI. These include ghee, coconut oil and essential fatty acids such as fish oils and borage oil. **See below** for my recommendations.

- *Repair your GI with glutamine:* Glutamine deficiencies have been associated with intestinal degeneration after times of stress, infection, surgery and radiation.[9] Glutamine supplementation has been shown to stimulate intestinal cell growth and repair the intestinal lining.[10,11] Glutamine is found in animal protein, beets, spinach and parsley. To get a therapeutic dose, take a glutamine powder supplement for three months. **See below** for my recommendations.

- *Repair with zinc:* Zinc is an important trace element, and is critical for immune function and the production of stomach acid.[12] Zinc deficiency goes hand in hand with malnutrition, especially protein deficiency, which is common in people with digestive disorders.[13,14]

Zinc deficiency is also common in people with hypothyroidism and chronic fatigue. Zinc has been shown to improve leaky gut in people with Crohn's disease.[15] **See below** for my recommendations.

Supplement Suggestions to Heal Your Gut

Remove the Bad Bugs

You can save time and money by obtaining a comprehensive stool analysis before self-prescribing herbal formulas to remove bad bugs. If you decide to self-prescribe, it's best to start low and go slow. Many of these formulas work well to kill the bad bugs but can also cause a Herxheimer reaction, sometimes referred to as "die-off." This results when the toxins released from dying pathogens overwhelm your body's capacity to clear them. If you start to feel sick or have uncomfortable symptoms such as fatigue, gas and bloating, or headaches, simply back down on the dosage or take a day off. The last thing you want to do is overwhelm your body and stress your immune system with too many dying bugs!

I prefer combination formulas over formulas that contain only a single herb, as they tend to be more effective.

- Artemesia (sweet wormwood) – 400 mg, take 1-4 capsules per day just before meals
- GSE – Grapefruit Seed Extract – drops or capsules, take as directed on the label
- Olive Leaf Extract – 100 – 250 mg, take 1-4 capsules per day, or as directed on the label
- Berberine – 200-400 mg, take 1-3 times per day, or as directed on the label
- Caprylic Acid – 500 mg, take 1-2 per day, or as directed on the label
- Pure Encapsulations A.C.® Formula II – This is a good combination formula. Take as directed on the label

Replace What's Missing

Enzymes are available in both plant and animal formulas. Pancreatin contains a blend of lipase, which digests fat; proteases, which digest protein; and amylases, which digest starch. Plant-based enzymes are a good alternative for vegetarians and can be derived from aspergillus, bromelain or papaya. If you are allergic to mold, avoid enzymes derived from aspergillus. Try one enzyme product at a time, and keep track of how you feel.

- Pancreatin 500 mg, take 1-2 capsules just before each meal
- ProThera Vital-Zymes™ Complete full-spectrum vegetarian enzyme formula, take 2 capsules just before meals
- Pure Encapsulations Digestive Enzymes Ultra, take 2 capsules just before meals
- Betaine hydrochloric acid (HCL) 600 mg, take 1 – 4 capsules (or to tolerance) with each meal. Don't take betaine HCL on an empty stomach and only use HCL that is intended as a digestive supplement.

Reinoculate with "Good Bugs"

When choosing a probiotic, look for refrigerated enteric-coated formulas that contain multiple strains of lactobacilli and bifidobacteria. While there are several great formulas on the market, I mention the brands that I have the most experience with and take myself. Ask your functional or integrative health practitioner for the brands they like best.

- Klair Labs® – Ther-Biotic® Complete, take 1-4 capsules with a light meal, or as directed by your healthcare provider.
- Klair Labs® - Saccharomyces boulardii, take 1-4 capsules twice daily, or as directed by your healthcare provider
- Pure Encapsulations Probiotic 50B (Soy and Dairy Free), take 1-4 capsules with a light meal, or as directed by your healthcare provider.

Fiber Supplements – (Try One Product at a Time)

- Vital Nutrients Arabinogalactan Powder, take one teaspoon 1 to 3 times daily
- Now® Glucomannan Powder, take as directed on the label
- PGX® (PolyGlycopleX®), take as directed on the label
- Organic India Whole Husk Psyllium 100% certified organic fiber – Take one tablespoon 1 to 2 times a day. Is best taken after dinner. Do not take within 4 hours of taking your thyroid medication as it can reduce absorption. If you are constipated, make sure to drink plenty of water and take extra vitamin C, preferably buffered C or Ester C to keep things moving.

Repair Your Inner Tube

- Omega-3 EPA/DHA Complex 1000 mg, take 1-4 capsules per day
- Borage Oil 1000 mg, take 1-4 capsules per day
- Coconut Oil, take one teaspoon twice a day
- Glutamine powder, take 3000 mg up to 3 times per day
- Zinc picolinate, take 30 mg per day
- Metagenics GI Sustain™ Leaky Gut Syndrome, take 2 scoops daily, or as directed by your healthcare provider
- Metagenics UltraInflamX® 360 Plus, take 2 scoops daily, or as directed by your healthcare provider

Heartburn Acid Reflux and GERD

Heartburn, acid reflux and GERD often go hand-in-hand with Hashimoto's. If you suffer from these painful disorders, I have great news for you. You can heal these conditions easily and permanently. Even if you take antacids or proton pump inhibitors, you can wean yourself off of your medication and prevent recurring painful and destructive symptoms by eliminating the root causes of your condition.

Many people think that heartburn, acid reflux and GERD are caused by excess stomach acid. It appears the opposite is true. Many medical experts now believe these conditions are caused by *low stomach acid* (a condition called hypochlorhydria), and typically accompany other conditions such as leaky gut, gluten intolerance, high carbohydrate diets and/or bacterial overgrowth in the intestines.

You might wonder how *low* stomach acid could cause that terrible burning sensation in your chest. The gateway to the stomach is the lower esophageal sphincter (LES). When it's working properly, it keeps stomach acid in your stomach where it belongs, and out of your esophagus where it burns. If the LES becomes loose, weak or subject to abdominal pressure, it allows acid (even low acid) and undigested food to escape the stomach and burn the esophagus.

A class of drugs called proton pump inhibitors (PPIs) such as omeprazole (Prilosec), lansoprazole (Prevacid), rabeprazole (Aciphex), pantoprazole (Protonix) and esomeprazole (Nexium) are designed to protect the lining of the esophagus by significantly reducing stomach acid.

But reducing stomach acid comes with its own risks:

- Stomach acid kills potentially harmful bacteria in our food and helps to break down large proteins that might later be absorbed into the blood through the GI tract.
- Low stomach acid retards the absorption of certain nutrients like B vitamins (particularly B12), folic acid, calcium, iron and zinc.
- Low stomach acid interferes with iron absorption and can cause iron deficiency anemia and low ferritin (iron reserve protein). Low ferritin is associated with hair loss.
- Low stomach acid can cause vitamin B12 deficiency related anemia.
- Studies have shown that people with low stomach acid absorb less thyroid hormone.[16]

Many people are unaware that PPI's are designed for short-term therapy. For example, the directions for one popular brand reads: "Use as directed for 14 days to treat frequent heartburn. Do not take for more than 14 days or more often than every 4 months unless directed by a doctor." Sadly, many people live on these medications for years, which put them at risk for dysbiosis, nutrient deficiencies, osteoporosis and bone fractures.

One study demonstrated that people taking PPIs, even those who didn't suffer from heartburn or GERD to begin with, developed symptoms after they were given PPIs for two months and then suddenly stopped.[17] In other words, PPIs create dependency and can give you heartburn, even if you didn't have it before!

Self-Healing Program for GERD

You can heal your heartburn, acid reflux and GERD problems, and help reverse your autoimmune condition at the same time, by eliminating the foods that cause the problem in the first place. I have found that the easiest way to accomplish this is by following the *"Eating for Your Good Genes"* and *"Sensitivity Discovery Program"* for 30 to 90 days. In fact, every single one of my clients who suffered from heartburn, acid reflux or GERD noticed an immediate (typically within one week) improvement in their symptoms, once they cut out irritating substances, grains and starchy carbs, and began eating healing foods!

More good news! Excess body weight often makes GERD symptoms worse. Some people only experience GERD above a certain body weight. Eating the right foods will help you lose weight and reverse GERD at the same time!

Things to avoid if you have heartburn, acid reflux or GERD:
- Stressful situations – Never eat when you're rushed or stressed!
- Grains (especially gluten) and starchy carbs
- Coffee and caffeinated beverages
- Alcohol (including beer and wine)
- Fried and processed foods
- Chocolate
- Citrus fruits and juices
- Tomatoes
- Carbonated drinks
- Fructose
- Artificial sweeteners
- Anything that triggers your symptoms, for instance, some people have trouble with spicy foods, certain meats, fried foods and mint.
- Poor food combinations such as fruit and meat together

Things to include:
- Peaceful environments – especially when eating!
- Non-starchy veggies
- Healing fat's – especially coconut oil
- DGL – Deglycyrrhized licorice
- Aloe
- Zinc

You can follow the GI self-healing program like everyone else but avoid:
- Prebiotics
- Soluble fiber

While I have found betaine HCL with pepsin is beneficial for most people, I don't suggest it for those suffering from GERD who take PPIs or other acid-blocking medications. They simply negate each other. Betaine HCL with pepsin therapy may be added once your GERD is under control, and you have weaned yourself off of acid-blockers. Begin with one capsule, and increase to two if you can tolerate that dose without developing a warm or burning sensation in your stomach. If you still experience burping, bloating and gas after taking two capsules for a while, you may consider upping your dose if you can do so without the burning sensation.

Caution! Betaine HCL with pepsin should NEVER be taken along with NSAIDs like ibuprofen, aspirin or corticosteroids like prednisone. These medications can irritate and even damage the delicate lining of the GI tract. Adding betaine HCL to these medications can put you at risk for gastric bleeding or an ulcer.

During the healing process you can benefit from supplementation with zinc, digestive enzymes and probiotics. Taking enzymes with meals assists in breaking down foods so the body can absorb nutrients. Probiotics restore the balance of good bugs in your GI, thus eliminating the problems caused by (bad) bacterial overgrowth. **See my recommendations** for good probiotics and digestive enzyme supplements in this chapter under the heading "*Supplements to Heal your Gut.*"

Traditional remedies that I've also found helpful are apple cider vinegar, lemon juice or tinctures of bitter herbs, 15-20 minutes before a meal. Avoid drinking a lot of fluids with meals as this dilutes the stomach acid. Hydration is important but is best between meals.

Homemade bone broth soup helps restore the mucosal lining of the stomach. Bone broth contains short peptides called glyprolines that protect the lining of the stomach and help heal ulcers.[18] The glutamine in bone broth fuels and protects the cells of the intestinal lining.[19] Bone broth also contains plentiful minerals and other healthful constituents. I have found this to be the top GI healing food. An extra bonus is that your hair and nails will grow in thick and strong!

Deglycyrrhizinated licorice (DGL) helps protect from the damage caused by NSAIDs like aspirin and ibuprofen and is also effective at healing ulcers without reducing stomach acid.[20] You take one to three 380-400 mg tablets of DGL 20-30 minutes before a meal. Ginger is another great digestive aid. It contains an enzyme called zingibain, which digests protein, and stimulates the activity of other enzymes like lipase.

GERD and the Stress Connection

Stress affects more that just your mind. In fact, studies have documented the link between stress and heartburn, acid reflux and GERD.[21] The research shows that stress, particularly prolonged intense stress, make the symptoms of these uncomfortable disorders worse. The scientists were surprised by one of their findings; even though stressed-out people experienced a worsening of their symptoms, their stomach acid wasn't any stronger.[22]

The researchers speculated that stress makes low-level symptoms feel much worse; in other words, everything feels worse when you are stressed out! While that is certainly true, I think this finding reinforces the alternative view that GERD is not caused by excess strong stomach acid. The studies also show that exhaustion, which is certainly a common form of stress, also makes these conditions worse.[23]

It's easy to connect stress with heartburn, acid reflux and GERD, in fact many of us feel a pit in our stomach when we're stressed out. Adding insult to injury, stress often inspires unhealthy coping mechanisms such as the overuse of over-the-counter painkillers, alcohol and smoking, which contribute to the development of ulcers, GERD and other GI conditions.

In Chapter 15, I review some techniques to help reduce stress. But just as a reminder, try to reduce the stress in your life and avoid eating when you are stressed-out or rushed. You can improve your digestion by chewing your food thoroughly. Gobbling your food down can trigger an acid reflux attack. Chewing your food well assists the digestive process by mixing your saliva with the food and breaking it down into smaller pieces. Not only that, eating slower gives you time to enjoy your food and gives your body a chance to recognize that you've had enough to eat.

The key to healing heartburn, acid reflux and GERD is eating the right foods and eliminating the foods that cause inflammation and bacterial overgrowth. Seriously, if you eat well for long enough, you WILL get better. The body is funny that way. If you give the body what it needs, it will bounce back from just about anything. It is a mistake to ignore the body's natural ability to heal itself.

When You Need a Practitioner – Test, Don't Guess!

If you have followed the recommendations above but still have symptoms, I suggest you get a comprehensive stool analysis to find out what's bugging you. You may have an infection such as H. pylori, or an overgrowth of bad bacteria or candida in your gut. **See below** for my suggestions.

H. Pylori

H. (Helicobacter) pylori is a spiral shaped bacteria that lives in the stomach and duodenum (section of intestine just below stomach). It is estimated that roughly 50% of the world's population is infected with the organism. H. pylori overgrowth may cause symptoms such as peptic ulcer disease, gastritis, abdominal pain and nausea. Many times there may be no symptoms at all. In a vicious cycle, H. pylori infection occurs in an environment of low stomach acid and then further suppresses stomach acid, which can contribute to acid reflux and GERD.

H. pylori infection can reduce thyroid hormone absorption, which is a concern for those on thyroid hormone replacement.[24]

There are several tests you can take to determine if you have an infection. Ask your practitioner which one is right for you:

- **Helicobacter Pylori Antibody Assay:** This measures serum IgG antibodies to Helicobacter pylori, using the **enzyme-linked immunosorbent assay (ELISA) method.**

- **Breath Test:** The highly accurate, non-invasive 15-minute Urea Breath Test can detect H. pylori infection. The Urea Breath Test has the advantage of detecting active infections while blood serology tests sometimes produce false positive results because of detecting antibodies from a previous infection. This test also doesn't involve poking you with any needles. For this test to be effective, you need to be off any antibiotics for 28 days and off acid-reducing medications like PPIs for two weeks before taking the test.

- **Stool Test:** The HpSA is an antibody-based, antigen-in-stool immunoassay to detect Helicobacter pylori. This test can also distinguish between an active and non-active infection.

Treatment

Conventional H. pylori treatment consists of a combination of 2 or 3 antibiotics and a proton pump inhibitor (PPI). Prevpac is a common

> combination and includes Prevacid (lansoprazole), amoxicillin and clarithromycin. Treatment with this combination is roughly 70-80% effective. Note: Saccharomyces boulardii is a particularly good probiotic to take if you are on antibiotics to kill H-pylori. Saccharomyces boulardii is a yeast that is resistant to antibiotics.
>
> I suggest trying a healing diet, mastic gum (Pistacea lentiscus), DGL (deglycyrrhizinated licorice), Zinc carnosine (PepZin-GI), lactoferrin and probiotics. Some people have had success combining mastic gum with Manuka honey and monolaurin – 1200 mg twice a day (monolaurin is derived from coconuts, you might just use a few tablespoons of Coconut oil) along with the probiotics.
>
> Another treatment that has been proven to be very effective is Matula Herbal Formula. It can be purchased at http://www.perfectly-natural-health.com/

The Science

If you have a hard time convincing your gastroenterologist that high carbs and low stomach acid are responsible for your symptoms, there are two small studies that validate what I've repeatedly seen with my clients. The research, conducted by Professor Yancey and his colleagues at Duke University, followed five patients with severe GERD that had not responded to treatment. They reported that they eliminated their symptoms within one week of eating a very low carb diet.[25,26] The second study observed the effects of a very low carb diet on eight obese patients with severe GERD. The researchers measured the esophageal pH of the patients before and after the study, using something called the Johnson-DeMeester score and the GSAS-ds questionnaire. Five out of the eight patients had abnormal Johnson-DeMeester scores in the beginning and all five of them showed a marked decrease in symptoms (similar to what could be expected with PPI's) after eating a very low carb diet. All eight had marked improvement in their GSAS-ds scores.

When You Need a Practitioner – Test, Don't Guess!

There is a lot you can do on your own to heal your gut, but if you follow the *Sensitivity Discovery Program*, try the suggestions above and you still have symptoms, it's time to find out what's bugging you. A functional stool analysis is the quickest, most effective way to do that. You will have to find a functional medical practitioner to order the test and prescribe any necessary treatment. You can find a functional medical doctor by visiting the Institute for Functional Medicine's website at www.functionalmedicine.org. Click on the tab "Functional Medicine Resources" and choose "Find a Functional Medicine Practitioner" to find someone in your area. If you find a practitioner in your area, be sure to ask if they offer functional stool analysis. Alternatively, we have compiled a list of practitioners on *The Thyroid Cure* Web site at www.thethyroidcure.com/practitioners

Functional Testing for GI Splinters

There are several labs that offer functional stool analysis including Metametrix and Genova (who have now merged), and Doctor's Data. Ask your integrative or functional medical practitioner about which tests are best for you.

Testing for GI Function

- **Metametrix GI Effects Comprehensive Profile (Stool Analysis):** This test uses DNA analysis to identify microbiota with 100% accuracy including anaerobes, a previously unmeasurable area of the gut environment. In addition to much more comprehensive bacteriology, mycology, and parasitology this test reports drug resistance genes, antibiotic and botanical sensitivities, Elastase1, plus other inflammation, digestion, and absorption markers. The GI Effects test goes further than the Doctor's Data Comprehensive Stool Analysis (CSA, outlined below) into identifying the actual DNA of the bacteria present, and will indicate the specific strain of clostridium that may be present. The GI Effects also offers a more extensive parasite profile when compared to the CSA. Both the CSA and GI Effects will test for inflammation, as well as digestive and absorption parameters.

- **Doctor's Data Comprehensive Stool Analysis with Parasitology x3 (Stool Sample):** This test evaluates digestion and absorption, bacterial balance, metabolism, yeast levels and the presence of parasites. This test is used to evaluate the cause of various gastrointestinal symptoms, or systemic illnesses, whose origins can be traced back to bacterial imbalance, parasites, or intestinal dysfunction.

Testing for Leaky Gut

- **Genova Diagnostics Intestinal Permeability Assessment (Urine Test):** This test analyzes urine for the clearance of two non-metabolized sugars, lactulose and mannitol. Identifies "leaky gut" and malabsorption.

Testing for H. Pylori

- **Doctor's Data H. Pylori Antigen (Stool Sample)**
- **LabCorp Helicobacter Pylori Urea (Breath Test)**

Celiac Testing

- **LabCorp Celiac Disease Comprehensive Antibody Profile (Blood Draw Test)**

Genetic Testing for Gluten Sensitivity

- **EnteroLab Gluten Sensitivity Gene Test (Molecular HLA-DQB1 analysis) (Mouth Swab)**

You can learn more about these tests by visiting the individual laboratory websites listed in the Resources section, or www.thethyroidcure.com/GItesting

In the next chapter I'll review your liver's key functions and why optimizing its function is critical to healing your condition.

CHAPTER 17

Restore Your Liver

"The liver is the foundation of health"
— A SAYING OF CHINESE MEDICINE

Throughout the ages, a healthy liver has been recognized as the key to vibrant health. After all, it's responsible for many of the vital functions in the body, including detoxifying chemicals and heavy metals, metabolizing drugs and hormones, breaking down fats, regulating blood sugar, synthesizing vitamins and minerals, and converting T4 into the more bioavailable T3.

Chronic stress, sugar, alcohol, nutritional deficiencies, trans fats, food additives, prescription drugs, hormones, xenobiotic compounds, environmental toxins and heavy metals all stress the liver and cause it to become sluggish. A sluggish liver can't perform effectively, and you can begin to feel sick, tired, bloated and fat.

Optimal liver function is important for everyone, but it's absolutely critical for people suffering with any kind of autoimmune condition. It's virtually impossible to remove your toxic "splinters" when your liver is sluggish. Unfortunately, most healthcare practitioners who treat autoimmune conditions are not aware of the importance of optimizing liver function, and many people are given drugs and hormones that only add to their liver's toxic burden.

Optimizing liver function is pretty straightforward for most of us. It involves eating the right foods, and avoiding stress and toxic substances; but it's not always that simple. Some of us are more sensitive than others, and may have a difficult time processing and eliminating all the toxins of our modern world.

Most people who follow the guidelines in the previous chapters begin to feel better within the first 30 to 90 days.

If you scored high on the *Toxic Stress Assessment*, or if you begin *Eating for Your Good Genes* and follow the *Sensitivity Discovery Program*, and you still have symptoms (or if you feel worse), you need to dig a little deeper to uncover the cause. Your body might be burdened from exposure to chemicals or heavy metals and you may have specific nutrient deficiencies or genetic variants that impair your ability to detoxify efficiently.

If you have been sick for a long time, suffered a serious toxic exposure or if you have a more serious autoimmune condition, I suggest that you skip the steps in "*What you can do on your own*" and begin to work directly with a qualified functional or integrative practitioner to get to the bottom of what is triggering your immune system. Again, this is where the "Function" comes into the *Functional Mind-Body Approach*. Remember, every second that you live with an autoimmune condition, your tissues are being attacked by your immune system. It simply doesn't make sense to "guess" about what the triggers are. Please pay special attention to the section at the end of this chapter entitled "*When You Need a Practitioner – Test, Don't Guess!*

Let's review some of the liver's key functions and two common causes of impaired detoxification. Then I'll explain what you can do on your own to improve your liver's function, and how to recognize when it's time to seek medical guidance.

Your Liver's Key Functions

Your Liver Purifies Your Blood

Your liver filters your blood, and keeps "bad bugs" and toxins out of your blood stream.

Approximately three pints of blood pass through the liver every three minutes. A healthy liver will clear roughly 99 percent of large toxins, endotoxins (toxins from bacteria inside the body), antigens and waste products from the blood. Keeping toxins out of your blood and away from an inflamed and confused immune system is critical for healing any autoimmune condition.

Your Liver Breaks Down and Neutralizes Unwanted Toxins and Hormones

As you have learned, toxic and hormonal stress is a huge splinter in many autoimmune conditions. Remember, your liver is responsible for breaking down and neutralizing "splinters" such as drugs, food additives, pesticides, environmental toxins (including molds) and other poisons from the GI tract. The liver is also responsible for processing and metabolizing all of your hormones—not just the ones you make naturally, but also the ones you are exposed to through birth control pills, hormone replacement therapy (HRT) and xenoestrogens. As I've discussed in earlier chapters, it does this in two phases, known as Phase I and Phase II detoxification. Both phases require a number of vitamins, antioxidants, minerals, amino acids and phytochemicals found in healing foods to work properly.

If you scored high on the Hormonal Stress Assessment, you will benefit from restoring your liver function!

In Phase I, fat-soluble toxins and hormones are broken down by enzymes (specifically P-450 enzymes) and transformed into substances called "intermediary metabolites" to be passed on to Phase II for further transformation and elimination. Intermediary metabolites are often more toxic than the original substance that was neutralized as they create dangerous free radicals that can damage critical parts of our cells such as the cell membranes or DNA. Important antioxidants such as glutathione, superoxide dismutase, beta carotene, vitamins C and E, selenium, copper, zinc, manganese, magnesium, CoQ10, bioflavonoids and indoles are required to neutralize the free radicals and clean up the mess.

In phase II, the intermediary metabolites are transformed by a second series of enzymes, called conjugases, into substances that can be excreted though the urine or feces. Phase II pathways are: glucuronidation, acetylation, sulfation, methylation, glycine conjugation, and glutathione conjugation. Phase II requires the amino acids glycine, taurine, glutamine, and methionine found in complete protein such as natural lean meat and certain dairy products such as whey protein.

Your Liver Converts T4 into the More Active T3

Your liver is responsible for converting the thyroid hormone T4 into its active form, called T3. It needs the proper nutrients for this conversion. If your liver is stressed-out and sluggish, or missing key nutrients, it can't do the job of converting T4 to T3, which means you won't have enough of the active thyroid hormone circulating in your body.[1] Consequently, you'll feel sick and tired even if you're taking T4 hormone replacement.

Your Liver is Your Fat Burning Machine

Your liver produces a degreasing agent called bile, which is stored in the gallbladder. A healthy liver will produce about a quart of bile per day. Bile breaks down fats, and emulsifies fat-soluble vitamins, increasing their absorption in the intestine. Bile is also responsible for carrying toxins out of the body and it acts as natural laxative. When the liver is toxic and the secretion of bile is inhibited, it can't break down fat, and toxins begin to accumulate in the body. This not only stresses your immune system but it leaves you looking and feeling sick, fat, bloated and toxic!

Your Liver Regulates Your Blood Sugar

After a meal, your liver will store glucose as glycogen, and then release it for energy as your body needs it.

Other Important Functions

In addition to detoxification, the liver is critical for many aspects of digestion (breaking nutrients down) and assimilation (supplying those nutrients to our cells). It stores many essential vitamins (B12, A, D, E and K) and minerals, such as iron and copper. The liver produces the red blood cells that carry oxygen around the body. Specialized immune cells in the liver, called Kupffer cells, destroy bacteria, small foreign proteins and old blood cells, helping the body to fight infections.

> **What You Need to Know:**
> What you need to know: Your liver plays a primary role in reversing your autoimmune condition because it processes and eliminates "splinters" such as toxins and unwanted hormones. If your liver is healthy, it can better convert the thyroid hormone T4 to the more active form of T3. Your liver helps you burn fat and maintain a healthy weight. Your liver helps control your blood sugar. Your liver requires key nutrients to function optimally. If you are deficient in any of the key nutrients, your liver could become sluggish, your detoxification will be impaired, and you would be at risk of developing a number of health conditions, including autoimmunity.

Detoxification and Your Unique Mind-Body Type

How well your body processes and eliminates toxins depends on several factors:
- Your age
- Your gender
- Your Mind-Body Type (your constitution)
- Your individual stress levels
- The foods you eat (the nutrients you give your body)
- Your individual toxic exposures, past and present
- Your individual genetics, which influence your ability to process and eliminate toxins such as heavy metals, exogenous and endogenous hormones, endocrine disrupting compounds (EDCs), plastics, petrochemicals, pesticides and other toxic compounds

The bottom line is that we're all different, and so is our ability to process and eliminate the toxins we're exposed to. If you're reading this book, you probably have an autoimmune condition. If you have an autoimmune condition, chances are that you are more sensitive than most people, and you likely need help to enhance your body's detoxification capability.

As you have learned, the liver requires specific nutrients to function properly. If you are deficient in any of the key nutrients, your detox ability will be impaired.

To complicate matters, some of us have certain genetic "personalities" that have a difficult time converting nutrients from food into the substances required for optimal detoxification. That's why some people don't get better in spite of eating the "perfect" diet and doing everything else "right."

Next I'd like to familiarize you with two important factors necessary for optimizing your detoxification:
- Improving your methylation
- Boosting your glutathione

Methylation

Methylation is a biochemical process involved in almost all of your body's functions.

Without getting too technical, methylation is the addition of a single carbon and three hydrogen atoms (called a methyl group) to another molecule. The removal of a methyl group is called demethylation. Think of billions of little on/off switches inside your body that control everything from your stress response and how your body makes energy from food, to your brain chemistry and detoxification; that's methylation and demethylation.

Think of methyl groups as the on/off switches for:
- The stress (fight or flight) response
- The production and recycling of glutathione – the body's master antioxidant
- The detoxification of hormones, chemicals and heavy metals
- The inflammation response
- Genetic expression and the repair of DNA
- Neurotransmitters and the balancing of brain chemistry
- Energy production
- The repair of cells damaged by free radicals
- The immune response; controlling T-cell production; fighting infections and viruses; and regulating the immune response

If you have a shortage of methyl groups, or your methylation cycle is interrupted, any or all of these processes can become compromised, and you will get sick. In fact, research has clearly linked impaired methylation with all autoimmune conditions![2,3]

> **Autoimmune Diseases and Methylation**
>
> An autoimmune process occurs when the body's own immune system errantly attacks healthy cells. Why would this happen? Let's find out.
>
> First, maybe those so-called "healthy" cells are not really so healthy. Maybe their cell membranes are inflamed. Maybe their membranes are damaged by free radicals. Maybe those cells have pesticides locked inside. Maybe those cells have damaged chromosomes from airport scanners and cell phones. If the cell is damaged, it can become aberrant and such cells are slated for apoptosis (self-imposed destruction), or destruction by the immune system.
>
> Of 155,000 scholarly articles on methylation and autoimmune diseases, most cite the lack of methylation to maintain the DNA integrity.[4] Methylation is the process whereby DNA is repaired, telomeres repaired, and it's the process where unwanted gene expressions are deactivated. This makes having ample methyl groups available, particularly as a person ages, essential to a healthy life experience.[5] – Dr. Jack Tips, N.D., Ph.D., C.Hom., C.C.N.

Chronic Stress in All its Forms Impairs Methylation!

Methylation is critical to life for many reasons, including repair and detoxification. We naturally use up methyl groups as we age, but chronic stress, poor nutrition, alcohol, smoking, low stomach acid, toxic exposures and nutrient deficiencies (especially of methyl donor vitamins B6, B12 and folate), use them up more rapidly.[6,7] This leaves us vulnerable to accelerated aging and virtually every kind of disease. People in a state of chronic *fight or flight* use up millions of methyl groups as a consequence of overactivating this survival mechanism. Remember, the fight or flight response overrides all other metabolic functions, which means it takes the energy away from our body's normal processes to enable us to move quickly until danger passes. It makes sense that if you're stressed-out all the time, you are using up methyl groups that might otherwise be used for important metabolic processes like rest, tissue repair and detoxification.

It's far beyond the scope of this book to discuss every process involving methylation and all of the ways that it can get disrupted. As Dr. Jack Tipps writes, "A molecular biologist could write a million pages on methylation and only touch on a small fraction of the subject."[8]

> **What You Need to Know:**
> Improving your methylation is necessary for reversing your autoimmune condition and staying healthy for life!

> **What is a Methyl Donor?**
> A methyl donor is any substance that can transfer a methyl group (one carbon atom attached to three hydrogen atoms) to another substance, making methylation possible. Common Methyl Donors are S-adenosylmethionine (SAMe), cysteine, taurine, folate, B vitamins and TMG trimethylglycine (betaine).

Methylation and Glutathione

Improving methylation is important for everyone, but it's especially important if you have an autoimmune condition. One of the reasons is the role of methylation in detoxification and in the production and recycling of glutathione, the body's master antioxidant and "splinter" remover. Glutathione directly neutralizes free radicals, reduces hydrogen peroxide into water (reducing inflammation), and assists in the role of other antioxidants like vitamin C, E and lipoic acid. Glutathione contains sulfur groups, which are sticky compounds that adhere to toxins and heavy metals and carry them out of the body.

Studies have linked impaired methylation and low levels of glutathione to every type of autoimmune condition.[9] I haven't met anyone (including me), with any type of autoimmune condition, that has adequate methylation and levels of glutathione!

In a perfect world, your body makes its own glutathione from the amino acids cysteine, glycine and glutamine, and then recycles it via methylation using methyl donors like vitamin B12, folate, betaine and other nutrients. Under normal conditions, your body makes and recycles enough glutathione to handle all the toxins that you're exposed to. However, if you have a high toxic body burden, or a part of the methylation cycle is disrupted, you can get very sick!

Consider some possible scenarios:

- Glutathione can become depleted due to a high toxic load – meaning it gets used up faster than the body can make it. There are many toxins that deplete glutathione: alcohol, cigarette smoke, petrochemicals such as MTBE, pesticides and herbicides to name a few.
- Poor nutrition, especially low protein or vegan diets, can leave you without the essential building blocks for glutathione production.
- Your unique "genetic personality" might have difficulty creating and recycling enough glutathione.[10]
- You could be lacking the important nutrients (methyl donors), such as B12, folate and betaine, which are needed to produce and recycle glutathione. If you lack enough of these nutrients, it could be due to a

deficiency in your diet, or low stomach acid or some other factor like drinking too much alcohol, which impairs your ability to absorb these nutrients.

- You could have toxins, such as heavy metals, blocking your methylation pathways.
- You could have a "genetic trait" that impairs your ability to process folate, which is necessary for methylation. It's estimated that up to 40 percent of Americans have the MTHFR "trait" and are unable to convert folate from food into its active form (l-methylfolate).

The bottom line is that there are several factors that can contribute to impaired methylation and low glutathione levels. If you have an autoimmune condition, chances are you have one or more of these disrupting factors.

What You Can Do on Your Own

In Chapter 19: Detox Your Life, I'll discuss the ways you can begin to eliminate excess toxins from your environment and I'll share some special detox treatments. For now, let's talk about some of the ways you can enhance your liver's detoxification, improve your methylation and boost your glutathione with healing foods and nutritional supplements. Some of the information in this section is also covered in Chapter 14.

Restore Your Liver

The most reasonable step to enhance your liver's detoxification capacity is to reduce the amount of toxins it has to deal with. Here are some common sense reminders about what to avoid:

- Chronic stress
- Alcohol (alcohol abuse alone can destroy your liver)
- Smoking
- Caffeine
- Sugar
- Trans fats – hydrogenated fats
- Artificial sweeteners and flavorings
- Processed and junk foods
- Over-the-counter medications, especially Tylenol (acetaminophen)

(don't exceed recommended dosage ever, acetaminophen is the leading cause of acute liver failure in the U.S.) and NSAIDs like aspirin, naproxen (Naprosyn) and ibuprofen (Motrin)
- Recreational drugs
- Chemical exposure
- Long term, daily high intake of iron (over 45mg unless directed by a doctor), preformed (retinoid) vitamin A (over 10,000 units), or Niacin (over 2 gms)

Warning: Don't stop taking prescription medications without first discussing it with your doctor. Still, it can be helpful to find out if you are on any medication that is particularly hard on the liver. This list is far from exhaustive, but some examples are: codeine (pain killer); corticosteroids (taken to reduce inflammation); Augmentin, isoniazid, nitrofurantoin, and tetracycline (antibiotics); benzodiazepines like Valium (diazepam) and Restoril (temazepam) (anti-depressant, anti-anxiety); Tacrine (Cognex) (for treating Alzheimer's disease), Disulfiram (Antabuse) (for alcohol abuse); Lamisil (Terbinafine) (for fungal infections); and statin drugs for heart disease.

Restore Your Liver with Food

Your liver's Phase I and Phase II detoxification process requires adequate amounts of vitamins, antioxidants, minerals, amino acids, and phytochemicals found in healing foods.

You can do a lot to boost your liver's detox ability simply by eating abundantly from the core *Eating for your Good Genes* foods. Obviously, avoid any foods on the list that you know you have a negative reaction to.

- Apples
- Blackberries
- Blueberries
- Raspberries
- Artichokes – steamed or cooked
- Arugula
- Asparagus - steamed or cooked
- Bok choy - steamed or cooked
- Broccoli - steamed or cooked

- Brussels sprouts - steamed or cooked
- Cabbage
- Cauliflower - cooked
- Chard
- Collard greens
- Fennel
- Kale - steamed or cooked
- Spinach
- Beets and beet greens - steamed or cooked
- Carrots
- Onions
- Radishes
- Watercress
- Bone broths – made from organic natural meat
- Organic lean meats, such as beef, lamb and buffalo
- Organic poultry: turkey, chicken, game hen, pheasant
- Wild-caught fish: salmon or trout
- Hypoallergenic rice protein powder, whey protein powder or medical food

Restore Your Liver with Live Organic Juices

Your liver loves the antioxidants found in live organic juices. I have found that adding one or two live juice drinks per day, **in addition** to *Eating for Your Good Genes*, to be very beneficial for restoring liver function.

You can try a combination of any of the following:
- Apple
- Carrot
- Beetroot
- Beet leaves
- Dandelion greens
- Red radish or daikon radish
- Fennel
- Garlic
- Ginger
- Parsley

Michelle's Liver Bliss Detox Cocktail

2-cups dandelion greens
3-large carrots
1-large apple
1-fennel bulb
4-celery stalks
1-cup fresh parsley

Process all ingredients in the juicer of your choice. Shake or stir, and serve with a squeeze of lemon! Makes roughly 14 oz.

For more delicious juicing recipes, visit www.thethyroidcure.com/juicing!

A word of caution: I don't recommend juice or water "fasting" (drinking only juices and not eating food) for anyone with an autoimmune condition or other chronic illness, unless prescribed by a qualified practitioner. While there may be some healthy Mind-Body types that do well with juice and water fasting, I have found that most people with autoimmune conditions usually have higher stress levels, sluggish adrenals, nutritional deficiencies and impaired detox abilities, which can be worsened by juice and water fasting. Remember, your liver needs all the amino acids in protein for efficient phase II detoxification. If you're only drinking juices, you'll ramp up your liver's phase I detox, but may not be able to transform and eliminate all the intermediary metabolites that you've mobilized. This creates free radicals, which can damage your cells.

Juice fasting can also be dangerous for some people who have an imbalance between an overactive phase I detoxification and a slower phase II detoxification. This can be due to toxic exposure, nutritional deficiencies or genetics, and such a person is called a *pathological detoxifier*. Juice fasting can make this scenario worse and cause intermediary metabolites to accumulate in your body, making you feel even sicker than when you started!

> **What You Need to Know:**
> What you need to know: It's important to make sure you're getting all the right nutrients for your liver to function properly. You need the right balance of vitamins, antioxidants, minerals, amino acids and phytochemicals found in healing foods for your detoxification to be optimal. You need the amino acids found in protein for your liver's Phase II process to work efficiently. Many liver detox programs, such as popular juice fasts, ramp up Phase I with tons of antioxidants, but if you don't eat some kind of complete protein, the toxins build up and you will feel sick and toxic. That's why many people feel lousy on the second or third day of a juice fast!

Restore Your Liver with Herbs

There are several herbs that are proven to assist the liver's detoxification and stimulate bile secretion. Many of these herbs come in capsules as well as in loose teas and tea bags. Choose organic!

Look for these ingredients:
- Artichoke
- Chicory Root
- Barberry root bark
- Oregon grape root
- Beet leaf
- Burdock leaf and root
- Dandelion leaf and root
- Milk thistle
- Nettle
- Red Clover
- Turmeric
- Yellow Dock

Michelle's Liver Bliss Tonic

2 parts dandelion leaf or root
2 parts nettle
1 part burdock root
1 part yellow dock root

Use 4 tablespoons of herb mixture per quart of water. Place herbs in small saucepan and cover with water. Simmer for 25 minutes. Strain and serve. The tea will be stronger the longer it simmers. If it's too bitter for your taste, add lemon, ginger or stevia to taste.

Improve Your Methylation

For many people, improved methylation is a natural side effect of *Eating for Your Good Genes, Reducing Stress, Healing Your Gut,* and *Restoring Your Liver*. New research in epigenetics and nutrition (nutrigenomics) shows that you can change how your genes express themselves by improving your methylation with nutrition![11]

Here are some ways you can take control of your methylation and your genes:

- ***Eat healing greens!*** Eating tons of dark leafy green veggies daily provides you with natural folate (a methyl donor), necessary for proper methylation. Make sure to get a minimum of 2 cups of these healing foods per day.

- ***Get B vitamins and folate!*** B vitamins are methyl donors, especially folate, B6, B12 and riboflavin. *Eating for Your Good Genes* approved food sources of B vitamins are: organic chicken and beef liver, fish, eggs, dark leafy greens, asparagus, almonds, sunflower seeds and walnuts. Even if we eat right, most of us still need to supplement with B vitamins. Make sure your B complex or multivitamin contains adequate amounts of these important methylation cofactors. Look for folate in the form of l-methylfolate as Metafolin. **Note:** Dosages of B vitamins vary from person to person – I suggest nutritional testing to make sure you're getting the right dose. If you suspect that you have impaired methylation, it's important to start low and go slow. Introducing high-dose B vitamins and folate (l-methylfolate) can improve methylation fast, which ramps up detoxification, causing pathogens to "die off;" they release toxins as they die and those toxins make you feel sick. This is called a Herxheimer (Herx) reaction, also known as a "healing crisis." Increased methylation may also mobilize toxins such as heavy metals, which may also make you feel sick if it happens too fast.

- ***Support methylation with supplements!*** Make sure you get adequate amounts of magnesium and zinc, which support methylation. Take TMG trimethylglycine (betaine). **Note:** Dosage varies from person to person.
- ***Replace stomach acid!*** Remember, low stomach acid can interfere with the absorption of important nutrients such as vitamin B6, B12 and folate. Follow the guidelines in Chapter 16: Heal Your Gut.
- ***Take probiotics!*** Remember, the good bugs help produce and absorb B vitamins and folate!
- ***Reduce stress, booze, smoking and toxins!*** These toxic "splinters" burden and poison your liver, and use up methyl groups!

Boost Your Glutathione

Glutathione is the body's master antioxidant and a major "splinter" remover! Again, *Eating for Your Good Genes, Healing Your Gut, Restoring Your Liver* and *Improving Your Methylation* will automatically help boost glutathione levels in most people.

Here are some additional things you can do to boost your levels of this important antioxidant:

- ***Eat healing proteins!*** Eating foods that are high in the glutathione precursors, cysteine, glycine and glutamate will boost your glutathione levels. *Eating for Your Good Genes* approved food sources of these important amino acids include organic omega 3 enriched eggs, safe fish and organic lean meats.
- ***Eat healing sulfur foods!*** Sulfur is a key component of glutathione, so eating enough sulfur containing foods is vital. *Eating for Your Good Genes* approved food sources include garlic, onions and cruciferous vegetables like kale, broccoli, cauliflower, cabbage, watercress and bok choy. **Note**: Several older resources on thyroid conditions recommend avoiding cruciferous vegetables, claiming they are goitrogenic (interfering with iodine uptake to produce thyroid hormone). Let me assure you the cruciferous vegetables are safe, healthful and even protective for those with thyroid conditions as long as they are cooked, and you aren't iodine or selenium deficient.

- ***Get more sulfur!*** Another way to get sulfur is by absorbing it through the skin by taking detox baths with Epsom salt (magnesium sulfate). Studies have shown sulfur baths are capable of boosting glutathione and reducing oxidative stress.[12]

- ***Take healing protein powder!*** Undenatured whey protein powder, has been proven to boost glutathione levels by converting cysteine into glutathione, and it has many other immune enhancing properties.[13] If you are allergic to whey (which comes from dairy), you can try a hypoallergenic rice protein powder. Rice protein contains cysteine, a glutathione precursor. Take 1-2 scoops of protein powder per day in water, juice or smoothie.

- ***Take selenium!*** Selenium plays an important role in the production of glutathione. Take 200 to 400 mcg per day.[14]

- ***Optimize your antioxidants!*** Vitamins, C, D and E all boost glutathione levels.[15,16,17,18] Make sure you're getting optimal values every day!

- ***Move your body!*** Besides supporting reducing stress and depression, exercise also boosts your glutathione levels and improves detoxification.[19] Just do it!

- ***Get enough sleep!*** Studies show that lack of sleep can deplete glutathione.[20] Individual need for sleep varies. Make sure your get between 7-10 hours of sleep nightly.

- ***Herbs to support glutathione*** Studies have shown that milk thistle (silymarin) can boost glutathione levels.[21] Take between 100 and 300 mg per day.

- ***Spice it up!*** Curcumin has been shown to raise glutathione levels in the liver; one more good reason to use this anti-inflammatory spice![22] You can also take a curcumin supplement. Individual doses vary.

- ***Additional supplements to boost glutathione:*** N-acetyl-l-cysteine (NAC) is a synthetically derived source of cysteine and a basic building block for glutathione production.[23] Most practitioners recommend 600 mg, 2 times per day. Alpha lipoic acid is a critical substance for many body functions and it works alongside glutathione in detoxification.[24]

Standard dose is 100 to 200 mg, three times per day. SAM-e is an important methyl donor that helps synthesize glutathione in the liver.[25] Start with 400 mg, once a day in the morning. **Important:** Dosages of these supplements vary from person to person. Please work with a qualified functional or integrative practitioner to find the right dose for you.

- ***Glutathione supplements:*** Glutathione supplements come in capsules and creams. The jury is still out on the your body's ability to use these supplements (known as their bioavailability), and whether they raise glutathione levels inside the cell where it's needed, but the research is promising.[26] Look for oral products that contain liposomal glutathione such as BioGlute™. We have less research on transdermal glutathione creams but many practitioners have observed their efficacy. Personally, I like Super Oxicell from Apex Energetics.

- ***Glutathione Rx:*** Glutathione can be administered via IV, or compounded by a pharmacist and taken via injection, nebulizer, transdermal gel, capsule or suppository. Ask your practitioner if any of these treatments are right for you.

Avoiding toxins, lowering your stress, healing your GI, and consuming foods and supplements that support methylation and glutathione can enhance your body's ability to naturally detoxify and heal.

For a safe 14-day liver restoration program, including meal plans, please visit www.thethyroidcure.com/14dayliverbliss

Many times, just following the guidelines in this and the previous chapters is enough to reverse your autoimmune condition, and keep you healthy and vibrant for life. But sometimes doing everything "right" is not enough. While the strategies above work well for the majority of people, there are still those whose don't feel good, or may even feel worse. It's beyond the scope of this book to discuss all of the nuances one can experience while working this program alone. If you don't feel well, it makes sense to take the guesswork out and work with a qualified medical practitioner who can order testing and guide you through the detoxification process. **If you scored high on the *Toxic Stress Assessment*,** you may benefit from functional medical and genomic testing. This advanced testing can help you and your practitioner figure out your specific nutritional needs, your toxic burden and even determine if your unique "genetic personality" presents challenges to your methylation and detoxification capabilities.

> **Do Frogs have Bad Genes?**
>
> When scientists report that a third of the world's amphibians are dying off and becoming extinct due to toxic exposures and reduced habitats, do they blame it on the animal's bad genes?[27] No! In fact, as Russell A. Mittermeier, president of Conservation International (CI) says, "Amphibians are one of nature's best indicators of overall environmental health. Their catastrophic decline serves as a warning that we are in a period of significant environmental degradation."
>
> Apparently some scientists understand that frogs are sensitive creatures, with permeable skins, that are unable to tolerate toxic chemicals. I'm not sure why the same wisdom doesn't apply to humans. I'm always surprised when I hear medical experts talk about "bad genes" and "genetic defects" in relation to chronic illness. It may be true that some people naturally have better detoxification pathways than others, but that doesn't mean that any of us are built to tolerate the insane levels of chemicals we're exposed to! If you live on planet earth, you have been exposed to far too many toxins, regardless of your genetics. If you have an autoimmune condition, chances are that you more sensitive than others and your illness serves as a huge wake up call for humanity!
>
> Genetic testing can be an invaluable tool that can help you discover how your unique genes may be affected by stress, poor nutrition and toxins, and can help your practitioner design a program to help you get better or avoid getting sick in the first place. But it's a mistake to see yourself as "genetically flawed" just because you're getting sick in our increasingly toxic world. Just like our amphibian friends, your body is designed to thrive in a healthy environment that includes clean air, clean water and clean food – don't forget that!

When You May Need a Practitioner – Test, Don't Guess!

As you have learned, lowering stress, eating for your unique Mind-Body, healing your gut and improving your detoxification are critical steps in reversing any type of autoimmune condition. It doesn't matter if it's Hashimoto's, or Graves'; the splinters have to come out for your body to heal. For many people, this is a fairly simple process and involves lifestyle changes, improved nutrition and taking the right nutritional supplements.

For others, it's not so simple. While the majority of autoimmune thyroid sufferers bounce back quickly after making lifestyle changes, it's my experience that some don't. I have also found that people with advanced autoimmune conditions have a difficult time navigating a detoxification program alone.

If you have been diagnosed with a more serious autoimmune condition such as lupus, multiple sclerosis (MS), Sjögren's syndrome or rheumatoid arthritis (RA), or if you suffer from chronic fatigue syndrome (CFS) or fibromyalgia, you most likely have some functional imbalances that need to be corrected, or "splinters" such as toxins or infections that need to be identified and treated. The best way to know for sure is by working with a functional or integrative medical practitioner who can review your life history and your unique symptoms, and then prescribe the appropriate tests and treatment.

If you don't already have a functional medical doctor, you can find one by visiting the Institute for Functional Medicine's website at www.functionalmedicine.org. Click on the tab "Functional Medicine Resources" and choose "Find a Functional Medicine Practitioner" to find someone in your area. We have also compiled a list of practitioners on *The Thyroid Cure* Web site at www.thethyroidcure.com/practitioners.

If you find a practitioner in your area, be sure to ask if they have experience with advanced functional medical testing and detoxification. At this point in time, you may have to travel out of your area to find a qualified practitioner. I see that changing in the next few years as more and more physicians realize the limitations of conventional medicine in treating autoimmune conditions. There are thousands of medical doctors, physician's assistants, nurse practitioners, chiropractors, doctors of oriental medicine, nutritionists and health coaches joining the ranks of functional medicine every year and the numbers are growing.

Mercury and Autoimmunity

As you learned in Chapter 9, mercury and other heavy metals are splinters in many autoimmune conditions. If you are concerned that you have a high heavy metal exposure, it's important to get tested for these toxins. If you have silver amalgam fillings in your mouth, consider having them safely removed. Ask your dentist if she is aware of the protocol to safely remove amalgam fillings or visit the International Academy of Oral Medicine and Toxicology at https://iaomt.org/safe-removal-amalgam-fillings.[28] Mercury was a huge toxic splinter in my autoimmune condition and in the conditions of many of my client's as well. I'm not sure why the human mouth is considered the only safe receptacle for mercury as it is so toxic that its use and disposal is heavily regulated otherwise.[29] Recent studies have shown that removing silver amalgam fillings alone can improve an autoimmune condition.[30]

Natural Detoxification Versus Chelation Therapy

Improving your methylation and boosting your glutathione will help your body mobilize and clear toxins and pathogens naturally. Chelation therapy is designed to help carry large amounts of built-up toxins out all at once. It's important to understand how chelation therapy differs from improving your body's own detoxification.

Imagine your body as the house you live in. You're continually tracking in dirt and making little messes during the course of daily life. Now imagine your vacuum is broken, and you've run out of cleaning supplies. Since you don't have the tools to keep your house clean, the dirt accumulates and before you know it you're living in filth! That's what it's like to have impaired methylation and detoxification.

Now imagine you hire a housekeeping service to come in and do a one-time rough clean to get the dirt that's piled up. They manage to clean up most of the accumulated dirt and scum, but they don't do anything to fix your vacuum or restock your cleaning supplies. Chelation is similar; it's a one-time or periodic therapy to clear the toxins that have built up over time. If you don't fix your vacuum, restock your cleaning supplies and make housecleaning a regular habit, the dirt will eventually pile up again!

Chelation might sound convenient, but it's only effective for certain toxins and it does nothing to improve your detoxification for the future. If you have a very high toxic load chelation can be used as a first aid treatment while you work to reduce your toxic exposure and improve your body's natural detoxification.

It's important to *Heal Your Gut*, and *Restore Your Liver* before considering a more intense detoxification program. It's possible to mobilize toxins and heavy metals but if you have a leaky gut, or your liver is compromised, you might just re-distribute those toxins back into your bloodstream where they can find their way into other organs like your brain! Nutrigenomic testing can reveal any genetic challenges that need to be circumvented to improve methylation and detoxification.

If you've ever cleaned a house that's been dirty for a long time, you know that sometimes things can look worse during the cleanup process. The same thing can happen when you restore your body's natural detoxification processes. You might feel worse for a time as the toxic dirt in your system gets stirred up. You might worry that you're having a bad reaction to your therapy or supplements. Functional tests can be useful to monitor the elimination of your toxic splinters, so that you know your detoxification is improving.

Functional Testing for Toxic Splinters

Below is a list of functional medical tests you can use to assess your health. Ask your integrative or functional medical practitioner which ones are right for you.

Heavy Metals:

- *Nutrient and Toxic Elements – Hair - by Metametrix*
- *Nutrient and Toxic Elements – Urine - by Metametrix*

Chemicals:

- *Toxic Effects CORE by Metametrix* – CORE stands for "Chemical Occurrence & Related Exposure" and assesses the body's toxic burden, particularly due to chemical exposures. The CORE tests of a wide range of chemical exposures such as Bisphenol A (BPA), Organophosphates, Phthalates and Parabens, Chlorinated Pesticides, PCBs, and Volatile Solvents

Nutritional Testing:

- *NutrEval® Blood and Urine by Genova Diagnostics* – This blood-and-urine combo test evaluates your need for antioxidants, B vitamins, amino acids, essential fatty acids, and minerals. You'll also find out if you have imbalances in the GI tract or problems with detoxification.

- *ION™ - Blood and Urine by Metametrix* – ION stands for "Individual•Optimal•Nutrition." This is a comprehensive test that measures levels of organic acids, fatty acids, amino acids, vitamins, minerals and antioxidants to help evaluate a host of body functions.

Genomic Testing:

- *DetoxiGenomic®* **Profile by** *Genova Diagnostics* – This genetic test identifies genetic variables that can indicate increased risk of impaired detoxification capacity, especially in concert with environmental toxins. The test also alerts individuals to potentially adverse drug reactions based on their genetic profile.

- *NeuroGenomic™ Profile by Genova Diagnostics* – This test evaluates single nucleotide polymorphisms (SNPs) in genes that modulate methylation, glutathione conjugation, oxidative protection and the potential to evaluate vascular oxidation

- *MTHFR Genotyping by SpectraCell Laboratories* – This test identifies variants of the MTHFR genetic coding which can interfere with the ability to process folate needed for methylation and can result in elevated levels of homocysteine, a risk factor in several serious conditions. Knowing if you have a MTHFR variant may help determine if taking folate (often in combination with vitamins B6 and B12) may mitigate the issues connected to MTHFR variants.

In the next chapter I'll review some common infectious splinters in autoimmunity.

CHAPTER 18

Clear Infections

"It is becoming increasingly acceptable and recognized that infections are probably an underappreciated cause of chronic disease."
– SIOBHAN O'CONNOR, M.D. Associate director of the National Center for Infectious Diseases at the Center for Disease Control, American Medical News, July 9, 2004

Infections and Autoimmunity

The relationship between infections and autoimmunity has been heavily researched and today there is no doubt that infectious inflammation is a "splinter" in many autoimmune conditions. Scientists have now observed several mechanisms through which viruses, bacteria and fungi can initiate or exacerbate an autoimmune condition.

There are several theories that make sense, here are just a few:

Molecular mimicry is the theory that infectious pathogens share structural, functional or immunological similarities to host tissues.[1,2] In other words, bad bugs and viruses can sometimes "look" the same as our healthy tissue. When we have an infection, our immune system can mistake healthy tissue (self-antigens) for the bad bugs and destroy our own cells by mistake.

Bystander activation is the theory that infections can non-specifically stimulate the immune system in a manner that misfires in autoimmunity.[3] Bystander activation doesn't require a similarity of self and pathogen as in molecular mimicry. Additionally, during an infection, healthy cells that are in the area of the infection can be caught in the crossfire and killed as a result.

Protein changes, cryptic antigens, is the theory that infections cause an inflammatory environment that can lead to cellular death, oxidative stress and free radical production, which can transform "self" proteins into "non-self."[4] In other words, inflammation can cause your healthy cells to mutate into non-self cells. In addition, proteins in the cells that are ordinarily shielded from the immune system become exposed to, and subsequently attacked by, the immune system.

Infections deplete glutathione: Researchers have found that certain bacteria such as *Borrelia burgdorferi,* the bacterium responsible for Lyme disease, can deplete glutathione, your body's master antioxidant.[5] As you have already learned, low levels of glutathione are linked with all autoimmune conditions as well as chronic fatigue syndrome (CFS). New research links glutathione depletion within the cells to the activation of latent viruses and chlamydia and it may also be responsible for reactivation of other latent bacteria within the cells.[6,7,8,9,10] According to independent chronic fatigue syndrome (CFS) researcher Richard A. Van Konynenburg Ph.D., glutathione depletion triggers the reactivation of latent Epstein-Barr virus, cytomegalovirus and HHV-6 in CFS patients.[11] This hypothesis makes a lot sense and likely applies to autoimmunity as well. Dr. Van Konynenburg also takes note of Taylor's paper that suggests that Coxsackie B3 viruses thrive by weakening the host's immune system through depleting the selenium needed for the body to make glutathione.[12] In other words, viruses can battle your immune system by depleting the resources your body needs to make the glutathione it needs to fight back.

Throughout the literature, researchers agree that while infections play a role in many autoimmune conditions, the "host environment" or "the state of your body" is where the real story is told. As Dr. Amy Yasko says in her groundbreaking book, *Defeat Autism Now, "It may not be enough to hunt down and kill an individual microbe. We may instead need to consider all of the factors that undermine health and balance in order to create an environment less hospitable to microbial overrun."*

The inconvenient truth is that numerous factors can contribute to an autoimmune condition. There is no single cause. While infections play a role, not everyone exposed to a virus or bacteria will become infected. Not everyone who becomes infected will be unable to fight it off, allowing a chronic or stealth infection to take hold. Finally, not everyone with a chronic infection will get an autoimmune condition.

Years of chronic stress, negative emotions, malnutrition, GI imbalances, impaired detoxification and disrupted methylation can trigger a cascade of events – a "perfect storm" so to speak – and an infection may be the straw that breaks the camel's back. Almost every article on autoimmunity and infections affirms that hypomethylation of host DNA plays a major role in the process.[13] In other words, scientists have found that the disruption of your body's natural healing and detoxification processes creates the conditions for immune system misfire.

The underlying mechanisms linking infections to autoimmunity is a fascinating topic and researchers are learning more everyday.

> **What You Need to Know:**
> Scientists have made amazing discoveries that connect the dots between infections and autoimmunity. If you have an autoimmune condition and an infection anywhere in your body, it's critical to strengthen your immune system by balancing your body's core systems. It's common sense really; infections = inflammation, and inflammation keeps your immune system on high alert!

The good news is that by optimizing your nutrition, *reducing stress*, getting enough sleep, healing your G.I. tract, restoring your liver and improving your methylation, you take a big step towards fighting any infection lurking under the surface that might trigger or exacerbate your autoimmune condition. In my experience, many infections clear up on their own when you restore your body's core systems to balance. In fact, many times improving your GI and liver function will start to clear infections and drive viruses into remission, *due to boosting glutathione and improving methylation.*

It's not always that simple though; some people have several infectious "splinters" burdening their system. Let me share Maria's story with you. At 64, she had been living with lupus for over 15 years. She had elevated liver enzymes, sore joints, aching muscles, GI distress and a malar rash (also called a butterfly rash) over her nose and cheeks. Her health history recounted a lifetime of numerous infections. A survivor of sexual abuse, she was diagnosed with herpes at 13 years old and had frequent outbreaks ever since. At 24, she was diagnosed with chlamydia. She explained that she probably had it for years before the infection finally caused fallopian scarring resulting in an ectopic pregnancy. She had two episodes of walking pneumonia, one while she was in college and the other at the age of 48, a year before she was diagnosed with lupus. She confessed to a history of drug and alcohol abuse and added that her "teeth started going bad" when she was in her late 20s. She had advanced periodontal disease and had lost several of her teeth due to infections. She had four failing and infected root canals. She also suffered with chronic sinusitis and recurring fungal infections.

I asked her if she remembered a point in time when she felt well, and when her health took a turn for the worse. Her eyes lit up and she said, "I never thought of this before but the last pneumonia really knocked me down. I haven't been the same since!"

Maria's case was far beyond my scope of practice as a health advocate. I explained that I could help her improve her nutrition and provide her with relevant research about the triggers in autoimmunity, but that her recovery would involve more than following an elimination diet and taking vitamins. I recommended she consult with a medical doctor and a dentist before moving forward. She was already under the care of a warm and compassionate rheumatologist who turned out to have a curiosity about the role of infections in autoimmunity. He was surprised to learn that she had suffered so many previous infections. Due to her history of walking pneumonia, he tested her for mycoplasma and sure enough, she had an active infection. He referred her to an ear, nose and throat specialist (ENT) who determined her sinus infection to be a fungus.

Both doctors agreed that the failing root canals would have to come out. She was treated for the fungal sinusitis and mycoplasma, and after 3 months her liver tests improved. She followed the *Sensitivity Discovery Program* and found that dairy, nightshade vegetables (peppers, tomatoes and eggplant but not potatoes) and all grains triggered her symptoms, especially the sore joints and butterfly rash. She began eating tons of healing veggies, healing fats and small amounts of lean organic animal protein. She started taking a good multivitamin, a B complex with l-methylfolate, essential fatty acids, magnesium, zinc, digestive enzymes and probiotics.

After 9 months, all her labs had improved and her digestion was "great." Her sore joints and rash were gone! She said she had more good days than bad ones and felt that a total recovery was possible. Convinced that the final piece of the puzzle would be to remove the infected root canals, she was saving up for dental treatment.

Unfortunately, Maria's story is not uncommon. She had other splinters in her condition but treating her infections took a lot of stress off her immune system and helped her heal.

Successful treatment of infections can be complex due to many factors. Your unique physiology (Mind-Body type), life circumstances and nutrition must be taken into consideration. *If you scored high on the Infectious Stress Assessment,* I suggest you work with an integrative or functional medical practitioner to get the right tests and treatment. Integrative and functional medical doctors can prescribe both natural and pharmaceutical agents to treat infections. They can also design a treatment plan to help boost your immunity and bring your body's core systems into balance.

Common Infections Associated with Autoimmunity

These infections may or may not be symptomatic, and include:

- **GI infections: bacteria, fungus, parasites**
- **Gingivitis and periodontal disease**
- **Infected root canals or dental implants**
- **Chronic sinusitis**
- **Chronic and systemic fungal infections**
- **Bacterial infections:** *Mycoplasma,* **chlamydia,** *Mycobacterium tuberculosis* **(TB),** *Klebsiella, Streptococcus, Staphylococcus aureus* **(staph),** *Brucella*
- **Viruses: herpes, human papillomavirus (HPV), Epstein Barr, hepatitis B, coxsackie B, carvovirus B-19**
- **Tick Borne Disease:** *Borrelia burgdorferi* **(Lyme)**

What You can Do on Your Own to Clear Infections!

There are steps you can take today to begin to clear up infections and reduce the bacterial and viral burden on your immune system.

- ***Clean up Your Mouth!*** If you have gingivitis or periodontal disease (gum disease), it's critical that you get treated immediately. If you're not on a first name basis with a dental hygienist, I suggest you get to know one right away. Many people don't realize they have infections in their mouth. You might not think twice if your gums bleed when you brush your teeth, but if your hands bled when you washed them, or your scalp bled when you brushed your hair, you'd be alarmed! Your gums are no different. If they bleed, you've got a problem. I used to work in dental offices that utilized dental microscopes; you would not believe the bad bugs that can wind up in your mouth! You can take huge load off of your immune system by keeping your mouth as clean as possible. Home dental care is easy and affordable; you need to brush and floss your teeth every day. You might be surprised to learn that flossing is more important than brushing.

If you have deep pockets or gingivitis, a dental water irrigator like a WaterPik® can be a big help; only use irrigation solutions that don't contain alcohol. Alcohol damages the mucosal tissue and can even help certain bad bugs populate. A solution of six or seven drops of grapefruit seed extract (GSE) by Nutribiotic® in water can be used in your WaterPik, or you can rinse your mouth with it. GSE makes a great toothbrush disinfectant as well – soak your toothbrush in it overnight. Make sure to change your toothbrush every 3 months or when the bristles begin to fray. I recommend using a Sonicare toothbrush if you can afford one. Don't ever use anyone else's toothbrush and store yours separately from the rest of the household! Additionally, buy mouthwashes and toothpaste that do not contain sodium laurel sulfate or fluoride. I like the Dental Herb Company. www.dentalherb.com.

The Ayurvedic practice of tongue scraping is quick and easy, and contributes to a clean mouth. One study showed that tongue scraping significantly reduced bacteria known to cause tooth decay (*Streptococcus mutans* and *Lactobacillus*) and also reduced bad breath.[14] Specialized stainless steel U-shaped tongue scrapers are inexpensive and available in health food stores and online. You simply start with the back of your tongue and slowly scrape to the tip five to ten times. The whole procedure takes less than 30 seconds. Another study confirmed that an added benefit of tongue scraping is an improved sense of taste.[15]

- **Clean up Your Nose!** If you suffer from chronic sinusitis, it's is a good idea to find out if it's due to fungus. Recent research indicates that chronic sinusitis is an immune disorder that arises when the immune system attacks fungi in the sinuses, causing damage to sinus membrane in the process. 75% of the patients improved when the fungus was treated.[16,17] Check the section at the end of this chapter, ***When You May Need a Practitioner – Test, Don't Guess!*** If your doctor determines that your symptoms are due to a fungal infection, it can be treated with a topical antifungal agent. You may need a prescription for this.

    My clients (and I) have had success combining a saline solution such as NeilMed Sinus Rinse with one or two drops of grapefruit seed extract (GSE). You can make your own saline solution and use a neti pot as well. **Caution:** Never use more than one or two drops of GSE and always combine it with the saline solution – otherwise it can really burn! Another effective sinus remedy is to inhale the essential oils of concentrated organic thyme, clove and cinnamon leaf extracts. You simply add a few drops of each to a bowl of steaming hot water, cover your head with a towel, and breathe in deeply for a few minutes. Believe me, this very effective! Make sure you use only high quality organic concentrates. I have used Sinus Doctor, available at www.sinusinfectiondiscovery.com.

    Almost all traditional medical systems connect the sinuses with the GI tract. Interestingly, many people notice that their chronic sinusitis disappears when they remove aggravating foods and heal their gut!

    Finally, studies have shown that yoga and pranayama breathing can help heal chronic sinusitis.[18] The positive health benefits of yogic breathing are scientifically documented and too numerous to list.[19]

- **Reclaim the Healthy Erotic:** Sex and making love can be some of our most pleasurable and transformative experiences. Great sex is our birthright! Whether you're in a monogamous partnership, have "friends with benefits" or are just "hooking up," having sex with another person means sharing that person's bodily fluids and their bugs. We humans, regardless of our sexual orientation or religious beliefs, have a lot of emotional hang-ups around sex. Personally, I feel that sexually transmitted diseases (STDs) are one of the symptoms of our collective wound of shame. That's a whole separate book. My point is; sex is still an uncomfortable topic for a lot of people (for every reason under the sun). Many of us don't talk about it enough, even with our partners. Unfortunately what happens in the dark stays in the dark – not just in Vegas – and the results can be harmful to the mind, body and soul.

Most of the women who have come to me for help with autoimmune conditions had a history of some sexually transmitted disease. While many were aware of their past infections, some didn't know if they had ever been infected and others were too afraid to find out. One client told me, "If it's going on below my waist, I don't even want to know about it!" My simple advice is this: Find a doctor or nurse practitioner that you feel comfortable with and get tested. Don't judge yourself. Instead, use this as an opportunity to take your power back. Part of reclaiming the healthy erotic is to become aware of your body and illuminate any darkness or confusion surrounding your sexuality. Establish healthy boundaries with your sexual partners. Don't assume anything! This might sound simplistic but make a point to talk about sex with your sexual partner. You have a right to know about their sexual history and whether they are, or have ever been, infected with an STD. They also have right to know your sexual history and status. Practice safe sex (use barriers). Change condoms when switching from oral or anal sex to vaginal sex, to prevent the introduction of harmful bacteria into the vagina. If your partner has an infection (of any kind) don't have sex, even oral sex, until the infection is cleared up. If your sexual partner has periodontal disease, gingivitis or any infectious disease (such as fungus or candida) they are contagious. You can't afford to kiss them until they cleanup their mouth. The same goes for oral sex!

Practice good hygiene; always wash before and after sex. If you are a woman prone to bladder infections or cystitis, always pee after sex and make sure you wipe from front to back when you use the restroom. For more information on home remedies for infections and irritations of the vagina and bladder, visit my website at www.thethyroidcure.com/yonihealth

- ***Eat for Your Good Genes, Reduce Stress, Heal Your Gut and Restore Your Liver!*** Honestly, if you follow the steps outlined in the previous chapters, you will naturally improve your capacity to fight infections. Eating for your good genes will starve out yeast and fungus (candida); following the GI healing protocol will control yeast and bad bugs. Restoring your liver function will improve methylation and boost glutathione, which are both proven infection fighters. Reducing stress and getting enough rest are classic no-brainers to boost immunity. I have seen amazing recoveries from all types of infections when people eat right, reduce stress and heal their gut!

- ***Get Vitamin D3!*** Vitamin D3 plays a major role in our immune response, defending against infections and bacteria by activating and arming killer T-cells. It reduces inflammation throughout the system and modulates the expression of important genes. Most people with autoimmune conditions are grossly deficient. It's impossible to get enough vitamin D3 through your diet. The body makes vitamin D3 mostly from our exposure to sunlight. Research indicates that 3 out of 4 teens and adults and practically all blacks and Hispanics don't get enough vitamin D3.[20] Getting more sun can improve your health and improve your mood at the same time. Try to get 15-30 minutes of unprotected sun exposure two to four times a week. Vitamin D3 supplementation is inexpensive and well worth it for significant health benefits. I recommend getting tested so you know how much you need. It's safe to start with at 2000 IU per day but research and my experience shows most people need twice that amount to raise their levels. Don't take more than 10,000 IU a day in order to avoid vitamin D3 toxicity.

- ***Sweat!*** Raising body temperature helps fight infections and fungus; our body develops a fever for that same purpose. Hypothyroid patients commonly have below-average body temperatures, which in turn creates an environment where infections (especially fungal) can thrive. Try a far-infra-red sauna or a detoxifying bath. I give more information on these therapies in Chapter 19: Detox Your Life.

> **A Word on Candida, Candida Related Complex and Systemic Candida...**
>
> There is fungus among us! Fungal infections are far more widespread than most people think. In fact, statistics suggest that over one billion people a year get infected with some kind of fungus and that number is growing.[21] Fungal infections may spring up on their own, but often arise from the vulnerability created by other diseases, or antibiotic or immunosuppressive drugs. For example, antibiotics kill many of the "good bugs" populating the GI tract and vagina, allowing the fungus *Candida albicans*, that is always present but held in check by those "good bugs," to proliferate and become an infection. 70% of women will get a vaginal yeast (*Candida*) infection at some point in their lives. Many people are susceptible to *candida* related bladder infections.[22] More seriously, patients with AIDs often die from fungal pneumonia. Cancer, TB and asthma often lead to serious secondary fungal infections.
>
> When I was diagnosed with Hashimoto's, I had positive antibodies IgM, IgG, IgA to *Candida,* indicating a current and long-term infection. I did not have any visible signs of fungus on my body but I did get recurrent UTI's (that never once tested positive for bacteria), and chronic sinusitis. I had to strengthen my immune system, and get fungus under control, for my health to get better.
>
> You can get a fungal infection just about anywhere in or on your body:
> - Skin and nails
> - Urogenital tract (yeast infection and bladder infections)
> - Mouth and throat (thrush)
> - GI infection
> - Sinuses
> - Systemic infection (fungus gets in the blood, potentially life-threatening)
>
> **What is Candida Related Complex?**
>
> Besides obvious and easily treated *Candida* vaginal yeast infections and deadly systemic blood infections, there seem to be low-grade, stealth *Candida* infections that often go undetected, leading to a condition referred to as *Candida* Related Complex (CRC) and a host of vague but persistent and unpleasant symptoms including fatigue, anxiety, depression and fibromyalgia. One theory suggests that long term *Candida* proliferation

burdens the immune system and another view proposes that *Candida* infections contribute to inflammation and leaky gut syndrome, in turn allowing foreign particles past the intestinal wall into the bloodstream, leading to multiple symptoms and potentially triggering autoimmunity. *Candida* related complex has been little studied and you will find that many mainstream medical doctors are more than skeptical that chronic *Candida* infections even exist, let alone that they can cause a systemic influence through *Candida* related complex.

If you suspect that you have a problem with *Candida*, it's important that you insist on being tested, even if your doctor is hesitant. You might have to find a new practitioner who will work with you to check for fungus. In my role as a medical advocate, I have met a number of doctors who didn't feel *Candida* was a possible problem but who nonetheless tested for it and found it in my clients after we insisted on the proper tests.

Fighting Fungus!

You shouldn't be surprised to learn that probiotics along with a diet low in sugar and processed carbs (that the fungus thrive on) will go a long way to keep fungus under control.

For those who need to treat fungus more aggressively, often with the help of a practitioner, here's an outline of the various conventional treatments for fungus:

Different antifungal medications are used depending on the type and location of the infection. There are topical over-the-counter medications for genital yeast infections. Tea tree oil is a wonderful natural topical antifungal. The oil can be diluted and used in a douche or topically for skin and nail fungus. *Candida* infections located in the gut or throughout the system are usually treated with prescription and natural anti-fungal medications. Some of the more powerful oral pharmaceutical anti-fungals can be hard on the liver and many practitioners will test for liver function periodically while the patient is on these medications. Intravenous medication is prescribed for the worst systemic infections that sometimes arise in immunocompromised people such as those with AIDS, cancer and other serious conditions. Oral thrush often resolves on its own, but is sometimes treated with antifungal mouthwashes or lozenges. There are countless alternative protocols for utilizing natural remedies for *Candida* but a discussion of all those options is beyond the scope of this book. My advice is that if you think you have *Candida*, get tested and treated!

Supplements to Fight Infections and Boost Immunity

We each have a unique Mind-Body Type so it's impossible to outline which supplements, at which dosages, will work for every infection, and for every person, every time. There are literally hundreds of natural remedies for almost every kind of infection. Remember that any plant or substance, whether used as food or medicine, externally or internally, can cause an allergic reaction in some people. Not only that, but some herbs such as echinacea, astragalus and green tea (to name just a few), can act as immune system modulators and influence both Th1 and Th2 responses. This can be a good thing, but it can also be problematic. It will save you time, money and aggravation to work with a qualified medical professional to get the right treatment for what ails you.

Below are some supplements that are very effective at fighting infections.

- ***Garlic***: Garlic has wonderful anti-inflammatory properties and has been used for centuries as an herbal remedy for infections. Garlic has anticancer, antioxidant, cardiovascular and antimicrobial properties. Garlic can be eaten fresh or taken in capsules, oils and tinctures. Garlic may also be used as a topical treatment for fungus such as ringworm and athlete's foot.[23]

- ***Grapefruit seed extract (GSE)***: Studies have found grapefruit seed extract to be an excellent safe antimicrobial, antifungal and antibacterial.[24] GSE can be used both internally and topically for both fungus and bacteria. I personally use GSE made by Nutribiotic.

- ***Olive leaf extract (OLE):*** Olive leaf extract contains oleuropein, which has antiviral, antimicrobial, antioxidant, anti-inflammatory, anti-atherogenic, anti-cancer and anti-hypertensive properties.[25] One study demonstrated that olive leaf extract was effective at selectively reducing H. pylori and Staphylococcus aureus (including MRSA) bacterium.[26] It has been reported to support natural killer cells and to be effective against viruses like HIV, hepatitis B and C, and herpes.[27] There are many brands of Olive leaf extract, liquid and capsules, with varying percentages of the active component oleuropein (look for 15-18%), so refer to the label for suggested dosage.

- **Neem**: Neem has been used in Ayurveda for its antifungal and antimicrobial properties for thousands of years. Many Indians actually use a twig from the neem tree as a toothbrush to control oral bacteria, and natural toothpastes made from neem are available. Studies have confirmed neem to be an effective antifungal.[28,29] Neem is available as a liquid extract, in tablets and capsules, and in topical creams, soaps and other products. Because of the wide variety of neem treatments, use as directed on the label.

- **Undenatured whey protein:** Undenatured cold processed whey protein may be the best food source for boosting your glutathione, and boosting your glutathione is a very powerful way to increase your body's natural healing and detoxification capacity. Undenatured whey protein contains the amino acids used for glutathione production (cysteine, glycine and glutamate) and studies confirm it raises glutathione.[30] Of course it is also a good source of concentrated protein. Immunocal is a quality whey protein powder that is listed in the *Physicians Desk Reference* (PDR) and has been subject to clinical trials that demonstrate its ability to boost glutathione.

We've all been conditioned to "take a pill" when we get sick instead of correcting the imbalances that lowered our immunity in the first place. It's true that sometimes we need help to fight off infections, but trust me when I tell you; an infection is not the result of an antibiotic, antimicrobial, antiviral or antifungal medicine deficiency! Remember, it's not just about "killing bugs" – it's about boosting your body's ability to fight infections, and that requires a personalized healing program.

When You May Need a Practitioner – Test, Don't Guess!

If you scored high on the Infectious Stress Assessment, or you have been diagnosed with a serious autoimmune or autoimmune related condition such as lupus, multiple sclerosis (MS), Sjögren's syndrome, rheumatoid arthritis (RA), chronic fatigue syndrome (CFS) or fibromyalgia, and you feel you might have an infectious "splinter", I suggest you make an appointment with a functional or integrative medical practitioner who can review your life history and your unique symptoms, and then prescribe the appropriate tests and treatment.

You Really Can't Afford to Guess About What Might be Bugging You!

If you don't already have a functional medical doctor, you can find one by visiting the Institute for Functional Medicine's website at www.functionalmedicine.org. Click on the tab "Functional Medicine Resources" and choose "Find a Functional Medicine Practitioner" to find someone in your area. We have also compiled a list of practitioners on *The Thyroid Cure* Web site at www.thethyroidcure.com/practitioners.

Testing for Infectious Splinters

The tests for infections splinters are standard tests that may be ordered by a licensed healthcare provider. Alternatively, you can order some of these tests without a doctor's prescription online through companies such as www.mymedlab.com or www.directlabs.com. I have given extra detail about the tests I feel may need more explanation.

Testing for GI infections: bacteria, fungus, parasites
- Refer to Chapter 16: Testing for GI Function pg. 311

Testing for gingivitis, periodontal disease, infected root canals and dental implants
- Make an appointment with a dentist for a physical exam and treatment plan.

Testing for chronic sinusitis
- **Candida IgG, IgA, IgM**, candida antigen, candida antigen/antibody complexes.
- **Sinus CT Scan** to check fluid levels, polyps or mucosal thickening.

Testing for fungal infections
- **Candida IgG, IgA, IgM,** candida antigen, candida antigen/antibody complexes.
- **Comprehensive Stool Analysis** – refer to pg. 311
- **Candida Intensive Culture by Genova** - This test evaluates blood and stool for immune reactivity to Candida albicans, using the Yeast Culture and Candida IgG Antibodies to create a comprehensive profile.

Testing for Tick Borne Disease: *Borrelia burgdorferi* (Lyme)
- Two primary antibody tests are used to diagnose Lyme disease, the ELISA and the western blot. Doctors commonly order an ELISA first to screen for the disease and then confirm the disease with a western blot. However, current ELISA tests are not sensitive enough for screening and may miss over half the true cases. Because of this, the best antibody test to use for diagnosis is the western blot. Two other tests that may be used to diagnose Lyme disease are PCR and antigen detection tests. A Polymerase chain reaction (PCR) test multiplies a key portion of DNA from the Lyme bacteria so that it can be detected. While PCR is highly accurate at positively detecting Lyme DNA, it produces many false negatives. This is because Lyme bacteria are sparse and may not be in the sample tested. Antigen detection tests look for a unique Lyme protein in fluid (e.g. blood, urine, joint fluid). Sometimes people whose indirect tests indicate negative come up positive on this test. To learn more about testing for Lyme Disease, go to www.lymedisease.org. **Note:** Treating chronic Lyme can be challenging and always involves boosting your body's natural defenses. Always work with a practitioner who has had experience with this condition.

Testing for bacterial infections
- **Mycoplasma:** *Mycoplasma pneumoniae* antibodies, IgG and IgM, Serum
- **Chlamydia:** *Chlamydia* Serology, Serum, tests for *Chlamydia trachomatis,* and *Chlamydophila,* which includes *Chlamydophila pneumoniae* and *Chlamydophila psittaci.*
- **Mycobacterium Tuberculosis (TB)** *Mycobacterium tuberculosis* Complex, Molecular Detection, PCR
- **Klebsiella:** *Klebsiella pneumonia*
- **Brucella:** *Brucella melitensis, Brucella abortus, Brucella suis, Brucella canis.*

Testing for Viruses
- **Epstein Barr:** The three antibodies the test looks for are viral capsid antigen (VCA) IgG, VCA IgM, and Epstein-Barr nuclear antigen (EBNA). The presence of VCA IgG antibodies indicates that an EBV

infection has occurred at some time (recently or in the past). The presence of VCA IgM antibodies and the absence of antibodies to EBNA means that the infection has occurred recently. The presence of antibodies to EBNA means that that infection occurred sometime in the past. Antibodies to EBNA develop six to eight weeks after primary infection and are present for life.

- **Herpes:** Herpes Simplex Virus 1/2 IgG, Type-Specific Antibodies (HerpeSelect®)

Testing for Methylation and Glutathione

Improving methylation and raising glutathione are important factors in clearing infections and boosting immunity. Here are a few tests to evaluate glutathione and methylation. Ask your functional medical practitioner about which tests are right for you.

- *Glutathione, Whole Blood*
- *NutrEval® Blood and Urine by Genova Diagnostics*
- *DetoxiGenomic® Profile by Genova Diagnostics*
- *NeuroGenomic™ Profile by Genova Diagnostics*
- *MTHFR Genotyping by SpectraCell Laboratories*

CHAPTER 19

Detox Your Life

"The best armor is to keep out of range."
— Italian Proverb

We are living in an increasingly toxic world. Even if we improve our nutrition, heal our GI tracts and support our livers, we're still exposed to over 70,000 chemicals in the surrounding environment. As I've said before, all environmental toxins are inflammatory. Even low doses of toxins can trigger your immune system and result in inflammatory autoimmune reactions. From heavy metals, petrochemicals, endocrine disrupting compounds (EDCs), herbicides, fungicides and pesticides, to volatile organic compounds (VOCs) and substances found in most commercial and home cleaning products; there is literally no end to the exposures we face. Many of them come from products that are legal, and are even mass-marketed as "safe and beneficial."

Despite this unfortunate state of affairs, there is a lot you can do to reduce your exposure, simply by sticking to choices that keep harmful chemicals out of your home and body wherever possible. While you may not be in control of what's in the environment outside your home, you are in control of what you bring into it. The first step is to learn more about what's in the products you use every day. The second step is to make sure you're eliminating the ones that could harm you.

There are healthier alternatives to just about every chemical solution you have in your home, office and garden. A comprehensive list of options, from natural product lines to homemade cleaning and personal care recipes, is far beyond the scope of this book, but you can use this information as a starting point. From here, you can take a closer look at the products you use and determine which ones you'll need to swap out for natural versions that will refresh your home and nurture your body, instead of contributing to its toxic burden.

I hope this section will get you thinking about healthier solutions for personal care products, cleaning supplies, and garden products. When you're ready, you can also check out the Resource section in the back of this book for a list of wonderful websites and books that will help you continue your journey to a cleaner, greener life!

I've also included some safe detox treatments that anyone can use; they're a great way to assist your body in safely removing toxins.

Clean Body—Revamp Your Personal Care Products

Your skin is your body's largest organ, and it absorbs a lot of what you put on it. Unfortunately, most of the personal care products that fill the shelves at the drugstore and supermarket are full of toxic chemicals such as phthalates, parabens and other endocrine disrupting compounds. You can dramatically reduce your toxic load right now, and save your body a lot of toxic stress over time, simply by being mindful of what you put on your skin.

Here are a few basic, easy-to-remember rules of thumb to protect yourself and your family from unnecessary toxic exposure from personal care products:

- *If you can't pronounce it, don't buy it!* Lotions, face creams, sun blocks, shampoos and other personal care products have the ingredients listed on the label. If a product has a long list of chemical ingredients that you can't pronounce, don't buy it!

- *Go fragrance-free!* Many products that you can smell contain phthalates. That goes for perfumes and colognes as well. Look for products that are either labeled "fragrance free", or contain natural fragrances such as essential oils.

- *Just say no to parabens!* Parabens are used as preservatives in many lotions and creams. Check all your self-care products for parabens (also known as ethyl paraben, methyl paraben, butyl paraben, propyl paraben, benzyl paraben, etc.) and toss the ones that contain chemicals with "paraben" somewhere in the name.

- *Avoid sodium lauryl sulfate!* (Sodium lauryl and laureth sulfate are toxic foaming emulsifying agents that cause irritation and build up in the body's organs and tissues.[1,2] Check all lotions, shampoos and personal care products for this nasty additive.

- *Use natural toothpaste!* Most popular brands of toothpaste contain fluoride, sodium lauryl sulfate and artificial sweeteners. Look for brands that are all-natural and fluoride free.
- *Use only natural deodorants!* Many of the antiperspirants and deodorants on the market contain parabens, endocrine disrupting compounds, petro chemicals and aluminum compounds. Look for deodorants that are all-natural and chemical free.
- *Use only natural sunblock!* Look for products that contain only zinc oxide or titanium oxide. Avoid products that contain endocrine disrupting compounds such as: benzophenone-3, octinotate, 3-benzylidene camphor, 3-(4-methyl-benzylidene) camphor, 2-ethylhexyl 4-methoxy cinnamate, Homosalate, 2-ethylhexyl 4-dimethylaminobenzoate, 4-aminobenzoic acid (PABA), oxybenzone, or retinyl palmitate.

Putting chemicals on your skin everyday might be worse than eating them! According to Dr. Joseph Mercola, "When you eat something, the enzymes in your saliva and stomach help to break it down and flush it out of your body. However, when you put these chemicals on your skin, they are absorbed straight into your bloodstream without filtering of any kind, going directly to your delicate organs.[3]" Yikes!

Do your body a favor and clean up your personal care act. Treat yourself to healthy personal care products: with a little searching, you can find affordable and deliciously indulgent personal care products with pure ingredients that you'll like much better than their chemical cousins!

Want more handy reference information about chemicals and the sneaky names they hide under? Check all your personal care products at the Environmental Working Group's page at www.ewg.org/skindeep for more on what they really contain.

Clean Home

Remember, whatever you can smell is entering your body and having an effect on your health. Smells are actually tiny particles of the substance entering your body! Knowing that puts the "new car smell" in perspective, doesn't it? In terms of the variety and amounts of toxins you're taking in on a daily basis, indoor air pollution is often much worse than outdoor air pollution.

Indoor toxins include adhesives, cleaning products, air fresheners, synthetic fibers, plastics, perfumes and anything that has a "new " smell. Take a sniff under your kitchen sink; if you can smell it, it's probably not good for you!

Allowing so many chemicals into our bodies and homes eventually lands them into the environment, where they contaminate the air and groundwater, blowing across the landscape and invading the water table, only to rain back down on us. Air and water are the most basic components of life on earth. We would quickly die without them. Our bodies are about 60% water, and we can't live for more than a few minutes without air.

Unfortunately, many of us take the purity of these basic elements of life for granted. Becoming more conscious of what we put in our bodies and our homes will ultimately impact our not only our health but our planet as well. Let's all do our part and reduce the toxic burden on our lives and our mother earth!

Drink Clean Water!

Clean water is one home improvement that's worth the investment. I would even say that it should be the main investment. Unless you live in a pristine rural area where the well water is untouched by industry and development and free of toxic natural elements, the only way to get clean water is to outfit your home water supply with the best filter you can afford. Tap water often has been dosed with fluoride, which we already know is a major problem for people with thyroid issues. To make matters worse, our water supply is increasingly tainted with pharmaceutical drug residue. According to the Associated Press, officials in Philadelphia discovered 56 pharmaceuticals drugs or drug byproducts in treated tap water, including medicines for pain, infection, epilepsy, high cholesterol, asthma, heart problems and mental illness.[4]

Water Filters

There are a number of options for filtering water, from reverse osmosis systems to systems that use carbon, ion, and sub-micron filtration. It might take some research to see what solutions fit your budget and living situation. If you're unable to filter all the water in your house, first and foremost consider filtering your drinking water, followed by the water in your shower. Many chlorine-removing shower filters can be purchased in the $30-to-$60 range. If you're not prepared to buy an expensive system, a water filter pitcher can be purchased for about $30 and is far better than nothing. An additional bonus of water filtration is that your water will taste better, so you'll drink more of it!

Billions of plastic water bottles are not only tainting the water inside them, but are clogging our landfills and oceans as well. One study found phthalate residue to be common in plastic bottled water.[5] Even low levels of phthalates can have an endocrine disrupting effect, which is troublesome for everyone but especially people with autoimmune conditions.

When storing water in the fridge or taking it with you, try to avoid using plastic bottles.

Buy water bottles, pitchers and containers made of glass, stainless steel or ceramic for storing water and other drinks. If you do need to use water in a plastic bottle, keep it out of direct sunlight and never allow it to get hot (like in your hot car), which accelerates the leaching of plastic chemicals into the water.

Breathe Fresh Air—Not Chemicals!

Fresh air is priceless and it doesn't come in a can! Home fragrances are a billion-dollar market; but most people don't realize that the commercial scents like 'Spring Rain' or 'Twilight Meadow,' are anything but fresh and natural. Air freshening sprays and 'plugins' usually contain volatile organic compounds (VOCs), formaldehyde, camphor, ethanol, phenol, benzyl alcohol and petroleum-based artificial fragrances. In other words, they're fast-evaporating invisible poisons. A 2007 study found that using air fresheners and spray cleaners as little as once a week increased the risk of developing adult asthma by 50%; four times a week doubled the risk.[6] To add insult to injury, these concoctions only mask household odors and do nothing to remove the source of the smell.

Want to know what's really in your air fresheners and home care products? Check the health rankings of air fresheners and a host of other household products using the guide published online by the Environmental

Working Group at http://www.ewg.org/consumer-guides.

There are lots of wonderful natural alternatives that smell even better than store-bought chemical scents! Try making your own natural air fresheners with essential oils, such as lavender oil in water or sage; you then disperse the scents into the air by boiling them with water in a saucepan, or by using a clay diffuser, a reed diffuser set or a ring diffuser that fits around a light bulb.[7]

Better yet, remove the source of any bad smells and consider an air filtration device. Our indoor air can carry mold spores, dust, pet dander, pollen and other irritants. Breathing allergens provokes the immune system and can be a splinter in the autoimmune process. There are a few technologies to choose from that have various costs and benefits: HEPA, activated charcoal and ionization. Consider your living situation and air quality, and investigate if air filtration could support your health and well-being. Most central heating and air-conditioning units have built-in filters. While these filters are rarely as effective as dedicated units, it's a good idea to remember to replace your filter periodically with a quality replacement. Many standard filters now use HEPA technology.

Clean Green!

When looking for ways to get toxins out of your home, don't miss the ones that are sitting in plain sight. Carefully review the household chemicals and cleaners that you use. Many times the clean-smelling product you spray your counter top with is worse for you than the dirt it's supposed to remove.

Consumer demands for green cleaning products have skyrocketed in the last decade making natural alternatives more available and affordable than ever! There are literally hundreds of all-natural home care product lines on the market: some of my personal favorites are Seventh Generation, Earth Friendly Products (ECOS), and Ecover.

Unfortunately not all products labeled as "earth friendly" or "non-toxic" really are. If you're unsure about an ingredient you see on any label, it always helps to consult the consumer guides published online by the Environmental Working Group at http://www.ewg.org/consumer-guides.

If you really want to know what's in your cleaning product, consider making your own. There are several recipes for all-natural home care products that you can make yourself, usually at a fraction of the cost of their commercial alternatives. Some people simply use vinegar and water, or borax to cut grease or as boosters for natural laundry soap. Baking soda and food-grade diatomaceous earth make great scouring powders, and gently break up the dirty and baked-on grease on your cookware. They are also good for scrubbing off soap scum and hard water deposits in the bath and shower. (Diatomaceous earth is available online or at some health-food stores; be sure it's food-grade!) Hydrogen peroxide is a great way to remove odors and stains, especially ones caused by many dark liquids, blood or bodily fluids, from laundry.

When making your own all-natural cleaners, it's important to know what you're doing, especially with bleach or ammonia, which should never be combined or mixed indiscriminately with other chemicals.

Mindfulness about chemicals should extend to your laundry detergent as well. Check the labels and look for health and earth-friendly products. Especially, beware of commercial dryer sheets and fabric softening sheets. One study found over 25 volatile organic compounds (VOCs) in the exhaust of household dryers using dryer sheets.[8] Try to find a brand that doesn't contain all these chemicals such as the ones made by The Honest Company.[9] Alternatively you can make your own natural fabric softener by adding a quarter-cup of baking soda or vinegar (but not both at the same time!) to the wash cycle.

Clean Up Electromagnetic Fields in Your Home!

There is another invisible splinter that needs attention in your home and lifestyle: electromagnetic fields (EMFs). One of the reasons EMFs are so important is that they, like endocrine disrupting chemicals, can interrupt and confuse your body's natural processes, with potentially disastrous results. Your body's cells communicate via bioelectromagnetic signals. Unfortunately, we are constantly bathed in a sea of foreign electromagnetic fields from cell phones, Wi-Fi and computers. These fields easily penetrate our bodies and can stress our natural balance. In modern life, it's almost impossible to live completely free from EMFs, but it's easy to drastically reduce your exposure. The longer you remain exposed to EMFs, the greater the cumulative stress on your system.

We spend much as much as third of our lives sleeping. Remember good sleep is *critical* for healing and detoxification. Consequently, the bedroom is the most important place to reduce EMFs. Studies indicate that people who sleep next to a cell phone have poor REM sleep, perhaps because EMFs might affect the pineal gland's secretion of melatonin at night. I suggest you use a battery-powered alarm clock and don't sleep next to a router or cordless phone base station. Sleeping under an electric blanket exposes you to electromagnetic fields right next to you body for hours at a time. One study linked sleeping under an electric blanket with a greater incidence of breast cancer.[10] Take a survey of where you sleep and then move or eliminate everything that generates electromagnetic fields.

Cell phones have become another major source of EMF exposure in modern life. The more you use them, the more careful you need to be. In 2011, the World Health Organization/International Agency for Research on Cancer (IARC) classified radiofrequency electromagnetic fields as possibly carcinogenic to humans.[11] If you are mindful, there are ways to reduce your exposure. Instead of holding the cell phone against your head, use the speakerphone function or wear a headset. Even an inch or two of distance between the phone and your head greatly reduces the EMF exposure. Not everyone has the willpower to use a headset for answering a quick call, but it's worth considering anytime you know you'll be spending a long time on the phone. Even though a Bluetooth headset emits some EMFs, at least one study showed them to be safer than holding the phone to the ear.[12] Even when you're not talking, your phone emits EMFs, so don't carry your cell phone next to your body when you have the option to leave it in your purse or briefcase. It's helpful to know that cell phones emit EMFs most powerfully when the reception is weak or when you are moving.

Give careful consideration to the electromagnetic fields around the rest of the house. Keep routers and base stations distant from where you spend the majority of your time, and turn them off when you don't need them. Keep laptop computers off your lap, and replace old CRT televisions and monitors with low-radiation LCD models.

The same goes for microwaves. The safety of microwaves is hotly debated, but rarely studied. The Soviet Union banned them in 1976, which should raise some eyebrows. If you do use a microwave, use good judgment and never cook in plastic containers! If you've got an autoimmune condition, it might be safer to get rid of the microwave, as it is a source of possible risk.

You'll also need to check the basement, and elsewhere, for another sources of harmful energy. Radon is a naturally occurring radioactive gas that the Surgeon General states is the second leading cause of lung cancer in the United States. The EPA estimates that radon causes 21,000 lung cancer deaths per year.[13] Low-cost radon test kits are available at hardware/home improvement stores and online. You can view radon risk zones on the EPA's radon map at http://www.epa.gov/radon/zonemap.html. If you find your house has elevated levels of radon, there are steps you can take to remediate and remove it; usually it takes a little remodeling, but there are a number of other ways to help reduce the risk. Even a ceiling fan can dramatically reduce your total exposure to radon.

Become a Mold Warrior!

Mold contamination can cause serious health issues for anyone, but people with allergies, asthma and autoimmune conditions are likely to be even more sensitive.[14] Being in a constant state of allergic aggravation places a huge burden on your immune system and may eventually trigger an autoimmune response.[15] Many people suffer intense immediate symptoms from mold exposure. I know because I used to be one of them. As soon as I entered a building that had mold I would suffer symptoms of foggy thinking and vertigo. If I stayed long enough (like overnight) I wound up with a rash. Now that I've healed, I'm much less sensitive and can tolerate moldy places much longer than I used to; but just like gluten, I stay away from mold!

Mold reproduces when its tiny spores are spread in the air, or by humans or animals, to some place with enough moisture for the spores to germinate. In other words, if you have mold, it probably came in through your windows and doors and found a damp place. Homes that have flooded are especially vulnerable.[16]

There are many kinds of mold: common household types include *alternaria, aspergillus, cladosporium* and *penicillium*, as well as the more rare and dangerous stachybotrys, known as "black mold." All of them need moisture to grow. Some species of mold are mild allergens while others can produce harmful mycotoxins. More research is needed to determine the direct affects of mycotoxins on human health, but it's clear from the research that toxic molds are implicated in many pulmonary, immunologic, neurologic and oncologic disorders.[17] Mold exposures puts people with compromised immune systems, or those with COPD and other chronic lung conditions, at risk for opportunistic fungal infections. It's important to talk to your health care provider if you feel you have symptoms related to mold.

The Centers for Disease Control recommends that all molds should be treated with the same care, regardless of the variety. Mold thrives on moisture, so the first step is to stop leaks and ventilate damp areas. Wiping moldy areas down with a bleach or borax solution can help. But if the mold has gone undetected and has had time to work its way into layers of construction, it may be necessary to contact a professional to have the mold remediated including removing drywall or flooring. Large infestations of mold can usually be seen or smelled, and may require substantial effort to clean up. If you suspect mold is an issue in your home it's a good idea to call a professional and have them investigate and clean it up if necessary.

Living with Pets

It's tragic to mention that some people are allergic to pets, more specifically to the proteins found in skin cells that animals shed, as well as in their saliva, sweat, urine and on their fur. If you moved into a place where the previous residents had animals and you developed respiratory or skin reactions, you may need to have everything thoroughly cleaned, and potentially replace carpets, bedding and other upholstered items contaminated with pet dander. If the pet belongs to you or your family, you have a difficult decision to face. The severity of your allergic symptoms will direct your action. You may simply need to sleep in a pet-free zone, filter their air and keep the animal well bathed (by somebody else). If your symptoms are more intense you might have to find a new home for your best friend while you're healing. I used to be terribly allergic to animals, especially cats. I'm happy to say that I can hug a kitty now without suffering a single sniffle! Once your autoimmune condition is reversed, you too may be able to live happily ever after with your beloved pets.

Warning: Most flea and tick control measures are seriously toxic to you and your pet's health. Flea collars and chemical spot-on flea and tick products contain dangerous pesticides, and should be considered a last resort for animals with severe flea allergies. According to a February 2002 article in the *Whole Dog Journal,* entitled, "Are 'Spot-On' Flea Killers Safe?" "All pesticides pose some degree of health risk to humans and animals. Despite advertising claims to the contrary, both over-the-counter and veterinarian-prescribed flea-killing topical treatments are pesticides that enter our companions' internal organs (livers, kidneys), move into their intestinal tracts, and are eventually eliminated in their feces and urine." Additionally, these chemicals easily transfer to human skin when the animal is handled. This can be particularly dangerous to people with autoimmune conditions!

> **What You Need to Know:**
> Autoimmune conditions, allergies and sensitivities often result from several "splinters" aggravating your immune system at once. If you are able to clean up your nutrition, heal your gut and remove other significant triggers, your immune system may calm down and your allergies may disappear. In some cases, you may be able to tolerate things you've been allergic to your whole life!

Are You Freaking Out Yet?

By now you might be asking, "How can everything be bad for me?" I feel your pain! At first, it might seem overwhelming to scrutinize all the products you use; especially when "normal" people all around you don't seem to be bothered. But to bring your immune system into balance, you need to ignore what the world says is "okay" and listen to what your body has to say. I hate to sound like a broken record, but remember that society suffers from epidemics of obesity, diabetes, cancer, autoimmune conditions and other chronic illnesses. Take a look at all the "normal" people and you'll find that many suffer a plethora of annoying symptoms.

It's true that many people seem to be able to get away with eating, drinking, and breathing anything, at least on the surface, but there is no telling what conditions are brewing below. If you have an autoimmune condition, you're likely to be more sensitive than most people and will likely have a stronger reaction to substances and circumstances that aren't good for anyone. It could be that the sensitive ones among us are sounding a warning about our toxic environment, giving humankind an opportunity to correct our course! Respect your innate sensitivity and take better care of yourself.

You may find that the process of eliminating toxins in your life comes with social challenges. Your friends and family might not appreciate your need to avoid products that are commonly taken for granted as "safe." Some people might feel threatened or offended when you ask them to switch to healthier choices. Don't let any skeptics get you down. If your friends and family begin to wonder if you've just joined Michelle's Hypochondria Boot Camp, just explain that you're more sensitive than most people and you need to give your body a break so it can heal.

Clean Garden and Garage

Your garden and garage are home to some of the most toxic and, luckily, the most avoidable chemical poisons. We have to be careful when choosing and using chemicals in the garden, and for home improvement and automotive maintenance. Try to choose products with the least impact on the environment and your health. When you need to use any product that could aggravate your lungs, skin or immune system, it's important to use gloves and a ventilator mask, available from your local home improvement store.

There is no such thing as a safe pesticide!

I recommend researching natural alternatives for keeping spiders and other creepy creatures out of your home. I use neem or orange oil mixed with water as natural insect repellants. Neem oil mixtures can also be used in the garden to control fungus, mites and other garden pests.

The fumes of the following products could be particularly aggravating to people with autoimmune conditions: lacquers, paints, solvents, glues, pesticides, pool and spa sanitization chemicals, paint strippers, wood stains and anything with a volatile smell or warning on the label.

No matter how careful we are about protecting ourselves during use, some products are just too toxic to risk using. Don't use paint strippers or other products containing methylene chloride, also called dichloromethane.[18] Keep an eye on labels to avoid xylene, trisodium nitrilotriacetate (NTA), toluene, ethoxylated nonyl phenols (NPEs), 2-butoxyethanol, hexane, tricholoroethylene (TCE), sodium or potassium hydroxide (lye), chlorinated phenols, diethylene glycol, nonylphenol ethoxylate, perchloroethylene, diethanolamine (DEA), triethanolamine (TEA) butyl cellosolve™, alkylphenol ethoxylates (APEs), formaldehyde and bisphenol A (BPA) in plastics. Be very careful if you need to use bleach (sodium hypochlorite).

I would love to provide a more comprehensive list, but there are at least 80,000 toxic chemical compounds and the number grows every day. It would literally be impossible to list them all. Even a thorough discussion of the alternatives to harsher chemicals and pesticides is beyond the scope of this book. Luckily, there are vast resources on the Internet dedicated to non-toxic alternatives to many chemicals. The main thing is to read labels (obviously, beware of "WARNING," "DANGER" or "POISON" on the container and look for words like "nontoxic" and "biodegradable.") Take a little time to research the healthiest way to take care of your home and garden. You may reclaim that time with better heath and increased longevity.

Of course, you can't believe everything you read on the Internet, so check the credibility of your sources and get a second opinion. There's new information emerging every day about all kinds of substances, their sourcing and what we know about their effects on the human body. No matter how much you already know, there could be a piece to the puzzle that you're missing. For example, I looked at one organic gardening page that recommended a variety of possible fertilizers including Chilean sodium nitrate, but then I discovered Chilean sodium nitrate has been found to contain perchlorate contamination, which blocks iodide from entering the thyroid gland where it's used to make thyroid hormone.[19,20] All we can do is keep our eyes open and engage in continual education, expanding our knowledge of health and awareness of health risks.

Clean Office

We spend a lot of our time at work. The health risks of the workplace are often similar to the ones we encounter at home: EMFs, cleaning supplies, air fresheners and office buddies tempting you with junk food. We don't all work in an office, and a discussion of all the possible scenarios encountered in different professions is also far beyond the scope of this book.

Again, it's up to you to investigate the possible risks and exposures that your work involves. You might uncover significant information that could change your life, or help you save it. I used to work as a dental assistant and was exposed to a lot of mercury in the process of mixing amalgam for filling teeth. There is a heated controversy about the danger of mercury in dentistry, so I'd like to state that I discovered my high mercury levels through testing, not guessing. Consider the exposures to EMF and chemicals that you face at work and ponder how those exposures could be minimized or eliminated.

Making healthy changes at home requires diplomacy and you'll need it in the workplace as well. If you need cooperation (or money to be budgeted), remember to bring a positive attitude to the discussion and remind management that healthy workers are better employees who don't call in sick or drive up insurance costs. If management takes the long view, removing chemicals from the workplace and reducing toxic and EMF exposure can be a win-win situation.

However, if diplomacy fails, you should know that if there is a clearly hazardous situation at work, or if your employer fails to provide sufficient safety equipment to protect you, that you have legal rights to a safe workplace. This is from the website of the Occupational Safety and Health Administration at https://www.osha.gov/workers.html:

> *OSHA standards are rules that describe the methods that employers must use to protect their employees from hazards. There are OSHA standards for Construction work, Agriculture, Maritime operations, and General Industry, which are the standards that apply to most worksites. These standards limit the amount of hazardous chemicals workers can be exposed to, require the use of certain safe practices and equipment, and require employers to monitor hazards and keep records*

of workplace injuries and illnesses. Examples of OSHA standards include requirements to: provide fall protection, prevent trenching cave-ins, prevent some infectious diseases, assure that workers safely enter confined spaces, prevent exposure to harmful substances like asbestos, put guards on machines, provide respirators or other safety equipment, and provide training for certain dangerous jobs.

Employers must also comply with the General Duty Clause of the OSH Act, which requires employers to keep their workplace free of serious recognized hazards. This clause is generally cited when no OSHA standard applies to the hazard.

Hopefully, you'll be able to take out any workplace splinters without creating an additional splinter of stress.

Safe Detox Treatments

While you are reducing your exposure to environmental toxins, there are special detoxifying treatments that you can do to help your body eliminate toxins you've already accumulated. These self-care treatments can be relaxing and help you feel good right away while improving your health in the long run.

Far-Infrared Sauna

The skin is the largest organ of the body and an important detoxification pathway. One way to stimulate detoxification through the skin is by taking saunas. I'm happy to say that I find that my time in the sauna not only helps clean my system but also gives me a time to unwind and release stress. I feel great afterwards. Getting a good sweat is particularly important during the part of the healing process where many people tend to lose weight. As you lose weight, your tissues release toxins bound in the fat and sweating helps clear them out of your body. Besides detoxing, raising body temperature helps fight infections and fungus; our body develops a fever for that same purpose. Hypothyroid patients commonly have below-average body temperatures, which in turn create an environment where infections (especially fungal) can thrive.

Not everyone can afford a sauna at home, so you might have to work with what's available at your local gym. If you have a choice, I believe that far-infrared saunas have significant advantages over traditional saunas. Infrared light is part of the invisible spectrum of light, and is capable of penetrating your body. The temperatures needed for an infrared sauna to be effective are lower than for traditional saunas, so it's a more comfortable way to get even deeper results. Just like the rays of the sun can warm you even on a cold day, infrared heats your body directly. You can purchase your own sauna for about $1,000-$4,000 and they require less electricity than regular saunas. Infrared saunas are also reputed to promote dilation of the capillary micro-circulatory system, improve lymph flow and relax muscle fibers. This reduces spasms and soreness in addition to the detoxification benefits.

Here are Some Guidelines and Tips to Help You Maximize Benefits from Your Sauna Treatment:

- It's best to use the sauna after you exercise.
- Don't eat for two hours before and one hour after using the sauna.
- Avoid alcohol and drugs before your sauna visit.
- Make sure you have regular bowel movements when you are focusing on detoxification. If you're not going at least twice a day, drink plenty of water and supplement with fiber to encourage the process.
- Have at least one tall glass of clean water before using the sauna.
- Drink water while sitting in the sauna, and drink even more afterwards.
- It's a good idea to talk to your practitioner about your sauna treatment, particularly if you take certain medications or are experiencing detox symptoms.
- Infrared saunas don't need to be any warmer than 140 degrees F (150 degrees max) to be effective.
- Dr. Mark Hyman recommends taking multivitamin and mineral supplements while doing sauna therapy. The minerals replace those lost in sweat and the vitamins help process the liberated toxins.
- Dr. Hyman also recommends taking two to six capsules of activated charcoal before the sauna to bind toxins released in the bile and help the body expel them.

- After using the sauna is a good time for another detox treatment: dry skin brushing (see below).
- Shower after your sauna to rinse off the toxins excreted through the skin.
- Try to sauna regularly, if not daily, while detoxing intensively; later you can scale back to once a week if you like.

Dry Skin Brushing

Another great treatment that aids detoxification is dry skin brushing. It takes just a few minutes a day, makes your skin look and feel better, and is practically free. All you need is a soft brush with natural hair. You may want to look for a long-handled brush so you can reach your back. Start at your feet making long strokes up your legs on both sides towards your heart. Then work from the tips of your fingers along your arms toward your chest.

This treatment exfoliates dry and dead skin, opening the pores for efficient detoxification. Dry skin brushing is said to aid the lymphatic system in its role of clearing toxins; it also stimulates your nervous system, bringing your awareness to every inch of your body.

Epsom Salt Baths

Epsom salt baths are a relaxing detoxification alternative, especially if a sauna isn't an option. They make a great addition to your routine. Epsom salt is made up of the minerals magnesium and sulfur, and is an old-time remedy for treating minor inflammation and muscle aches. Both minerals are readily absorbed through the skin.

The magnesium ions absorbed through the skin regulate the activity of hundreds of enzymes, help reduce inflammation, relax muscles and may even help to prevent hardening of arteries. The arterial benefits arise because the body cannot assimilate calcium without sufficient magnesium; otherwise the calcium accumulates in your vessels. Magnesium also plays a role in preventing metabolic syndrome, which increases risk for heart disease and diabetes. People with low serum magnesium levels are 6-7 times more likely to have metabolic syndrome. Studies indicate that healthy women who get higher levels of magnesium through diet and supplements have a 27% lower risk of developing metabolic syndrome.[21]

The other component of Epsom salt is Sulfur. Sulfur is the third most common mineral in the body and necessary for the liver's phase II detoxification process. The body needs sulfur to synthesize cysteine, which is stored in the body in form of glutathione (GSH), one of the most important antioxidants in the body.[22] Science has documented that sulfur baths reduce oxidative stress and reduce LDL and total cholesterol levels.[23] You can also get Sulfur benefits when soaking in hot springs baths rich in sulfur.

Epsom salt increases osmotic pressure on the skin (in other words, it draws fluid out of cells) which helps bring toxins to the surface and out of your body.

Beside the physical benefits, a nice warm bath before bedtime helps you unwind and reduces stress. It also softens skin and reduces wrinkles, and the magnesium contributes to relaxation for a good night's sleep.

Epsom salt costs just a couple of dollars per pound. You just need one or two cups, added to a hot bath in a standard-size bathtub. I recommend a hot 15-minute bath, 3-4 times a week, although you can take daily baths during detoxification. If you are bathing before bed, keep the lights low, perhaps using candles, to prepare your body for sleep and reduce stress.

Beyond Clean EDTA Bath

For an even more potent mineral bath that's formulated especially for those who have been exposed to heavy metals, "Beyond Clean with Zeolite" by Longevity Plus is a bath treatment made with calcium EDTA and zeolite.

The manufacturer states, "Calcium EDTA is known for its ability to help remove heavy metals, such as lead, from the body. It works by binding and holding onto (chelating) minerals and metals such as chromium, iron, lead, mercury, copper, aluminum, nickel, zinc and other metals. When they are bound, they can't have any effect on the body and they are then removed through the body's natural excretion process.

"Zeolite is a mineral that allows some molecules to pass through and others to be excluded, or broken down. The results show that zeolite can be used effectively for the removal of metal from water supplies."

The directions suggest, "Add 2-6 tablespoons to bathwater to prevent absorption of toxic metals found in most water supplies. Soaking for 20-30 minutes may have anti-aging benefits on skin." Beyond Clean maybe used along with Epsom salts and the combination of magnesium and calcium may be symbiotic. If you're aiming to remove heavy metals from your system, try both!

Conclusion

This information may seem overwhelming at first, but I hope I've got you thinking of ways you can reduce your body burden and ultimately take some toxic splinters out of your system. Remember, your autoimmune condition is a natural response to an increasingly unnatural world. While you don't have control over everything in your environment, you do have some control over your body, home, garden and office. As you make more conscious choices for yourself and your home, you help to lighten the load for the planet. Thank you for doing your part!

CHAPTER 20

Putting It All Together

"If someone wishes for good health, one must first ask oneself if he is ready to do away with the reasons for his illness. Only then is it possible to help him."
— HIPPOCRATES

I know this book contains a lot of information. It helps to review the sections that apply the most to your condition and your life. Don't be discouraged if you don't remember all of the information. Use this book as guide and return to it as a resource.

Here are some reminders of the key points.

Get passionate about getting better! Remember your compelling reasons for reversing your condition and living the life you were born to live.

Step out of the victim role and take responsibility for your health! An autoimmune condition can make you feel like a victim. It's ok to grieve the loss of your health, but don't allow yourself to get trapped in self-pity! Become empowered by accepting control over your life and your health! Love yourself enough to make your health a priority.

Take action by challenging the system! Understand that our current medical system is designed to treat *symptoms* and rarely addresses the underlying causes of chronic illness. Become your own health advocate and learn what your doctor may not even know about reversing disease and restoring health!

Become your own health advocate! You have the highest stake in getting well. Become a scientist with your own body and hire the right practitioners to help you get better!

Make the necessary lifestyle adjustments to heal! Getting better takes action! Resolve to heal your life!

Reframe the autoimmune process! Think of autoimmunity as a reversible condition instead of an incurable disease! Autoimmune conditions are the result of too much stress!

Your genes are not your destiny! 70 to 90 percent of chronic illness results from how our genes interact with our (inner and outer) environment! Your diet, emotions, lifestyle and product choices shape that environment. You have control!

Understand the physiology of stress! Allowing yourself to remain in a chronic fight or flight state will wear you out and make you sick! You have control! Remove the physical, emotional and environmental factors that trigger your autoimmunity and you will get better!

Uncover the splinters that trigger your autoimmunity! Use chapter 9 and the personal assessments to help you discover the factors that combined to trigger your autoimmune response.

Find a practitioner! Find a functional or integrative practitioner, or at least a practitioner who is willing to consider your condition is reversible. Finding the right practitioner will save you time, money and frustration while you're healing. Be willing to spend money for what insurance won't cover!

Feel better fast! Eat for Your Good Genes and follow the *Sensitivity Discovery Program* for 30 to 90 days, or until your symptoms disappear!

Reduce stress and support your adrenals! Get proper sleep and exercise! Practice mindfulness! Try to cultivate joy! Cultivate these changes and you'll be amazed as how much better life can be. The better you get, the more energy and happiness you'll have to thrive and get well.

Heal your gut! G.I. infections and leaky gut are huge autoimmune splinters. Work with a functional or integrative practitioner to get the right tests if necessary.

Support your liver! Restore the healing powers of your body by improving your detoxification. If you improve methylation and boost glutathione, your body will fight off diseases and infections and protect you from toxins in the future. If you suspect that you have some toxic splinters, work with a practitioner and get tested!

Clear infections! If you feel you have infectious splinters, review chapter 18 and test don't guess! You can't afford not to know what's bugging you!

Detox your life! Drink clean water, breathe fresh air and learn about which toxic chemicals you may have in your home that can be replaced with healthy alternatives! Try some detox treatments!

Give some thought to Part Three: *The Mind-Body Connection* and explore if negative emotions are influencing your health.

Remember, the successful treatment of autoimmune conditions always includes:

- Recognizing each individual's unique biochemistry and life circumstances
- Empowering wellness through proper nutrition, exercise and rest
- Enhancing the body's natural detoxification capacity by supporting the liver and healing the gastrointestinal tract
- Finding and removing pathogens (i.e. bacteria, fungus, viruses, heavy metals and chemicals)
- Cultivating happiness and a sense of purpose!

It's my wish that you take this information to heart and find your own path to health. I believe you came here to heal yourself and to be a source of healing for all of us.

Namaste!

PART THREE

The Mind-Body Connection

"Your psychology becomes your biology."
– CAROLYN MYSS

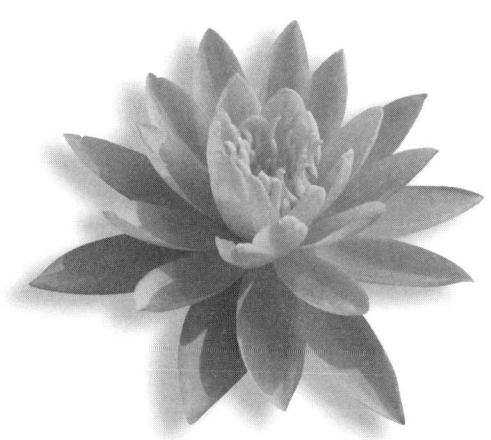

Connecting Emotions and Your Health

"For this is the great error of our day: that the physicians separate the soul from the body."
— HIPPOCRATES

My next book is going to be called *You're Not Sick, You're Unhappy!* I'm not kidding. That's how intimately I feel our emotions touch our health.

I am not pretending to be a psychologist or an expert on emotional health. I am a person who has learned through personal experience and independent research how to reverse my autoimmune condition and heal my life. I have validated my conclusions through helping several other people transform their health and their lives. While there are always multiple factors involved, I've observed over and over that there is a strong emotional component to virtually everyone's autoimmune process.

It's really quite obvious why: emotions are visceral sensations felt in the body. When we are stressed, our neck can get sore, we may get knots in our shoulders, and as the pressure builds, we may develop a headache. When we are anxious, we may feel like our stomach is in knots, and we may feel nauseous or have diarrhea. When we are grieving, we may feel a deep ache or emptiness in the middle of our chest.

Humans have recognized the link between emotions and health since ancient times. Traditional healing systems such as Ayurveda and Traditional Chinese Medicine have taught the interrelatedness of the mind, body, and spirit for thousands of years.[1]

In the last 20 years, we have seen considerable growth in the science of psychoneuroimmunology (PNI), which explores how our psychology affects our neurological and immune systems. Studies continue to demonstrate how chronic negative emotional states play a key role in the development and exacerbation of inflammatory diseases such as heart disease, diabetes, multiple sclerosis, Alzheimer's, and autoimmune disorders. I believe we can no longer deny the clear chemical links between our emotions and the regulatory function of the endocrine and immune systems through the central nervous system.[2]

Your physical condition cannot be separated from your life circumstances! In fact, it has been demonstrated that traumatic life experiences are one of the most fundamental causes of physical illness.

While there are hundreds of studies that explore the emotional roots of disease, the most insightful place to start may be the breakthrough ACE Study.[3]

Kaiser Permanente conducted a significant academic study that illustrated the destructive effect emotional traumas from childhood can have on subsequent health. The "Adverse Childhood Experiences (ACE)" study looked at 17,000 middle-aged, middle-class participants. Study director Dr. Vincent Fellitti published the findings in the *American Journal of Preventive Medicine* in 1998. Kaiser carefully interviewed participants to determine if they had experienced dysfunctional family behavior or abuse before they were 18 years old. Researchers identified eight categories of dysfunction or abuse, which constituted an "adverse childhood experience" or "ACE."

Half of the participants reported at least one adverse childhood experience. Those who reported one ACE were at least four times—and as much as 50 times—more likely to have a disease or other serious health issue, compared with those who didn't suffer an ACE. These dramatic statistics indicate that childhood trauma clearly correlates with compromised adult health.

Childhood trauma and the resultant chronic negative emotional states that ensued played a pivotal role in my own autoimmune process. I have found this to be the case with a majority of the clients I have worked with as well. I will share my experience, as well as a few case histories in this section that will point to the interconnectedness of trauma, negative emotions and illness. If you are interested in learning more about the ace study you may visit their website at www.acestudy.org. To find your ACE score check the Resources section at the back of this book.

It's important to remember that no matter how difficult your past experiences may have been, you can heal these wounds and, in doing so, benefit your health and wellbeing for life.

Chronic Negative Emotions: Melissa's Story

Chronic emotional negativity is toxic. It wreaks havoc in our lives and on our immune systems. In fact new research shows that proinflammatory cytokines produced in chronic illnesses such as autoimmune conditions can be directly stimulated by negative emotions and stressful experiences.[4] Overcoming our chronic negativity not only facilitates physical healing, but also enhances our quality of life.

There is a difference between having occasional negative reactions to the challenging experiences that are naturally a part of life, and harboring *chronic emotional negativity*. Strong feelings such as guilt, anger, resentment, and sadness are a part of the human experience.

While our feelings influence our body as we are having them, denying or repressing feelings can compound the problem and internalize the negative state. That's how emotional negativity can become a part of our psyche and poison us from within. Toxic negative states and situations can be the main cause of physical stress. Severe emotional trauma and turmoil put the sympathetic nervous system on high alert and launch us into fight-or-flight mode. In time, this chronic state can break down our bodies at the cellular level.

Take Melissa, a 34-year-old, drop-dead gorgeous movie executive from L.A. who was suffering from Graves'. Tall and thin, with a perfect olive complexion and luxurious black hair, she looked like she had stepped out of the pages of *Vogue* magazine in a sleek, black Channel suit, a pair of Ferragamo stilettos, and a Cartier tank watch.

Melissa's manner was very distinct and memorable. She glanced at her watch as soon as she stepped into my office and seemed to almost vibrate with a sense of urgency. I imagined a corporate jet, fueled up and idling outside in my driveway. She had a rapid, staccato style of speaking. Encoded in every sentence was an urgent message: *I don't have time for this. I don't have time for what I'm going through!* She filled out her application lightning-fast, her Mont Blanc pen blurring with speed. In the section on family life, she wrote, "We'll talk." And talk she did.

Her symptoms—high anxiety, diarrhea, palpations, and feeling hot all the time—had appeared eight months after a terrible family quarrel about her deceased father's estate.

Melissa revealed that she had not really known him because he left her mother when she was six years old. Shortly after his death, she received a phone call from an attorney who explained that she was the sole beneficiary of the estate. She could not understand why the man who had abandoned her so long ago would leave her everything. When I asked if she was sad that he had passed away, she replied with distracted indifference, "He wasn't a good person, so I really couldn't care less." Her two older sisters demanded that she split the estate three ways, which she agreed to do.

The trouble started when another woman came forward, claiming to be her father's daughter and wishing to be included in the estate. Melissa, who turned out to be a highly principled woman, felt this woman should be considered and told her sisters as much. Her decision enraged not only her sisters, but her mother as well.

Melissa's mother wrote her a letter indicating that Melissa was no longer part of the family, and should never contact any of them again (other than to write them their inheritance checks, of course). Unlike the staccato indifference of most of her testimony, this part made Melissa's eyes fill with tears, and she began blinking rapidly as she spoke about her mother. When I passed her a box of tissues, she said, "Excuse me, I seem to have something in my eye."

Melissa did, however, admit to being devastated by her mom's threat to disown her. She was angry and deeply hurt that her mother and sisters could be so cruel.

Melissa was married to a man who treated her reasonably well (according to her), although he hadn't held a job in six years and had accrued over $40,000 in unsecured credit card debt. She was buckling under the financial pressure of being the sole breadwinner. After the attorneys were paid, her share of the inheritance would just about cover her husband's debt.

As a movie executive at a top-flight studio, Melissa worked for a very demanding, narcissistic boss who was always making passes at her. In addition to her commitment to an intense hot yoga practice, Melissa followed a rigidly strict vegetarian diet. She said her health had been excellent until this point and was angry that the body she worked so hard to keep up was now betraying her.

Every woman with Graves' I've ever worked with had an illness onset that correlated with an acute emotional trauma. When I asked her if she felt the situation with her family played a role in her condition, she stoically said she was "handling everything just fine."

I suggested testing for some common underlying "splinters" such as GI imbalances, infections, and heavy metals. She agreed. To my surprise, her tests weren't too bad; she had mild intestinal imbalances, no leaky gut, no infections, and no significant heavy metals. The significant imbalances were in the comprehensive NutrEval test, which showed numerous vitamin and amino acid deficiencies.

I suspected that her acute emotional stress, compounded by her stressful lifestyle, was the last straw. It appeared that chronic emotional stress had depleted her B vitamins, and antioxidants. And her vegetarian diet caused her to be deficient in protein and several amino acids. She did not eat soy, legumes, nuts, or seeds because they made her feel nauseous. Her diet consisted primarily of fruits, vegetables, grains, and starchy carbohydrates like potatoes.

I suggested she remove gluten, nightshades, and citrus and add soaked and sprouted nuts and seeds, as well as more non-starchy veggies such as kale, asparagus, collard greens, broccoli, etc. I asked her if she was open to adding some animal protein in the form of fish and she agreed. I suggested my Women's Empowerment Formula, omega-3 fish oil, borage oil, extra vitamin C, alpha lipoic acid, CoQ10, digestive enzymes, and a good probiotic. I also recommended a medical food that supported liver detoxification and included many of the amino acids she was deficient in.

I proposed that she skip the hot yoga, because it was increasing her internal heat, and try a more relaxing or cooling form of exercise like swimming, restorative yoga, Pilates, or simply walking on the beach. I also suggested she speak to a life coach or psychologist to work through the challenges she faced at home and at work. I showed her some breathing exercises and suggested she try doing them for a minimum of five minutes, three times a day.

Three months into the program, she wasn't improving and her anxiety symptoms had worsened. She was angry and frustrated and ready to give up and start taking beta blockers for her hyperthyroid symptoms. She was under the care of an open-minded endocrinologist who was monitoring her closely, and he felt it was time to help her feel more comfortable.

Of course I agreed, but I was puzzled… I knew there had to be more to be more to the story. What were we missing? I suggested an appointment with a functional medical doctor to see if he could provide more insight. Melissa got very upset at the suggestion. She was sick of going to doctors and was ready to radiate her thyroid and be done with it. I conceded that the treatment was up to her. She would think about it and let me know.

Two weeks later, I received an urgent, after-hours call. Through her hysterical tears, Melissa said she might know what caused her autoimmune condition, and admitted to having a three-year affair with her boss. She said the guilt was "eating her alive." It had started as innocent flirting, but then one evening it went too far. She had tried to break it off many times, but had fallen in love. He was married with two young children, and although he said he loved her, he refused to leave his family. Melissa suspected that his wife knew about the affair and had somehow accepted it. She explained how she felt that her family blowout was a sign that she was being punished. She felt ashamed and unworthy of love, and now believed she would end up sick and alone like she deserved. She wept for over ten minutes while I listened.

When she calmed down, I remarked, "What an amazing ally your body has been. It's saying 'no' because you haven't been able to. Your body is simply telling you to wake up and make conscious decisions about your life." Suddenly, I felt her energy shift. She said, "I've never thought of it that way. You might be right." I asked her what action she could take now for her highest good and to advance her health. She said, "I want to break it off with my boss and divorce my husband. I can't take this anymore. I feel like dirt." I suggested that now might be a good time to call that life coach for some direction, and she agreed.

Five months later, Melissa had made some pretty significant changes in her life. She had broken it off with her boss and left her position for an even higher-paying job. She had told her husband everything. At first, he did his best to shame and blame her for being a cheat and a horrible wife. However, after a few couples coaching appointments, he came clean and confessed that he had had several flings over the course of their marriage.

He admitted that he had not been supportive emotionally or physically, and didn't blame her for seeking attention elsewhere. After a brief, three-week separation, they both decided to forgive each other and work toward a closer union. He started a new job and was working to pay off his debt and contribute to the household.

When Melissa's mother found out how sick her daughter was, she called and wanted to make amends. They decided to go to coaching together to resolve the hurt from the past. Mellissa's mother confessed that she had known about her ex-husband's other daughter, Melissa's half-sister, because she was the child of the woman he had left her for. He had not been able to commit to that woman either, and had walked away when the baby was three years old. Melissa's mother realized that she was punishing innocent people (Melissa and her half-sister) for a hurt that had been inflicted on her by a man she had deeply loved. She had been unable to forgive him all these years, and had unconsciously misdirected her anger toward Melissa and her half-sister.

Melissa's radical lifestyle changes had a major impact on her health. She did take the beta blockers when her symptoms became intolerable, but after two months, the "storm blew over" and she stopped. Her coach taught her techniques to calm down with meditation and breathing. When I spoke with her, she had been symptom-free for roughly twelve weeks, and her antibodies had dropped by 70 percent. She recognized that she had more emotional and physical healing to do, but was determined to stay on the path.

Two years later, after managing her stress and eating a diet that includes adequate protein, vibrant fruits and vegetables, and probiotics, she has completely healed. Her blood tests indicate no antibodies—her autoimmune thyroid condition was cured! She and her husband are now expecting their first child. She says that the whole experience has made her stronger, wiser, and more resilient. She looks forward to having all three of her sisters and her mother with her at home for the birth of her baby girl.

Melissa's story illustrates how our bodies communicate with us. Her choices caused her profound emotional confusion and cellular chaos. She realized that her unresolved feelings of shame and worthlessness stemmed from feeling that her father had abandoned her. This prompted her to act out choices, which made her feel even more ashamed and worthless. If she hadn't listened to her body's messages, the outcome could have been dismal.

Like Melissa, I needed a big bump over the head to wake up. Before I got sick, I was numb—the unconscious queen of denial. I might have stayed that way, but my body forced me to listen. When we get sick, we might feel that our body is betraying us, but the opposite is true. Our bodies are on our side when they say, "NO!" for us.

Summon the courage to examine how you feel and why. If you are sick and suffer from painful emotions, I believe it's critical to look for the roots of your pain and listen to what your body is telling you.

Forms of Chronic Negativity

"My research has shown me that when emotions are expressed—which is to say that the biochemicals that are the substrate of emotion are flowing freely—all systems are united and made whole. When emotions are repressed, denied, not allowed to be whatever they may be, our network pathways get blocked, stopping the flow of the vital feel-good, unifying chemicals that run both our biology and our behavior."

— CANDACE PERT, author of *Molecules Of Emotion: The Science Between Mind-Body Medicine*

Chronic emotional negativity seems to play a role in many illnesses, including autoimmunity.[5] If you have an emotion that makes you feel stress and discomfort in your body, it's affecting your health. Think of chronic negative states as the saber-toothed tiger that you're running from in your mind. Remember, your body can't tell the difference between a real or perceived threat. The stress of chronic negative emotions keeps you in constant fight-or-flight and puts stress on all of your body's cells, including your immune cells.

There are many forms of emotional negativity that can affect your health. I'm going to give special attention to shame and hostility in this section, because they tend to be chronic and thus are more likely to be a "splinter" in chronic illness.

Remember this basic principle: whatever you feel bad about affects your health, and the longer and more intensely you feel it, the more likely it is to be a factor in any condition you have.

Guilt

Guilt is a feeling of self-condemnation over our actions or circumstances. Any feeling that makes us feel chronic negativity within affects our health because our body follows along with the bad feeling. Guilt differs from shame as we feel guilty when we believe we have *done* something bad. We feel shame when believe we *are* bad.

Guilt can be a helpful wake-up call that we have acted out of integrity. That is called "appropriate guilt." One the other hand, people often suffer "inappropriate guilt" over events that they had no control over, such as hitting an animal that dashed in front of the car. None of us has psychic vision foretelling how every event will unfold so it's pointless to feel guilty for not making the perfect move every time.

Some people even feel guilty about the blessings of their lives such as love, family and financial abundance. This can be due to a sense of unworthiness in having more than our loved ones. Another face of guilt is survivor's guilt, which occurs after living through a disaster, accident or the deaths of friends or family.

It's important to become aware of the extent that you feel guilt so that you can address those feelings as part of your healing process.

Take a look at the guilt in your life. If your guilt is inappropriate, let it go and free yourself from needless pain and its attendant health consequences. If you feel rightly guilty, use it as a call for action to make amends, seek forgiveness, or simply resolve to act with integrity in the future. Bludgeoning yourself with negative guilty feelings serves no one and only punishes yourself and damages your health.

Grief

It's not surprising that prolonged sadness and grief can compromise the immune system and weaken our health. It is natural to mourn loss, but the body suffers along with us in the process. It's important to wisely cope with the challenge of grief. Denying the pain is worse than expressing feelings, but clinging to grief is self-defeating. The key is to move through the sad feelings without getting lost or stuck in them. Sometimes we even feel a moral duty to be depressed and unhappy about a loss. There are ways to honor our loss without remaining in an emotional hole indefinitely.

Feel and express your emotions without becoming addicted to the feeling of sadness, or wallowing in despair. "Poor Me," however justified, is self-punishing and self-punishing attitudes are contrary to reversing your autoimmune condition. Respect your sadness, feel the emotions, but don't get stuck and don't chew endlessly on the sad story.

Science has observed that grief can create inflammation in the brain.[6] Particularly challenging is Prolonged Grief Disorder (PGD), which is a pathological reaction indicated when an individual experiences severe grief for at least six months and is stuck in a maladaptive pattern.[7]

I don't blame those who grieve, and I don't want you to blame yourself. Still, if sadness and grief are setting the stage for your autoimmune condition, it's important to work on moving through your feelings, perhaps with the help of a therapist, or a grief counselor.

Shame and Hostility

Many healing books illustrate the autoimmune process as "anger" turned inward. I disagree. I see the self-destructive feelings that accompany shame and hostility as more fundamental to the autoimmune process because they are such intense, prolonged emotional negative states and tend to be chronic.

Now let's discuss how these forms of negativity arise in our lives, and how they can be transformed with understanding, forgiveness, love, and self-acceptance.

Shame

*Guilt is what we feel when we believe we have **done** something bad. Shame is what we feel when we believe we **are** bad.*

I have repeatedly witnessed chronic shame as the emotion that does perhaps the greatest damage to people's health and their lives. Shame is not the guilt that comes from hurting someone or having a moral lapse, nor is it the embarrassment that comes from looking foolish in front of others. Shame is the feeling of unworthiness, inadequacy and self-condemnation that we internalize when we believe that we are fundamentally flawed or worthless. We might use guilt about our actions as evidence to justify our shame, but many punish themselves with shame in the absence of any guilt.

Societies often use shame as a control mechanism to motivate conformity, but what might be considered "shameful" in one culture might be normal in another. Some cultures feel it's normal and acceptable for someone to walk around nearly naked, while other societies believe it is shameful for a woman to even reveal her ankle. Obviously, what constitutes "shameful" is subjective. It is often based on societal conditioning, rather than on a universal "truth."

The tactic of shaming or humiliating a person as a consequence of a violent, indecent, or unacceptable act might seem appropriate, but shaming often fails to bring reformation. Society uses the punishment of shaming to ensure that people follow the rules of the "tribe." Unfortunately, this tortuous approach rarely *inspires* anyone to change or evolve. In fact, people often just become cleverer at concealing their actions to avoid further shaming. In the worst cases, they become perpetrators of shame or abuse. Studies have shown that men who commit abuse as adults were more likely to have been abused as children. The cycle of shame perpetuates itself.

Worst of all, shame is often internalized by the victims of abuse, who did nothing to deserve their trauma but nonetheless often feel damaged, or even responsible. Adults are godlike to young children, who often blame themselves for the abuse they suffer. For example, it's common for children to blame themselves when their parents split up. Even kids from relatively healthy families may suffer shame when they fail to match expectations for their performance in school or sports. As children get older, they suffer by comparing themselves to their peers. There is always someone prettier, more popular, skinnier, or smarter.

Toxic Shame: the Cycle of Self-Loathing

"Shame corrodes the very part of us that believes we are capable of change."
— Brené Brown

Shame is toxic. Shame is our negative judgment of ourselves, making us our own enemy. It is self-punishment. We doubt we are worthy of Love. We question if we are "good enough." We feel insecure about our validity and doubtful about our place in other people's lives. We despair that we're damaged goods, that we don't deserve love, abundance, or wellness. Ultimately, shame can make us wish we were dead.

Shame is so uncomfortable that most of us prefer to ignore it. It's not even easy to read about shame. We pretend it's not there. We tell ourselves stories that it's okay to avoid looking at it, yet however subconscious the feelings may be, we often find ourselves apologizing for our existence. We strive to "be somebody"—to achieve and be the most ideal person we can imagine—in the hope that it may release us from the shame we hold ourselves in. While people who have suffered challenging childhoods or abuse often have a more intense struggle around shame, it appears to be a natural consequence of human conditioning.

Exploring the Origins of Shame

We come into life innocent. Seemingly all-powerful beings—our parents—orient us to this strange world, sharing what they believe we should think and know. Without them, we would be helpless and lost. They encourage, even pressure us to aspire to their values and follow their guidance. Seeking security, love, and acceptance (and in some cases our very survival), we try to meet their expectations. In so doing, we begin judging ourselves about the ways in which we feel we don't meet the idealized criteria.

Shame is born from the friction between who we think we are and who we think we should be.

"Who we think we are" is a self-referential pattern of thoughts, our self-image, which incessantly regards our history, our faults, our hopes and fears, and how the world treats us and forms opinions about us. Our minds swim in a stream of thoughts about ourselves. We create this self-image with our thinking, and we can reform it and heal it; each of us can become our own champion rather than our own worst critic.

"Who we think we should be" is a product of the conditioning we receive from society and our parents. Most of us try to be a perfect self that is unattainable and impossible. We believe we "should" be intelligent, attractive, talented, gracious, generous, creative, hard working, self-sacrificing… and the list goes on forever.

It's bad enough that shame is an issue for "normal" people. Shame becomes dramatically more toxic if a vulnerable child suffers abuse at the hands of a powerful adult. In this case, someone the child looks to for love and security instills fear and vulnerability instead. The child innocently believes they must have deserved the ill treatment, and later feels damaged. This can be so disturbing that the child locks the memory away in denial, but the shame of it still festers beneath the surface, polluting emotional wellbeing and eroding health.

While early childhood is a particularly vulnerable time for developing shame, it's certainly true that disturbing or traumatic events later in life can also bring shame, such as rape, impotence, bankruptcy, or unemployment. A person may also feel ashamed of their family, sexuality, culture, or country, or of being adopted. Shame can be passed down through generations, leaving us with a subliminal sense of self-loathing for the transgressions of our ancestors.

People who carry toxic shame have low self-esteem and believe that they are seriously flawed. They may fall into the role of either the victim or the perpetrator in an abusive relationship. Toxic shame accompanies many psychological disorders such as narcissistic and borderline personality disorder, eating disorders, and addictions. It is also at the core of many violent behaviors, such as rape and child molestation.

Toxic shame undermines intimate relationships. People often experience repeated patterns in successive relationships. Usually the patterns reflect wounds that we unconsciously re-enact, hoping for a better outcome, but somehow always choosing the partner who can't respect us, can't commit, can't be faithful, or even lashes out violently. Subconsciously, we think that's what we deserve, and we become accustomed to it.

We may pretend to be admirable instead of acting like who we really are. We may become perfectionists, or people pleasers. This is an attempt to compensate for our inner chaos and turmoil. We create an idealized false self, and then frantically work to maintain that image, because we believe, deep down, that we are ugly and unlovable. We may be hypercritical of others and ourselves. Even arrogance and megalomania can be signs of overcompensating for inner shame and self-doubt. We might want to hide or disappear. We might withdraw from the world. We don't dare to imagine the full expression of our innate brilliance.

Brené Brown, Ph.D., spent over a decade researching shame. In her book, *I Thought It Was Just Me (but it isn't): Telling the Truth About*

Perfectionism, Inadequacy and Power, she describes shame as a "full-contact" emotion because we feel it viscerally in our bodies.

She writes, "Shame is the intensely painful feeling or experience of believing we are flawed and therefore unworthy of acceptance and belonging. Women often experience shame when they are entangled in a web of layered conflicting and competing social-community expectations. Shame creates feelings of fear, blame, and disconnection…(It) can make us feel desperate. Reactions to this desperate need to escape from isolation and fear can run the gamut from behavioral issues and acting out to depression, self-injury, eating disorders, addiction, violence, and suicide."

No one likes to talk about shame, not even doctors, psychotherapists or healers. But however uncomfortable the subject, it is essential to examine the shame in your life, because the persistent feeling of unworthiness, of being down on yourself or even against yourself, is bound to take a toll on your health and wellbeing.

How Shame Leads to Chronic Illness

On the physiological level, shame can resonate through the cells of your body and cause inflammation. In fact, the 2004 study, "Immunological Effects of Induced Shame and Guilt," found that just writing about traumatic experiences in which the subjects blamed themselves for three 20-minute sessions resulted in alterations in the immune system, particularly activation of pro-inflammatory cytokine activity.[8] Imagine what effect chronic internalized shame could have over time!

I have regularly seen shame and its attendant self-destructive thoughts and unhealthy coping patterns playing a major role in many people's autoimmune processes, including my own. While it's clear that other underlying causes combine to trigger the autoimmune process, we must look within and work through any shame we find so each of us can become our own greatest supporter rather than our own worst enemy.

An Experience of Shame: My Story

"Owning our own story can be hard, but not nearly as difficult as spending our lives running from it. Embracing our vulnerabilities feels risky, but is not nearly as dangerous as giving up on love, belonging, and joy—the experiences that makes us the most vulnerable. Only

when we are brave enough to explore the darkness will we discover the infinite power of our light."

— Brené Brown, *The Gifts of Imperfection*

I know how scary it is to face your shame head-on, because I've spent most of my life running from mine. Looking back, I can see how much shame shaped my life and squashed my spirit.

Nothing was off-limits in my family. Even adult family members thought nothing of ridiculing anyone who was hurt or insecure. I remember one summer day when I was about nine years old. My aunt had picked up my two younger siblings and me to spend the weekend at her house. I sat in the front seat, wearing my new, white, stretchy dolphin shorts. I remember looking in the mirror at home and thinking that I didn't look *that* fat for a change. (I was always a little chubby as a kid.) My aunt got in the car and shrieked, "My goodness, you should be ashamed of yourself, young lady. If I had legs like yours, I wouldn't leave the house, let alone wear shorts! Your legs are so disgusting!"

I was so ashamed. I felt like I had been kicked in the stomach. I wanted to hide, to disappear. Actually, I wanted to die. When we got to her house I changed into long pants, threw my new shorts away, and climbed up into the walnut tree. Part of me hoped that I would fall down and crack my head open on the brick patio. I stayed up there for hours, until my uncle finally came home and coaxed me down. From that day forward, I was convinced that I was hideous, fat, and disgusting. Those negative feelings became the backdrop for an eating disorder that eventually contributed to an autoimmune condition. It's taken years to overcome the shame I had around my body.

Identifying Shame

It's easy to pinpoint obvious shaming experiences like the one above, but many people are unaware that they harbor subtle forms of shame.

Shame may be present behind feelings of insecurity, self-consciousness, fear, confusion, anger, shyness, or depression. We might end up judging others to project our shame away from ourselves. We might apologize for minor mistakes as if we were supposed to be perfect. We might fear that people don't really want us to be there—that we're secretly unwelcome and unaccepted.

Shame can make us act and feel "crazy." We may not even know why. We might lash out at someone else because we feel bad about ourselves.

I used to have a "crazy" reaction every time my ex-husband would suggest that we play volleyball, surf, or go to a pool party where I would have to wear a bathing suit. I would get very confused and experience a "spacey" feeling, then anger. I knew he hadn't done anything wrong, but I couldn't help but pick a fight. He would eventually go alone or stay home. I wasn't aware of it at the time, but just the suggestion of wearing a swimsuit triggered the shame I had about my body, and I would do anything to avoid that feeling.

Shame can keep us in isolation. We may forego social events. We may refrain from meeting new people, going to school, trying new things, or following our dreams. Shame can hold us prisoner and keep us from living authentically.

How do you know if toxic shame is affecting your life and your heath? Ask yourself the following questions:

Do you frequently feel worthless, ugly, stupid, or unlovable?

Do you feel like you're a bad person?

Were you shamed about anything as a child—perhaps your body, your intelligence, your behavior or your sexuality?

Do you feel shame around a traumatic experience such as childhood abuse or rape?

Do you hide the "real" you so that people won't suspect the truth about you?

Do you lie, cover up, or exaggerate about the details of your life to appear better, smarter, and more successful than you really are?

Do you have secrets about your past or current situation that you would be mortified if someone found out about?

Do you tend to be hypercritical of others and yourself?

Do you lash out inappropriately at others for no reason?

Do you find yourself chastising yourself constantly over the state of your work, body, finances, or relationships?

Do you find yourself apologizing for yourself over trivial matters?

Is it hard to look in a mirror?

Everyone feels some of these feeling from time to time, but it's important to identify if these feelings are chronic and making you feel miserable.

Transforming Shame

"Shame derives its power from being unspeakable."
– Brené Brown

Transforming shame is a journey that requires strength and courage. We must be willing to shine a light on the darkest places in our lives and in our psyche—the places that make us cringe with fear and disgust. We must go down to the basement and face the scary monsters we've been hiding from. We must be willing to name our shame and recognize it as the parasite that is sucking us dry. We have to observe how we let our own personal demons possess us.

Conscious awareness has the power to transform our emotional wounds once we bring them to light, much like a properly functioning immune system has the power to recognize and eradicate disease in our physical body.

Dr. Brown suggests that to transform shame, we must first identify and name it. We then summon the courage to reach out to others. Finally, we find our own voice to speak about our shame.

I was able to heal from the episode with my aunt by telling my story to a coach, 20 years later. It wasn't easy. As I related my experience, my heart started to race, and I felt a wave of heat wash over my chest and face. I got dizzy and nauseous. She kept reminding me to breathe. As I did, I began to sob. I re-experienced the pain and hurt of that day when I was nine. I mourned for the little girl who had been so deeply hurt by someone she loved and looked up to.

My coach related a similar story from her own past, then suggested that my aunt must have felt ashamed of her body in some way, and that my exposed legs triggered her own body image issues. Suddenly, it dawned on me that I had never seen my aunt in a bathing suit or shorts. In fact, I remembered seeing a picture of her when she was in her twenties at the beach, and everyone was in a bathing suit except her. She was wearing pants. In that moment, I was overcome with an incredible feeling of compassion for my aunt, and for myself.

That day was the beginning of a transformation for me, because I had taken the risk of telling my story. My coach related her own story of shame, which helped me to see that not only did she understand my feelings, she had similar feelings of shame about her own body. I wasn't alone!

Sharing our stories of shame and listening to the stories of others helps us develop empathy and compassion. Dr. Brown describes empathy as the antidote for shame. Compassion for ourselves goes hand in hand with compassion for others.

Ultimately, it is self-acceptance and love that transforms our shame. When you learn to love yourself, your whole life feels better. To heal your autoimmune condition, you need to develop compassion and love for yourself. You must wish yourself well, truly, from the heart.

Anger and Hostility

"Holding on to anger is like grasping a hot coal with the intent of throwing it at someone else; you are the one who gets burned."

– BUDDHA

Anger needs little introduction. You have been angry, or you haven't been human. Despite our common experience of anger, few people realize that it is a "secondary emotion." We get angry in response to a primary emotion such as fear, frustration, humiliation, or hurt. The pain of rejection is unbearable, so we react with anger to avoid the hurt. Our fear is too threatening, so anger surfaces in an attempt to protect us. We feel upset when something doesn't go our way, but instead of facing the frustration, we get angry. If you repress your anger when your spouse forgets your anniversary, you might wind up lashing out at the dog or the kids over some minor issue. Repressed anger can fester within and erode your health. Anger can become a habitual state of negativity that makes you routinely cynical and disparaging of others and the world. This chronic anger is called hostility, and you pay for it with your happiness and your health.

Hostility: Gina's Story

Hostility comes from the Latin word *hostis,* which means enemy.

When we are hostile, we see enemies everywhere—at the office, at the store, on the freeway, even in our own homes. We can become distrustful of others and of life itself. This becomes a self-fulfilling prophecy as others sense our hostility and thus are more likely to avoid us, reject us, or mirror our negativity. We can begin to view the world as a dangerous place where everything is a fight for our very survival. In fact, anger invokes our fight-or-flight response, which you have already learned is inflammatory. Chronic hostile negativity can be a potent cofactor in provoking an autoimmune response when other splinters also burden the system.

Take Gina, who came to me for help with rheumatoid arthritis and Raynaud's disease. Her hostility was palpable during her first visit. She sat across from me, stewing in disgust, as she ranted about how she disliked most people. "Everybody I know is a jerk," she said. "I've been screwed over so many times I can't even count anymore." She went on to reveal how her mother had betrayed her. Her husband left. Her kids wouldn't talk to her. Her boss was a bloodsucking vampire. She had been screwed over by a contractor, who ripped her off for $10,000, and even the police and judge in her town were corrupt because they had sided with him. As she was speaking, her cell phone buzzed. She became furious as she scrambled to the bottom of her purse to find it. "What the hell does this person want now? Can't I get a frickin' break?"

I excused myself and went to the ladies' room. I closed the door, leaned back, and thought, "What am I going to do with this person? She's so angry. She scares me!"

Then, I did what I always do when I don't have the answer: I prayed.

In a few moments, I began to wonder if Gina's hostility was covering a deep hurt, perhaps many deep hurts. I wondered if she had chosen hostility to defend herself from the deep pain of betrayal. One thing was clear, her hostile attitude was costing her life force energy. The constant stress of her fight-or-flight response was breaking her body down. I didn't see her as angry at herself; she was hurt and using hostility as a defense mechanism.

Gina's hostility had become chronic, and consequently fed a vicious cycle of stress hormones and neurochemicals that perpetuated yet more stress and more negative outcomes. I could tell that she wanted help, but I had to wonder if she was "addicted" to the stress on a physiological level. Hostility = stress hormones = negative expectations = negative outcomes = more hostility. It's a vicious and unhappy cycle, but I know from personal experience that it's habit-forming. Helping Gina reverse this pattern would be the key to helping her get better. I could tell that this wasn't the time to suggest that her attitude could be affecting her health. I didn't want to put her on the defensive. It takes diplomacy and a timely opportunity to bring up something so personal to make sure it isn't received as blame.

I walked out of the ladies' room and sat next to Gina, who was scrolling through her text messages. As I reviewed her health history and diet, I noticed that she was eating quite a bit of sugar. Her typical breakfast was a pastry or doughnut with coffee. Lunch was pasta, meat, and a Coke. Dinner was pasta, mac-n-cheese or a hamburger, bread, potatoes, fries, or sometimes a bowl of cereal, ice cream, and a Coke. She listed that she drank 3-4 Cokes a day. The other piece of the puzzle was clearly a sugar addiction. I explained that autoimmune conditions always have multiple factors. If she wanted to get better she would need to cut out sugar, gluten, and all refined carbs in order to heal her GI tract. Hoping she wasn't going to freak out, I bravely explained the connection between GI imbalances, unstable blood sugar, and explosive anger and hostility.

She asked, "Are you telling me that I'm pissed off because I eat sugar?" I replied, "Well, it certainly hasn't turned you into Mary Poppins. Why don't we try taking it out, balancing your blood sugar and your brain chemistry, and see what happens?" She laughed a little, and agreed to try the elimination diet. As she walked out the door, she remarked over her shoulder that she was going to be *really* pissed off if it didn't work.

I suggested my regular list of supplements: Multi-vitamin with B complex, selenium, magnesium, zinc, extra omega-3, extra vitamin C, digestive enzymes, and a good probiotic. I also suggested she start on a medical food for liver detoxification and suggested GABA for her irritability and sugar cravings.

The first week was awful. She was irritable, had headaches and anxiety, and described herself as "a bitch on wheels." After three weeks, though, she felt better. She e-mailed me that she had lost weight and her moods were more stable. It felt safe to face her again, so we scheduled a follow up on her 23rd day on the program.

She had picked up a handout from my waiting room, "Connecting

Emotions and Your Heath." She pointed to the section on anger and hostility. It explained how these emotions were connected to heart disease and stroke, and how suppressed anger may be connected to cancer. She said, "Maybe I *am* really pissed off! I don't have cancer or heart disease, but this autoimmune thing is just as bad, right?"

I said, "Well, if you really want my opinion, I feel that shame and hostility are two of the emotional components of many autoimmune conditions." I explained my view that we often choose hostility when the pain of a deep hurt is unbearable. I confessed how I had chosen hostility over vulnerability many times, and that it follows a predictable pattern. The more hostile we are, the more isolated we feel, the more we expect hostility from others, the more hostile they become… It's a vicious cycle that feeds on itself.

I explained that while some of us suppress our feelings when we are hurt, others feel safer getting angry and even staying angry. I reminded her that our Western culture encourages repression of emotions like sadness while encouraging the expression of hostility and aggression. We've all heard the sayings: "Boys don't cry," "Keep a stiff upper lip," and "Don't get mad, get even."

I explained that the first step in transforming hostility and its underlying sense of powerlessness involves detoxing our bodies and our minds. When our bodies are clear, our minds become clear. We become more conscious of our thoughts and how they drive our behaviors. We need to take out our inner trash so that our true essence can be revealed, but when the body is toxic, it's an impossible task.

After nine months on a good nutrition program Gina's autoimmune symptoms had all but disappeared. She's currently working with a HeartMath® therapist on letting go of rage and anger. When I last saw her she had a huge smile on her face and greeted me with a bear hug. (I suspect she's on the right path!)

If you feel that hostility is slowly poisoning you, make a point of working on this issue, perhaps with a therapist or coach. Resolving hostility will not only uplift your health but may improve your social life and relationships.

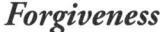

Forgiveness

"Miraculously, we often find that once the hatred is out of our own hearts, others can no longer sustain the negativity they have for us either."
– Karl Baba

Many of us feel that when we forgive somebody, we're doing them a favor. Perhaps they've changed, or apologized, or maybe we feel that we've made them suffer enough.

The reality is, the main beneficiary of forgiveness is the forgiver.

Holding on to the past and the wrongs done to us keeps us in fight or flight mode and drains our precious life energy.[9] Choosing to relive our negative experiences over and over, without resolving to learn and grow from the experience keeps us in the powerless position of the victim.

On the other hand the process of forgiveness liberates us and brings us peace. Releasing anger, hostility and the need for revenge has positive health benefits.[10] Witness the negative charge within you, without obsessing over its dramatic story, and let it go. By forgiving others, we forgive ourselves. When Jesus said, "Judge not, lest ye be judged," he was not dispensing morality. He was illustrating the process by which we condemn ourselves. The judgments and grudges we hold against others create the framework for our judgment against ourselves. Negative feelings within us contaminate our state of mind, and are in turn reflected in the world around us.

Taking the leap to forgive others releases negativity within us, makes us whole, and automatically begins to heal the grudge that we have with ourselves. It weakens our bondage to our pettiness, and makes a space for love. The most important person to forgive is yourself. It's simply contradictory to seek healing with one hand and punish yourself with the other.

Does forgiveness mean we have to resume or maintain the relationship with the ones we forgive? No, forgiveness is an inner state of releasing negativity. It is for your own good. If expressing that forgiveness will subject you to further abuse, you don't have to communicate it. Forgiving the violent ex-husband doesn't excuse his actions, nor does it mean you have to take him back. It just means that you aren't holding a place of darkness within yourself that ties you to your past wounds and suffering.

You don't have to resume sending money to your wayward child so she can finance her alcoholism. You don't have to dismiss charges against the violent criminal so he can go find another victim. You can speak out against injustice, protect yourself or the weak and exploited. Just don't allow any grudge to fester within. Don't suffer the same wounds for the rest of your life. Forgive and be free.

Blame vs. Responsibility

"In our ignorance we are innocent; in our actions we are guilty. We sin without knowing and suffer without understanding."
– Sri Nisargadatta Maharaj

There is an old Cherokee story of an elder teaching his grandson about the battle within. He said, "My son, there is a battle between two 'wolves' inside us all. One is Evil. It is anger, envy, jealousy, sorrow, regret, greed, arrogance, self-pity, guilt, resentment, inferiority, lies, false pride, superiority, and ego.

"The other is good. It is joy, peace, love, hope, serenity, humility, kindness, benevolence, empathy, generosity, truth, compassion, and faith."

The grandson thought about it for a minute, and then asked his grandfather: "Which wolf wins?"

The grandfather simply replied, "The one you feed."

To heal, you must choose to follow the voice within that wishes you well, that chooses healing, and forgoes self-pity in favor of empowerment. You begin to walk in a good way towards balance and healing.

That walk begins with taking responsibility for your own health. I would like to stress that this is not the same as being "to blame" for your illness. Blaming yourself just adds guilt to your list of problems. Blame is negative. It implies that someone is at fault, or that we willfully caused ourselves harm.

Taking responsibility doesn't mean that we are "to blame" for our illness. We did not consciously choose to be sick.

Responsibility means taking conscious action, stepping outside of the story of our lives and impartially observing how we live. When we do this, we notice how our actions and patterns of behavior create our current reality. When we become aware, we can say without judgment: *"Oh boy, I see how my pattern of x, y, and z, which started when I was little, is causing the stressful situation in my life now. What can I do to get better results?"* Or, *"Wow, I'm stressed-out all the time. How is that affecting my health?"*

When we were children, we didn't get to choose our circumstances. We instinctively learned to react to our parents and our environment to get our needs met. Many of us with autoimmune conditions grew up in stressful homes; some of us endured physical and emotional abuse. We developed "coping" personality strategies in order to survive, such as being "perfect," "a pleaser," "always being nice," "never getting angry," "taking care of everyone else first," "never saying no," or "making others' problems our own." Many of us have weak personal boundaries and an underdeveloped sense of self.

We had no choice, really; we learned coping personality traits for survival.

I was beaten and endured sexual abuse as a child. From an early age, I also had the responsibility of "making sure the house was perfect…or else!" I was told that children should be seen and not heard, so I learned to be silent. I refused to cry when I was beaten. I learned to always say, "Yes, Papa!" even when I really wanted to say "No!" I learned to be helpful, organized, and clean—always. I learned how to act "perfect" to avoid trouble and gain acceptance.

I developed these personality traits to navigate the treacherous waters of my violent family life. As I grew older, the coping mechanisms that saved my life as a child landed me in relationships that ultimately made me sick. I chose codependent relationships, personally and professionally, because I didn't know how else to relate to the world.

I was drawn to relationships where I couldn't express my true feelings. If I did, they were dismissed with anger, even violence. I chose relationships where I paid most of the bills and did all the housework while my partner went off to play. There I was, like Cinderella, silently suffering and cleaning, feeling sorry for myself all the while. " Woe is me. I never get what I want. Nobody cares about my feelings." Because I didn't love myself, I was repeatedly attracted to commitment-phobic men who didn't know how to love themselves, and were consequently incapable of loving me. I made unfulfilling career choices because I lacked the self-esteem to pursue my dreams.

Was I creating my own reality? Yes. Was I responsible or to blame? No, because I was not conscious of what I was doing. I was recapitulating dysfunctional patterns from my childhood because I didn't know any better.

The shift came when I got sick. I was forced to look at every area of my life, including my emotions. I had to be honest with myself and admit how unhappy I was. I asked myself *without judgment,* "What am I doing to contribute to my illness? What patterns am I repeating from the past that cause stress in my life? What am I still holding onto from childhood? Who would I be without this sob story? Am I ready to drop it, move on, and heal?"

The answers were easy to identify with the help of a good coach, but only when I was completely honest with myself. To find your own answers, start with the things you complain about the most. See if you have been complaining about them for a while (like most of your life?). We tend to re-enact the dramas and traumas of our childhood. Look for repeating patterns in your relationships. Usually, the common thread is within us if we are honest enough to recognize it.

Is the Imbalance in Your Mind or Your Body?

"The root of all health is in the brain. The trunk of it is in emotion. The branches and leaves are the body. The flower of health blooms when all parts work together."
– Kurdish Saying

Do toxic emotional states lead to ill health? Or does ill health contribute to a chronic state of unhappiness? The answer is both. Our chronic negativity can make us sick, and then our poor health inspires more negativity. They reinforce each other.

The New Age concept that "our thoughts create our reality" contains a wisdom that is often misinterpreted. Many people have turned that wisdom into more of a New Age Guilt Trip. I see a lot of people struggle needlessly when they mistakenly blame past traumas and negative thinking *alone* for their chronic illness. I've seen many clients who have spent hundreds (if not thousands) of dollars on therapies such as counseling, psychotherapy, neuro-linguistic programming, bio-feedback, hypnotism, and spiritual healing with the hope of turning their health around only to see very little, if any, improvement. While these therapies can have tremendous value, they focus on the cognitive, spiritual or emotional aspect of health and typically gloss over, or worse, totally ignore the physical imbalances.

Many people ignore the negative influence that excess caffeine, sugar, carbs, drugs (even prescription and over-the-counter drugs), and alcohol can have on our brain. These poor coping strategies disturb the clarity and peace of mind that can be the foundation of a flourishing life. The bottom line is that the huge toxic load we're exposed to in modern life affects our brain chemistry and our moods.

The point is: work on healing your emotions to heal your body, but also work on your body to heal your mind. Otherwise it's like learning to dance while carrying a bowling ball: grace will be difficult to achieve.

Sarah came to see me one month after her 38th birthday to lose weight. Within the first minute or two of talking to her, I felt a wave of compassion because, frankly, she seemed to be a mess on so many levels. Her face was puffy and she was borderline obese. For the young wife of an affluent doctor, her appearance was frumpy and disheveled. She was wearing a men's pair of black, elastic-waistband sweatpants and an oversized t-shirt with running shoes. She was frazzled and forgetful. For example, I poured each of us a cup of tea, and three times she accidentally drank from my cup and then, in a state of flustered embarrassment, apologized profusely. She began almost everything she said with some sort of apology. She spoke in run-on sentences while gesticulating nervously with her hands.

She was the mother of two toddlers, who weren't with her, but she had lugged a large, plastic diaper bag with diapers and baby bottles spilling out of the side pockets into my office. This bag was also her purse, and at one point, like a magician pulling a white rabbit from a hat, she yanked out a skinny, white cotton sun dress and waved it dramatically in the air.

"Just look at this!" she said. Her voice, which had an edge of hysteria, went up an octave or two. "This used to fit me! I used to fit in this dress!" She shook the dress in her fist as if it were evidence of a cosmic injustice. "Now look at me!" She gestured toward her t-shirt and sweat pants and it became obvious that she was very aware of her frumpy attire and appearance. "I wear sweatpants every day because I refuse to buy fat clothes!" The nervous, run-on monologue suddenly paused, and her eyes welled up with tears. "If I gain any more weight, I know my husband is going to leave me!"

I comforted her as best I could, and once she calmed down there were more revelations. "To hear me talk, you would probably never guess that I have a Ph.D., and before my first child was born I was a researcher at [a major university]. I can't even read anymore! Even a romance novel is too hard for me. I just read the same paragraph over and over again. With each pregnancy I gained 20 pounds, and I can't get an ounce of it off!"

I questioned her more about some of her symptoms and found out that she was constipated, fatigued, cold all the time, and had foggy thinking and memory problems, transient rashes, miserable hay fever year-round, low energy, crying spells for no reason, chronic yeast infections (every month), and zero desire for sex. Her doctor had tested only her TSH (thyroid-stimulating hormone), which was 4.7, and told her that her thyroid was "fine" and that she needed to eat less, exercise more, and go to a stress reduction class.

Sarah had been seeing a psychologist since her first child was born 4 years ago. She revealed that she had been sexually abused as a child and was an active member of an adult survivor of childhood abuse support group. "But now that I have children, the abuse seems more current somehow and bothers me more!" I told her that this was common for abuse survivors raising small children. As their own children pass through the ages that they were at when the abuse started, it brings the horror of the past to the forefront. They can't help but to think how horrible it would be if the same thing happened to their kids, and have a difficult time wrapping their heads around how any adult could hurt such an innocent child.

Attempting to work through her childhood trauma, Sarah had tried a smorgasbord of therapies: biofeedback, cognitive therapy, stress management classes, art therapy, and some sort of expensive encounter sessions that sounded very dubious. Summing up this work on herself, Sarah said, "I realize that I'm creating my own reality and that the thoughts I'm thinking are making me sick, but I can't seem to stop them. I never smile or laugh anymore. I don't even remember what it feels like to laugh. I try really hard, but I just keep getting worse. I think there is something really spiritually wrong with me. I've been praying really hard and doing all the right things, but nothing works. I must not be a good person, or maybe I just have bad karma." She had been referred to a psychiatrist for antidepressants. She was considering that as her last option, but had held off because she had read about the weight gain side effects of many antidepressants.

I asked Sarah if she was open to the idea that there might be more to her symptoms than past traumas and negative thinking, and that perhaps there were some major physiological imbalances in her body that warranted deeper investigation. She was open, so I sent her home with some blood test recommendations for her physician, as well as a test for heavy metals. Unfortunately, her doctor refused to order the blood tests, so rather than taking the time to find a new doctor, she decided to have her lab tests performed by MyMedLab.com. The results were astonishing. Her T4 and T3 were far below the functional range, her TSH had risen to 6.2, and her TPO (thyroid antibodies) were 274. The high antibody count indicated the autoimmune thyroid condition known as Hashimoto's. Her other test results indicated inflammation and high cholesterol and triglycerides, and elevated antibodies pointed to a systemic Candida infection. Her heavy metals test revealed elevated levels of mercury, lead, and cadmium.

I suggested she start *eating for her good genes* and follow phase I of the *Sensitivity Discovery Program* to remove dietary toxins and food allergies. I also recommended a medical food supplement to support her liver detoxification, along with the Women's Empowerment Formula, additional omega-3 fish oil, borage oil, extra vitamin C, and a good probiotic. I suggested she talk to her physician about thyroid hormone therapy and antifungal treatment. I explained that she needed to heal her GI before considering a heavy metal detox to avoid the risk of the body reabsorbing the toxins. She could begin detoxification, however, with Epsom salt baths and far-infrared sauna sessions.

Her doctor was surprised at her test results and apologized for not taking more time with her at her last visit. (This poor doctor sees over 25 patients a day in a very busy OBGYN facility.) He wrote her a prescription for a compounded T4/T3 sustained release combination through The Compounding Pharmacy of Beverly Hills, as well as a 3-month round of Diflucan for the chronic yeast infection.

After 11 weeks on the program, Sarah had completely removed gluten and all refined carbs, dairy, and sugar from her diet. She had finished the antifungal therapy and had been taking the supplements and probiotics. She was taking Epsom salt baths 4 times a week and did a 30-minute far-infrared sauna 5 days a week. She upped the dose of thyroid medication initially, but was feeling a little overmedicated and had dropped it back a bit. So far, she had lost 29 pounds, which was only 10 pounds from her wedding weight. She had not had a yeast infection, UTI, or rash since she first came to see me, and she was sleeping "mostly" through the night (meaning she only woke up if the kids woke her up).

One of the most profound transformations was in her mood, which started right around 21 days into the program. She was able to laugh and experience joy for the first time in years. She told me, "I woke up one day about 3 weeks into the program and my head was clear. My little girl came in with her daddy's shoes on and I couldn't stop laughing. It was like a mountain of weight had been lifted off of me. I can think clearly, and I feel hopeful for the future. I still have my bad moments for sure. But now, when those negative thoughts come, I know they will pass and I can breathe through them. It's like all of the tools my therapist has been trying to teach me for 4 years sunk in all at once!"

At her 18-week blood check, her TPO had dropped to 27 (indicating her Hashimoto's condition was reversed) and her IgM antibodies to Candida were gone. Her cholesterol and other blood test results had also returned to normal.

Sarah stopped psychotherapy because her psychologist said she was ready to live her life on her own. She is now going back to school to become a counselor for women who have been abused. She credits healing her body with healing her mind. "I see now that my physical body was so out of whack that it was preventing me from improving my emotional life. I just want to help other women make the same connection between their physical bodies and their emotional states."

Admittedly, Sarah's case is a dramatic one, but in many ways, it is still representative of what many women with autoimmune thyroid conditions go through. She's also a perfect example of how balancing the body helps to balance the mind. I'm certain that had she not addressed her physical symptoms, she would have wound up taking an antidepressant and progressing to an even worse condition. Who knows how long it would have taken for her doctor to discover the autoantibodies and infection, if ever? How long would she have struggled for answers in psychotherapy? More importantly, what would her quality of life have been like while she was in therapy? Is there any chance that she could have overcome her emotional imbalances without addressing the physical ones? I don't think so.

My point is that it's simplistic to think that it's our thoughts *alone* that create our illnesses, because there are always underlying physical issues that need to be addressed. Whether it is the body or the mind that erodes our physical health, once our body is affected, it will exert a negative influence on the mind. We need to address both to heal both. The best psychotherapist in the world cannot correct nutrient deficiencies, GI function, an immune system imbalance, low thyroid hormones, gluten sensitivity, toxins or an infection. Yet any one of these imbalances can profoundly influence your emotional state.

Inspiration and Motivation Empower Healing

I was giving a lecture to a group of physicians when someone asked, "What is *the most* important aspect of recovering from an autoimmune disease? Do you have to go totally Paleo? Do you have to practice yoga every day? Do you have to spend a ton of cash on supplements? Do you have to meditate, or become a more religious person? Do you have to move to the mountains? What is *the* key to optimal wellness?"

My answer was that initially I had believed that recovery began on the physical plane, and that if a person could simply balance nutrition, detox, knock out infections, and exercise, then they could reverse and prevent illness. However, in my research and interviews with people who had reversed disease, I discovered that quite a few had experienced a " spiritual awakening" of some kind, and as a consequence had healed their physical body. This got me wondering if addressing the emotional or spiritual aspect of illness was the first step in reversing it.

Finally, I asked myself, "What does everyone who has healed have in common?"

What I realized is that whether their process started in the physical body or in the spiritual/emotional realm, each had learned to let go of fear and negative thoughts, and assume responsibility for their lives and their health. They each had expressed a true desire and passion for getting better. They wanted to be healthy so much they could taste it!

What I witnessed is that the more *responsible, loving, and forgiving* people became, the healthier they grew. In some cases, they had even escaped dreadful diagnoses like cancer and lupus. Even though these folks had be diagnosed with "incurable diseases," once they stepped out of the victim role and took responsibility for their health, they got better and stayed better.

These empowered people also seemed to possess a peace of mind, an ease that was missing in the ones who didn't get well. They appeared to be engaged with life and living from their hearts. They had found the courage to stop pretending to be what others wanted them to be, and as a consequence, they could finally relax. They had accepted themselves and their gifts. Operating from that place of acceptance gave their bodies enough energy to not only heal but to thrive.

One woman explained it to me this way: "My lupus has given me a choice—to be authentic or die."

I noticed that people who had made these emotional shifts had also learned healthier coping mechanisms for stress. They tended to drink less caffeine and alcohol. They stopped smoking. They reported fewer aches and pains and needed fewer over-the-counter and prescription drugs. They chose healthier food, and exercised more because they had the energy to do so. They tended to be forgiving, compassionate, and joyful; they possessed a healthy sense of self and good boundaries; they enjoyed loving relationships.

What I have learned is that healing from any chronic condition takes all the enthusiasm and energy you can muster up. If you're sick, you can't afford to lose energy to negativity. You simply don't have the luxury.

It doesn't really matter how you get there, but you must come to the fork in the road where there is no other choice.

Your desire to get better must be so compelling that you will do

everything in your power to reverse your condition.

Take Back Your Power and Express Yourself

"Never be bullied into silence. Never allow yourself to be made a victim. Accept no one's definition of your life; define yourself."
– HARVEY FIERSTEIN.

There seems to be some tragic, divine poetry in the body attacking its own thyroid gland, seated in our throat. My repeated observation after having interviewed hundreds of thyroid patients is that many of us feel disempowered. We have lost our "voice." We are holding back our feelings, restraining our self-expression, and sacrificing our needs. When you feel "choked up" and hold back your expression out of fear, unworthiness, or insecurity, you feel the pain and constriction in your throat.

To heal, you need to take back your power, to say what you feel, to quit being invisible.

Pay attention anytime an emotion or situation creates a visceral feeling in your throat. Look for a way to express what is provoking that feeling. Act as if you count just like everyone else…because you do!

Years of holding feelings and expressions within may have built up a good deal of emotional water behind the dam in your throat. In the beginning, you may need to be careful not to hurt people or be callous. You may even choose to begin speaking out loud by yourself, clearing the pent-up emotional charge.

Remember, the goal is to be yourself, express yourself, and take your place as an empowered human among your family, friends, and community. You are have a place and you are welcome here!

Conclusion

Your journey of psychological and emotional healing is as complex and individual as life itself. It is far beyond the scope of this book to provide the answers that our hearts and souls need to mend. The best I can do is point out the importance of discovering our unhealed wounds so we can begin our healing process.

I want to honor the unique challenges of your life—the traumas and experiences you've been through. That journey has brought you to this book. I can't tell you what path of transformation will work best for you. I can tell you, from personal and clinical experience, that it will take courage. You will need the collective powers of your mind, heart, and intuition to complete this journey. You will need to question assumptions, question authority, and question yourself.

Only you can persist on the healing path. Never give up. I hope this book helps light the way, but there is much you will have to investigate, consider, and practice on your own.

I salute all of you who engage in the courageous challenge of life transformation and healing. You are on an epic journey that can involve great difficulties, uplifting experiences, and personal discovery. Although the goal is healing, the journey is as important as the destination. You'll learn about yourself in the process. It's a worthy adventure. Give it everything you've got. That's what it takes.

There's a traditional prayer that suggests that when you are praying for your own healing, you also pray for all others who are similarly afflicted. Part of what helped me heal was that I wanted one day to help heal others. It helps to have a great aim or purpose that reaches beyond your own condition. A great purpose is what summons the deep moral courage to face a great challenge. People who have the will to heal almost always have a will to be a healing presence in the world.

Many call this sort of will by a one-syllable word: Love.

PART FOUR

Interviews with Doctors Who Are Curing Autoimmune Disease

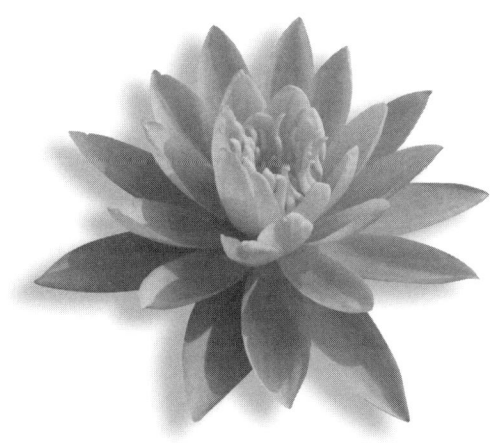

Dr. C. E. Gant

Dr. C. E. Gant has practiced Integrative, Complementary/Alternative and Functional Medicine for over three decades. Dr. Gant also teaches mindfulness-based meditation and incorporates Gestalt, REBT (Rational Emotive Behavioral Therapy), Transpersonal and other mindfulness-based psychotherapies into his medical practice.

His doctorate thesis research in the 1980's predicted that mindfulness-based therapies should evoke consistent neurophysiological changes in brain function (especially frontal lobes), which should be measurable with brain neuroimagery. This has essentially been proven in the last decade in functional Magnetic Resonance Imaging (fMRI) and Positron Emission Tomography (PET) research.

Dr. Gant is also Medical Director of the Academy of Functional Medicine & Genomics (www.academyoffunctionalmedicine.com), which provides webinar-based training for clinicians who wish to expand their skills into functional medicine and genomics (gene testing).

Dr. Gant received his B.S. degree in chemistry from Hampden-Sydney College and his medical degree from the University of Virginia Medical School. Dr. Gant pioneered many of the nutritional and detoxification protocols for the treatment of substance use and other mental disorders while serving as the Medical Director of Tully Hill Hospital, medical consultant at Syracuse Behavioral Healthcare and as a psychiatric consultant at numerous substance abuse and mental health clinics throughout central New York.

Dr. Gant currently practices at National Integrated Health Associates (NIHADC.com), where he provides the latest, cutting-edge, diagnostic, functional laboratory testing for his patients to define the root nutritional, hormonal, toxicological, allergic, metabolic and genetic causes of symptoms which can then be targeted in an individualized manner to optimize brain health and general wellness in his patients. This science-based approach can reverse the biochemical roots of aggression, addiction and mental disorders, as well as many medical disorders.

Q: There are roughly 70 million people in the United States with autoimmune disease, 70 percent of which are women. Can you tell us what may be causing such an epidemic?

A: I think the main cause is an unprecedented exposure to toxins, heavy metals, petrochemicals, and solvents, largely due to 200 years of an industrial revolution. Our immune systems and our abilities to detoxify are overwhelmed. Part of the cleaning up of the garbage is the immune system's responsibility. White blood cells, for instance, grab toxins, burn them and help to transport them. Our systems are being pushed to the limit. It's one of those realities that people are going to wake up to one of these days and basically say, "We have to constitute a more organic, respectful approach to life and our environment or we are going to be in big trouble."

These are part of many other astonishing statistics: over 100 million Americans are chronically disabled now, which significantly impacts their occupational, social, interpersonal and academic performance. 1 out of 2 Americans will have a serious mental illness in their lifetime. At any one time, 1 out of 4 Americans does. The brain is at least 10 percent white blood cells. It's a giant lymph node that's monitoring the immune system. It's no wonder that with all the stress we are under from toxicities that our systems are breaking down.

Q: Do you have an opinion on why women are affected more by autoimmune disease than men?

A: I don't know why that would be, and am not sure if there is good scientific data to explain it. I could offer speculations. I suppose if you look at the epidemiology you could probably come up with some ideas. Perhaps lower testosterone is a factor. Women athletes have higher rates of joint disease; testosterone supposedly protects men's joints from the battering of athletic sports competition.

Actually women, because they have more DNA, are tougher than men in many circumstances. There are a lot of ideas about this. Women endure the stressors of pregnancy and childbirth. They may need to have a more responsive immune system to protect the unborn child, so there might be factors along those lines. The fluctuation of hormones that happens more in women contributes stress, such as so-called PMS. Any kind of stress makes one more vulnerable to immune disturbances. You can get into all kinds of psycho-social factors too. I ask men how they would feel if the other sex was bigger and stronger? There are the stressors of a sexist society, stressors women face that men don't. Many men may have autoimmune disorders but they may be less inclined to seek assistance. They have to be "tough," and denial may more closely fit their stereotypic social expectations. It's a "guy thing" to not ask for directions. Women seem to show up more in doctor's offices willing to admit that "something's wrong" with my body. Perhaps because women are more naturally in a position of being healers and caring for children, they are more cognizant of health care matters. Men may be walking around with fibromyalgia or Hashimoto's but they don't get the help for it. All of this is of course speculation, but the statistics are accurate.

Q: What is your approach to treating people with autoimmune disease?
A: To turn off the immune system's aggressive nature, by removing the challenge to the immune system instead of injuring the immune system with drugs. The problem is not the immune system. The disease model says that when someone has autoimmune disorder the immune system is the problem. The immune system is actually doing too good a job. The problem is that the immune system is challenged by something that it is responding to in either an adaptive or a maladaptive way, and then once the immune system is aggravated enough, it often starts to bully different parts of the body and normal tissues.

The immune system needs to be treated like any other part of the body. If it's aggravated, you don't kill it with chemicals. That's stupid. It's like if I slugged you and you got mad and went and slugged someone else. That doesn't make any sense. You would want to address the problem where the problem is. The problem is that there is a reason that the immune system is aggravated and we need to turn that off. That's all.

The three most common areas are challenges in the gut (irritable bowel), challenges in the sinuses (chronic sinusitis) and challenges in the dental infections (cavitations). Usually that's where there is a toxic foci, a focus of toxicity where the immune system is working extra hard and begins to be suspicious of everything else it encounters. The other term for it is Chronic Systemic Inflammatory Syndrome (CSIS), which is often used to refer to respiratory inflammation, but I use it signify a "whole body challenge."

There are many reasons why we become chronically inflamed. We become inflamed if we get infected with a germ. That's a normal response, so the first thing that can be done is to find out where the germ is, and 90 percent of the actual cells of the body are the cells in the intestines or the tiny "germs" that live in the gut. Only 10 percent of the cells of our body is our body.

That's a huge ecosystem in which to go looking for unfriendly flora—60 to 80 percent of the body's immune system lives in or around the intestines to keep unfriendly flora in check. That's the first place you look for a systemic challenge, which could be igniting an autoimmune disorder, because that's simply where the immune system lives. If the immune system is over challenged then it probably has something to do with the gut. You have to do good stool cultures. You have to find out what the good flora is and put it back if it's missing. You have to take out the bad flora, replenish digestive enzymes, and repair the lining of the intestines. Take care of food allergies and then help the liver in its detoxification process. In fact, when my colleagues just get going and they are learning how to be authentic healers, I tell them to focus on learning how to heal the GI tract. If they can learn how to fix the GI tract they'll make marvelous gains in helping a lot of people.

The next step is to make sure you're working with a good holistic or biological dentist. They can take care of what's happening in the mouth. That's a huge area of infection.

If you Google "Mayo Clinic and sinusitis," you will find out what the Mayo Clinic essentially proved about the actual cause of chronic sinusitis in tens of millions of Americans: this is a fungal infection that lives in the sinuses. The way to treat it is to use topical antifungals or nebulizers and destroy the fungus, which produce mycotoxins that challenge the immune system and could be the agents that set off the autoimmune problem.

More about the toxicity: toxins can bind to normal body proteins so that certain proteins no longer look normal to the immune system and instead look like foreign protein such as that which might be in germs. One of the jobs of the immune system is to identify what is foreign protein and differentiate it from what is self. When thyroid tissue gets a little bit of mercury stuck in it and its protein starts to look foreign, it's very easy for the immune system to begin to say, "Well, I'm not sure that's normal thyroid tissue. That looks a little weird to me." Then the immune system starts to attack it.

I had a colleague look up approximately 400 different autoimmune disorders and he concluded they are all actually the same disorder. It's just a different part of the body that gets picked on by the fickle immune system so we give it a different name. With the thyroid, it's thyroiditis; the lung, sarcoidosis; fascia and the skin, it can be lupus; if it's the joints, it's rheumatoid arthritis; if it's the brain, it's multiple sclerosis, and so on. All these different names just confuse the issue—a left over from the disease era where you have to diagnose the disease to differentiate it from other diseases without actually knowing its cause. But it's all the same disease—all the same problem. Once you understand that it's all the same disorder, and that the thyroid and the joints are the two most common places the immune system picks on, then the solution is obvious: simply turn off the aggravating causes that the immune system is reacting to.

Q: As patients, we're told by our doctors, "Forget about it, autoimmune disease is incurable. Don't waste your time. It cannot be cured."

A: We are taught in medical school that everything is incurable. There is a total distrust of the capacity of the body to heal itself. It's like when someone gets a cut, the skin heals. Obviously healing happens. How can you ignore it? It's happening all the time. It's almost as if they are saying, "That's never going to get well. That wound in your skin is going to stay open forever." Because it's on the skin where everyone can see it, you can't pull the wool over the eyes of people. But if your thyroid is damaged, you can't see the thyroid. You can get away with convincing the patient that their thyroid can never get well and who are they to object to this assertion—they can't see it.

The notion that chronic illnesses like autoimmune thyroid disorders are incurable, and that all you can do is manage "irreversible" problems with expensive chemicals, requiring you to fork over a fifth of your equity over most of your lifetime to pay for it, is called "the accepted standard of care." The objective of the FDA then is to make drugs as expensive as possible so that they can be taxed and the government can make more money to fund mega-institutions like the FDA. That then supports the regulators and everybody is happy. The whole system is based on keeping people sick so that they can be manipulated and controlled and money can be made off of them. There's little money to be made in making people well because they go on with their lives and don't purchase health care products and services. The objective is to make people sick and keep them sick so that they depend on caregivers, manufacturers and the government and convince them that they're going to have to depend on the "altruistic care" for the rest of they're lives. Therefore, there's a relationship that's built up that has a dire economic consequence for the patient but a very lucrative consequence for the health care system. That is the health care crisis right there!

Q: It's the opinion of many doctors, including alternative and integrative physicians, that once the genes for autoimmune disease are turned on they can't be turned off.
A: That's so ridiculous! What genes are they talking about?

Q: I'm not sure. They don't say the exact ones.
A: Of course not; it's a hokey excuse when clinicians are too lazy to actually investigate what the actual causes are of their patients' problems. I test genes all the time. So anybody who gives me that kind of bologna I want to know what genes they're talking about because I test them all the time. The genes we test for are modifiable (you can do something to change their expression); important (they can do bad things); measurable (we can measure improvements in gene expression); and common (why test for rare genetic quirks?). The big excuse used to be viruses. "I don't know what's wrong with you and I'm too incompetent to figure it out, or too lazy to care, so it must be a virus." But now it is, "I don't know what's wrong with you; it must be your genes." Well, then find the gene, and

change its expression to make symptoms go away.

Q: So your answer is that it is not really scientific to say that the genes for autoimmune disease cannot be turned off?

A: Of course not, I do it all the time. For instance, read about one of the gene panels we routinely test for, the Immunogenomic panel from Genova Diagnostics. This bologna is simply a way to manipulate people with fear. If you can keep people ignorant and fear-based then you can control them and profit from them. I, as the God-almighty healer, can stay in control because you must depend on me completely for all the answers for anything that could happen to you, rather than you being empowered with knowledge so you can take responsibility for your life and make the positive changes needed to get well.

Q: So then your official opinion as far as autoimmune thyroid disease goes, is it can be reversed as long as you can find what's causing it.

A: Certainly. If you find the cause, then you can entertain the possibility of rationally targeting the intervention. However, if you've had severe Hashimoto's and Graves' for a long time, and you've had a lot of injury to the thyroid, the thyroid may be too damaged to make a full recovery despite everything we try. It's a battleground scene where there's been a lot of death and destruction. Luckily, the bio-identical hormone therapies are exactly that—they're bio-identical so you don't have to treat an irreversibly-damaged thyroid gland with drugs. You can treat it by adjusting the levels of the thyroid hormone and then over time following the TSH, the T4, and the T3 to maintain normal levels. If the thyroid is damaged enough it's sometimes impossible to bring full repair even after the antithyroid antibodies normalize, indicative that an ongoing autoimmune process has cooled down. The thyroid is like any organ that gets too scarred—it may not recover its full function—so we provide the bio-identical hormone to help it along.

Q: But at least you can stop the process?

A: Yes, in 1000's of patients over almost 4 decades of practicing integrative medicine, I cannot recall a single patient who followed my suggestions and was not able to stop the autoimmune process from ravaging their bodies. If you have an autoimmune disorder, a word of caution: don't dilly-dally. Autoimmune disorders, although they commonly express themselves as thyroid- or joint-related symptoms, are never just a single autoimmune disorder. It's always a "mixed connective tissue disorder." There's no autoimmune disorder that strictly fits the textbook definition. There are always other problems associated with it so if you don't remove the immune system's reason for why it's so aggravated then it can very easily start picking on some other part of the body resulting in more disability.

Q: That starts to cover my next question: do you feel that a diagnosis of an autoimmune disease can be the beginning of a more serious autoimmune process?

A: Oh, certainly, I've seen it a lot. You want to put the fire out as soon as you can so that it doesn't spread. When it does, you're dealing with that many more problems, lurking in the background. If the immune system is distracted with an autoimmune disorder, then it has to divide its resources and it's supposed to be devoting some of its resources to killing cancer cells. You don't want it distracted and not doing one of its primary objectives, which is to handle the number two cause of death—cancer.

Q: In your opinion, how important is nutrition in our health, and are there any specific foods that seem to be troublemakers for people with autoimmune diseases?

A: You have to nurture and feed your immune system, a living entity, for it to be healthy. You don't want to eat foods that have certain toxins that can distract it or cause it to go off the deep end. You want to eat as organic and wholesome a diet as you can. You want to avoid complex carbohydrates, which often feed yeast and Candida. Those mycotoxins commonly aggravate the immune system even more. You basically want to follow the guidelines of a low carbohydrate diet with essential fatty acids, good oils, and good proteins, and take lots of digestive enzymes to digest your food so that your immune system doesn't have to fight off food allergies too, which is another aggravating factor. Use lots of digestive enzymes and eat foods like papaya and pineapple because those good enzymes will help you digest food. The main thing is to keep yourself healthy despite the immune problem that's going on because immune stress can wear you down. It's like having a flu that never goes away. Your body's going to need more nutrition than ever to keep up the fight because it's tearing itself down catabolically; it's eating itself up so you've got to do more repair to regenerate tissue because there's degenerative inflammation happening, you see. Nutrition is very important.

Q: Gluten, nightshades and dairy seem to be aggravating to a lot of individuals with autoimmune disease. Can you speak about that?

A: Preferably, simple testing for IgG antibodies in the blood to various foods will help to identify the main offenders. If you were to examine 1000 people with the same autoimmune disease, like Hashimoto's thyroiditis, they're all going to be completely different from each other. They all have different food allergies, different biochemistries, toxicologies and genetics, so the idea is to get tested so you know exactly what caused the problem and specifically where to focus your energies to turn the immune system off.

The chronic systemic inflammatory syndrome, the inflammation, can be down regulated with anti-inflammatory herbs. Turmeric, ginger and green tea generally turn down the immune response. Make sure you have omega-3 and omega-6 fatty acids, for instance, because these create the immune modulators that are anti-inflammatory. You may want to cut down on animal fat because that's the precursor for the pro-inflammatory immune modulators.

The idea is to keep backing down the immune system and little by little you change genetically and your epigenetic response down regulates over time.

The same is true with food allergies. You can't assume you have gluten or dairy or nightshades allergies. The idea is to actually test for the food allergy via IgG or there are even more expensive, more refined, food allergy tests that test the cellular response or lymphocyte reactivity. The idea is to find out what is aggravating your immune system, such as allergic foods. Some factors are connected to others, so food allergy is a symptom of a more basic problem, leaky gut, caused by unfriendly parasites, bacteria or mold living in the intestines. You have to heal the gut no matter what because normally foods wouldn't do that to you unless it was leaking through a damaged intestinal lining. If there are allergies, then there's something going on in the intestines, which is allowing that to happen.

You have to remember that our ancestors were eating foods that were in season or foods they could scavenge. We've only been farmers for a mere several thousand years but we haven't changed genetically for 100,000 years. The vast majority of that time we were eating seasonal foods or foods we could go out and hunt or find so we were constantly rotating different kinds of proteins.

Our ancestors did not eat the same proteins every day like wheat, dairy, eggs or peanuts—constantly putting the same proteins in front of the immune system for it to start to develop reactions to. Our ancestors were eating things that were fermented. Before refrigeration, many foods were fermented and all that good flora was constantly being inoculated. Less foods were cooked and more were raw, so our ancestors got more benefit from the enzymes in the food to help them digest their food.

The epidemic of autoimmune disorders is simply the consequence of deviating far from a diet and a lifestyle that sustained humanity for eons. That's all it is, and those most genetically vulnerable and damaged by modern-era toxins will be more likely to suffer. It's the natural outcome. People don't know that we've deviated so far because it now looks like the norm of society, but if you take what we're doing and compare that to what our ancestors did, we've veered so far from basic, commonsense strategies to be healthy that it's no wonder that those who are most genetically vulnerable are so susceptible to such disorders.

Q: A lot of people aren't sure what came first, the chicken or the egg. Is it the food that's causing the leaky gut or is it the leaky gut that's causing the food allergy, and if a person's allergic to a particular food do they have to eliminate that for their whole entire life?

A: No, they only need to eliminate it until their gut heals. So the acronym is the 5 R's. You have to remove the bad flora that's causing inflammation in the intestines, which you find through stool cultures and other tests. You have to Re-inoculate the good flora so that that lining of good flora that we get from mother's milk is restored. You see we've destroyed it with fluoride and chlorine in our drinking water. We've destroyed it with preservatives and mercury that's used to kill bacteria that cause tooth decay. We've killed it with antibiotics that we either take or that get into our food. When we don't have that protective layer of good flora, then the unfriendly flora in the intestines starts to attack the lining of the intestines and causes inflammation. When the immune system starts fighting back and the lining of the intestines gets caught between these two warring parties —the immune system and unfriendly flora—then leaky gut and food allergies ensue.

So you need to remove the bad flora, re-inoculate the good flora, replenish digestive enzymes, repair the lining of the intestines and restore liver detoxification. Once that's done in a logical, straightforward way, every autoimmune disorder is completely reversible. I've never found one that isn't…yet.

Q: That's good news!
A: It's very straightforward really. Like I said, you could have so much damage that you may not regain full function of an organ. That's possible. Like with Hashimoto's, you may have to be on thyroid hormone the rest of your life. That's possible, but at least you put the fire out, and it's possible to put the fire out in every single person—no exceptions. Absolutely no exceptions!

Q: In conclusion, what advice do you have for a person who has just been diagnosed with autoimmune thyroid disease?
A: Empower yourself with knowledge, like this book. We're in the information age, so you don't have to swallow the "expert" opinions, which clearly are motivated by people who don't know what's really going on, or they are afraid of regulators so they need to keep things hush-hush. I got really good at memorizing things so I could get A's in college, and I memorized stuff right through medical school. I could parrot everything. We basically get brainwashed into a way of looking at the disease model and the idea is to not get caught up in the fear. You've got to become your own expert: empower yourself with knowledge, start collecting the facts and get to work on this. Once you do, there is clearly an answer.

You may need an expert to test you to find out what's going on through functional and genomic testing, but even then, I encourage patients to get other opinions.

I like to consult with other doctors because I like to teach them and they can always teach me a thing or two. I've made a lot of mistakes in 35 years and I can help clinicians save a lot of time by not having to figure out the solutions the hard way.

The idea is to empower yourself. You have to become your own physician. There's no other way around it. If you want to find people helpers, you have to find people helpers who see you as a co-equal in the journey, not as a child in a parent/child relationship where the parent tells the child what to do.

In transactional analysis terms, you want an adult/adult relationship, a co-equal relationship where the healer is just as willing to learn as you are about new things and about what's going on. You can always solve it. The immune system is not supposed to do this, but the problem is not the immune system. The immune system is only reacting aggressively because it's being triggered to do so, and you have to find out what those triggers are and take those triggers away so that the immune system will calm down and won't be so aggressive anymore.

Q: That's wonderful! Thank you so much for your time and this interview. I'm sure this will be very empowering for my readers.

You can learn more about Dr. Gant at his Web site http://cegant.com. You can learn more about the Academy of Functional Medicine & Genomics at http://www.academyoffunctionalmedicine.com.

Dr. Susan Blum, M.D., MPH

Dr. Susan Blum, an Assistant Clinical Professor in the Department of Preventive Medicine at the Mount Sinai School of Medicine, has been treating and preventing chronic diseases for the last decade. Her passion and dedication for identifying and addressing the root causes of chronic illness through the groundbreaking, whole body approach known as Functional Medicine, is helping to transform our health care system.

As the Founder of Blum Center for Health, Dr. Blum's crusade for personalized medicine is paramount for treatment and prevention. A Preventive Medicine and Chronic Disease Specialist who has appeared on The Dr. Oz Show, Fox 5 News and ABC Eyewitness News, and is regularly quoted in *Real Simple*, *Harper's Bazaar*, *Redbook* and *Martha Stewart's Whole Living*, Dr. Blum's mission for the center is to facilitate a personalized healing experience by creating a healing partnership with her patients, providing cutting-edge Functional Medicine, and teaching self-care skills for changing health habits.

Through Dr. Blum's medical practice, education efforts, writing, research, and advocacy, she empowers her patients to strive to stop covering up symptoms, in order to actually treat the underlying causes of illness, thereby combating—and most often curing—the chronic-disease epidemic.

Dr. Blum completed her Internal Medicine training at St. Luke's Roosevelt Hospital, her residency in Preventive Medicine at The Mount Sinai School of Medicine in New York City, and is Board Certified in Preventive Medicine. She received her Masters in Public Health at Columbia University, and her training in Functional Medicine from The Institute for Functional Medicine in Gig Harbor, Washington. She is also a member of the Senior Teaching Faculty at the Center for Mind-Body Medicine in Washington, D.C., where she has been sharing her knowledge and insight for over a decade, while teaching their training programs throughout the country.

Dr. Blum practices what she preaches. Ten years ago, she was diagnosed with Hashimoto's thyroiditis, an autoimmune disease where the body attacks the thyroid as if it were a foreign tissue. By following the same Functional Medicine and lifestyle principles she prescribes for her patients, Dr. Blum has cured herself of this serious condition.

Q: There are roughly 15 million people in the United States who have been diagnosed with an autoimmune thyroid condition, 70 percent of which are women. Can you tell us what may be causing such an epidemic?

A: I think you're going to get the same answer from everyone you speak to, especially if they're seeing a lot of autoimmune patients and if they are practicing functional medicine. We all have genetics, and yes, there have always probably been people that have genes susceptible to autoimmune disease. Developing an autoimmune disease is an interaction between whatever your genes are, which is how you come into this world, and then whatever your exposures are to the environment. We have come to understand there are a lot of environmental triggers for autoimmune disease such as mercury, which is a very important one for the thyroid.

The other really important aspect as to why we have so much autoimmune disease now is that our guts are just a mess. We overuse antibiotics, antacids, alcohol, Advil and medications. Our kids are starting their early years, and growing into adults, with a lot of antibiotics, and they have a lot of stress. A lot of people have intestinal dysbiosis, which is an imbalance of the flora in their gut. Seventy percent of the immune system lies right underneath the intestinal lining. Because of what's happening to our intestinal flora, there is a concern about the evolution and the development of children and developing adults. There are some theories, such as the hygiene hypothesis, which postulates that our children are too clean, but at the end of the day, we know our flora is not in balance anymore.

Imbalanced intestinal flora promotes a situation called leaky gut syndrome, which is increased intestinal permeability. The immune system—like I said, the intestinal lining houses the largest immune organ in our body—is being exposed in ongoing ways to environmental insults and toxins that are coming in through the foods we eat. That is what is disrupting the system.

This gene-environment interaction and our gut-environment interaction is really causing our immune systems to get out of balance. When I think about the epidemic, I link increased environmental toxins, our digestive system and how our flora and fauna is completely out of balance as the cause.

Q: Do you have an opinion on why women are more affected than men?
A: There are a lot of medical theories and they seem plausible to me. I've been reviewing the literature and it's thought to be associated with estrogen and what is called "estrogen detox pathways." Some people are very susceptible to accumulating toxic metabolites of estrogen in the body. There's a lot of evidence about the different estrogen pathways through the body and the ratios of the good to the bad estrogens. The liver has two different detox pathways by which to detox estrogen. This is again, in a way, toxin and environmental exposure (and the way we are eating), affecting the way women are metabolizing estrogens in the liver, your body's main detox organ. There is an association between the bad estrogens and lupus.

Q: You were personally diagnosed with an autoimmune thyroid condition. Can you briefly share your story with us?
A: In a way my story is very similar to yours. When it initially happened, I was actually feeling really healthy. It was around 2000, I had had all my children and felt healthy and great, but a friend of mine said my hands looked yellow. Although we know that can be from just eating too much colored vegetables, I went and got a checkup, and my doctor found that my beta-carotene levels were very high.

Thyroxin, a thyroid hormone, is one of those hormones that helps you make vitamin A out of beta-carotene, so a high beta-carotene level is a good reason to look at your thyroid. He checked my thyroid and I was a little hypothyroid, and he found thyroid antibodies. I was shocked, because I was at a good weight, I had good energy, and I felt really healthy and well, but I was definitely hypothyroid.

I tell my patients there are two parallel processes going on. On the one hand, you have this brewing immune system inflammation and immune activation going on: it's the part of the iceberg that's under the water. You don't know it's happening. It's attacking your thyroid without you knowing it. Eventually your thyroid gland itself will be damaged enough that you will then become a little hypothyroid. Then you will see that in routine blood work.

I was already above the surface. My blood work showed that my thyroid was damaged, so I know I had been brewing that for a long time. Nobody knows how long that takes. For some people it can be a few years; for other it can be 20 years. There are no studies or evidence that show how long we can brew antibodies for any autoimmune disease before the disease shows up. But for me, when I was first diagnosed, I was already hypothyroid and my doctor put me on medication for that.

I was just starting to learn about functional medicine, and I decided to use it myself. Just like you did, I went on a fact-finding exploration. I kept a journal, and I wrote down all the people I saw. I went to see an acupuncturist, a top Chinese medicine guy in New York City who was known for cancer. I did homeopathy. I went to a naturopath. I had someone look at my red blood cells under a microscope. I did everything I could think of, that I thought was available around me, anything that was called "integrative," to try to see who could help me figure out why I had antibodies. I wanted to know why. I knew I did have issues in my family history. My grandmother had lupus, I have cousins with lupus, my father has Hashimoto's—so I have the genetics. I still wanted to know how and why.

None of those people helped me but the naturopath, who did functional medicine with me. (This is before I went and got my functional medicine training, which I did then the following year.) The naturopath was great; he got me started, but my gut was a mess. I had high mercury, and when he started doing chelation therapy with me I got really sick. I got headaches, and I couldn't tolerate any chelation pills that he gave me. So I stopped seeing him, because there was clearly something missing. He couldn't guide me through the process that I personally needed. The way he was approaching it, it wasn't working.

So I jumped into functional medicine with both feet and practiced on myself. After I did AFMCP, the main eight-day training, I came home from the training and I did the detox elimination program with the gluten, dairy, corn, soy, and eggs. I started doing detox with the detox shake, and I had intense detox reactions. The inside of my mouth felt like it was on fire for three days. I'm convinced there was metal coming out. Over the course of a year I got my silver fillings out of my mouth, went on a gluten-free diet and I healed my gut. I took herbs, fixed the bacteria, got the flora in balance, cleaned out the bad stuff. A year later, I tested my antibodies and they were gone.

That's the process I do with everybody. At that point I was immersed in mind/body medicine. I've been working with the Center for Mind-Body Medicine since 1998, and I teach their training program here, and outside the country. The mind/body medicine is important also. Stress, understanding the adrenals and how they influence the immune system—that's the baseline background that you have to be working to help everything stay in balance.

Q: Do you feel there are emotional/spiritual components to autoimmune conditions?

A: Absolutely. It's always that interplay, intersection, with your emotions, thoughts and feelings, and your spiritual journey. What is your experience on a daily basis? How are you bringing that into your body, or aren't you? Is that making you sick? If there are some things troubling you that you are bringing into your body, the place you're bringing it is your stress system.

There's definitely a very important connection between sympathetic fight-or-flight, as well as adrenal and cortisol, with the immune system that is causing imbalances in TH1 and TH2 (which we'll talk about next). The immune system is absolutely affected by that. My personal opinion is that I think an acute trauma, or an acute stressful event, or severe ongoing stress or emotional trauma—intense anything that is disruptive—can be a trigger. But those other things are in place already. You might have the genetics or some sort of environmental toxins. There are other things that are off and you might have been hanging in there, but the emotional/spiritual piece puts you over the top.

On the flipside—for healing to take place—reversing autoimmune disease, treating your antibodies and helping your immune system come into balance, you absolutely must address the mind/body/spirit aspect. There's a saying in functional medicine, "When you're sitting on a tack, the answer is to get rid of the tack." Right?

That chronic stress, the chronic emotional spiritual disease that you have, can still be a thorn in the side of your immune system. You need to find balance. Reversing autoimmune disease is about balance, balancing all these systems so the stress system needs to be balanced too.

Q: I want to quickly go to a question on genetics since we've talked about that so much. There are a lot of experts that make the claim that "once the genes for autoimmune disease are turned on, they cannot be turned off."

A: That makes absolutely no sense to me. With everything we know about nutrigenomics and epigenetics, we know that's not true. Genes are turned on and off all the time.

Now, what kind of genes are we talking about? Let's do the genetic tests. I've done all those panels on myself. I attended the advanced practice detox module and Ken Bach was up there showing the DetoxiGenomics results for all of the autistic kids. Mine are worse than theirs. I know why I got sick: I cannot clear metals. I cannot clear mercury out of my body. I have no glutathione. My whole panel is completely bad. I should have breast cancer too (I have terrible genetics on that). We know that you can modify it. I did my inflammation panel too, and I do have a susceptibility to making more TH1.

Genetics give you susceptibility, so the genes can be activated and the genes can be turned back off. Anybody who says that they can't, well they're not reading any of the newest studies of epigenetics. That's what this whole new field of epigenetics is—how the environment modifies genetic expression. It affects it in a negative way and it can affect it in a positive way.

Q: There are alternative health clinics popping up all over the country, and they're stating on their Web sites, "Autoimmune thyroid conditions are always caused by an imbalance of the immune system pathways, specifically TH1 vs. TH2." They go onto say that if you have an autoimmune condition, you have one dominant pathway, and they claim that in order to manage the autoimmune condition, the dominant pathway must be modulated.

I'll share a little bit of my story about this: I had symptoms that reflected dominant pathways on TH1 and TH2, so according to me, I was all over the map with dominant pathways.

A: This is a very simplistic view. They're trying to make something very complicated sound very simple. It's just not as simple as that. When you read all the literature about TH1 and TH2, you'll know there's another one called TH17. The TH17 is actually thought to be a driver for autoimmune disease, when it's activated. So there's now this evolving "next bad one" that's TH17.

In general, when you read the literature, they're trying to make groupings. As you know, TH1 is cytotoxic T-cells. Those are the TH1 cells that are driving increased cytotoxic T-cells. Whereas the TH2 cells are the ones that are bumping up and activating the plasma cells to make more antibodies. They're trying to break things down into lists of TH1 diseases and TH2 diseases, which is nice for general categories, but some of them cross over.

In general, TH1 are all the organ-specific diseases, like thyroid and MS, which are attacking one organ. TH2 is thought to be more systemic.

But rheumatoid arthritis for example, crosses over to both. It's systemic in some ways, because there's so much antibody activity, but it's also in the joints, which makes it organ-specific and the cytotoxic T-cells are involved. Rheumatoid arthritis is a perfect example of a condition that has both systems activated.

I would reframe the way I view this: I would say that while it looks like most autoimmune diseases are shifted toward a dominant pathway, where one is overactive and the other is underactive, the answer is not about suppressing anything. The answer is to go to the naïve T-cells, and help them make more T-regulators that regulate these processes.

So you go back to the root of the immune system and the T-cells where they're developing. Because there are these naïve T-cells they can go to one of four places: to a TH1, a TH2, a TH17, or become a regulator. The idea is to help those naïve cells make more regulators, and not just be driven down one pathway or another.

The way you make that sound, it's almost like those clinics claim we have to shut down or modulate the dominating pathways. Rather, I would look at it as you're trying to help all those helper cells be in better balance. And I think that is true regardless of whether you believe it's too much TH1 or too much TH2. There's a fundamental issue that you have too many affecter cells and the regulators aren't working properly. The answer is to help the regulators work better, because they will help, and as the TH1 or TH2 get activated, the regulators help turn them off.

Q: *How do you help the regulators become informed?*
A: There's multiple ways to help the regulators. One is by having good bacteria. That's why cleaning up the gut is so important. The probiotics, the friendly flora in the gut, help boost the whole T-regulator population.

And then there are a whole lot of other things, which I'm accumulating in my book, like balancing the stress system, because cortisol and sympathetic nerve terminals push to TH2. That's why when you get really stressed, you get sick easier, because your cytotoxic T-cells go down and you're shifting to TH2. You have to remove all that stress and bring it into balance and it will help take the pressure off pushing one way or another.

But, most specifically, probiotics improve T-regulators. That's what specific, direct studies have shown. So, in addition to removing toxins that are pushing things in one direction, if you also support the T-regulators and the T-regulator cells, you can help that process. You can read in the literature that green tea and vitamin D increase T-regulators. It's not about shutting one side off or not, it's about supporting T-regulator cells starting with the very naïve T-cell population and helping that not get pushed in one way or another.

I think we would all agree that in autoimmune disease, you definitely have an overproduction of either TH1 or TH2 and maybe sometimes both. And now they're talking about this new helper cell called TH17, which makes a lot of other inflammatory cytokines that seem to drive the autoimmune process. Since there's a third one there now, that sort of helps shut down the TH1/TH2 hypothesis. It's not that simple—I think we all have multiple pathways that are activated.

But it is important to keep in mind. For example, I have a lupus patient, and she's got terrible trouble with Epstein Bar chronic viruses, because she does have a big shift towards TH2. Her TH1 is under functioning and her cytotoxic T-cells are not so good, which are the ones that kill viruses (hand-to-hand combat).

Q: As patients, we are told by our doctors that autoimmune thyroid conditions cannot be cured and that the best we can hope for is to manage our condition with thyroid hormone replacement.

A: It absolutely can be cured, and it actually makes me sort of angry sometimes. I feel a lot of frustration around this issue. The worst actually, is when people are diagnosed and the doctor says, "Oh you're fine. There's nothing you can do, we're just going to watch and wait." And they waited and they waited, and four years later they were hypothyroid. If you do nothing, you will develop a problem with your thyroid gland.

I do antibody screenings on everybody. It's a part of my new patient panel. It doesn't matter what your TSH is, I pick up antibodies all the time in people with a normal thyroid function. But, remember, there are two processes here. There's the autoimmune condition, which is the part of the iceberg under the water, and then there's the actual hypothyroidism, which is the part of the iceberg you see above the water. If I catch a patient when they're still subclinical, when there's no problem with the thyroid gland yet—they just have antibodies—I can fix those antibodies and they can never end up hypothyroid.

I don't believe that "there's nothing you can do" and it's very frustrating when people are told that. I'm really not a judgmental person (I work very hard at that), and I understand because I come from the conventional medical world. We're just not taught in the conventional medical world that there's anything that can be done about it. The problem is that to be a specialist, or to be practicing the best medicine, you have to be reviewing the literature. I'm spending hours and hours reading the current literature on autoimmune disease. There's a lot of evidence for how you can bring things in balance. So I don't know why some of my colleagues are not reading the literature.

Q: In your opinion, how important is nutrition to our health, and are there any specific foods that seem to be troublemakers for people with autoimmune conditions?

A: It's the whole field of nutrigenomics, and when you talk about genetic expression, there you go. Like what we were talking about before—"once genes are turned on, they can't be turned off"—it's completely not true. Food has the power to turn your genes on, because food is information. It goes to your cells, it goes to the nucleus of the cells, it sends in these phytochemicals and the DNA gets transcribed differently. We know that food has a very powerful effect on genetic expression and on how the cell behaves. In the literature, the most important food is gluten. There's abundant literature on gluten and its affect, not just on celiac disease but on several other autoimmune diseases that gluten has an association with. It's in the literature; this is all autoimmune thyroid diseases—both Graves' and Hashimoto's, and rheumatoid arthritis and MS.

What I tell my patients is this: everybody with an autoimmune disease goes on a gluten-free diet. I test everybody for celiac, and sometimes people have just an anti-gliadin antibody. They don't have celiac disease, and they're told, "You can go eat gluten. You are fine even though you have anti-gliadin antibodies." This is another big frustrating moment for me.

There's something called latent celiac disease, and if you have a positive anti-gliadin antibody (even if you don't have damage to your small intestine yet), you have potential celiac disease. If you do nothing, you will probably end up with full celiac disease later, and you may develop a different autoimmune disease first from the gluten. That's for the group of people that have those positive anti-gliadin antibodies. So everybody should get tested, and even if you don't, you still need to be gluten-free.

Part of the issue, really, is that everybody needs to understand what a lab test is. A lab test is asking a question of the body, and modern medicine only has a repertoire of 10 questions it knows to ask. Just because we don't have the right test to measure it, doesn't mean we're not having a bad reaction in the body. Gluten is such a culprit for all these autoimmune diseases that I just tell everyone to go on a gluten-free diet. Gluten is the big one.

Q: What is your approach to treating people with autoimmune thyroid conditions? If I was someone coming in to you, and I have my Hashimoto's, what is your next step?

A: You go on a gluten-free diet, you go home with a stool test and you go home with a heavy metal test. We look at cleaning up your gut, cleaning up your diet (gluten-free), checking out your gut, starting that process of cleaning that up, checking your metals, and seeing what needs to happen with that.

With metals, I'm specifically looking for mercury. If you come up high in mercury, then I don't just jump to chelation at all. I actually work to support the liver, and do a whole lot of metabolic detoxification work for a three-month minimum before I do any chelation. And then I give people selenium. That's what I do at the first visit—it's a process. Then we keep going.

Q: A lot of practitioners feel comfortable trying the functional approach with Hashimoto's, but when it comes to treating a Graves' patient, they immediately refer a person to an endocrinologist, which as you know typically leads to treatments that permanently damage the thyroid gland. There seems to be a real sense of urgency with hyperthyroid symptoms, and I know a lot of clients that come to see me, they're scared to death. So is your approach different with treating Graves'?

A: Actually, my approach is not different. What I do is this: I sit with the patient and we make a decision. I'm not afraid. It depends on how hyperthyroid they are. It's just a fork in the road; it's how bad are your symptoms? Do you have terrible insomnia? Do you have palpitations? Is there anything life-threatening or risky about how you're feeling right now?

Usually the people who come to see me, they're somehow tolerating it already, because they've already said, "no" to their endocrinologist. They've already said, "No, I don't want you to give me terrible medication to kill my thyroid. I want another opinion," and they'll come to see me. And at that point, if we agree together that the symptoms they are having are ones they can bear, they're ok and there's no life threatening nature of it, we'll work together. That's really a clinical judgment of me, as a doctor, and the opinion they already have from their endocrinologist. They're usually told how urgent the situation is.

So, if the situation isn't urgent or life threatening, and we have two months that we can work together, we can have buffer time to do a little work first. People can usually feel better pretty quickly. So I treat Graves' exactly the same way I treat Hashimoto's. Maybe I'll be a little more aggressive at the beginning; I won't wait for a test to come back—I might just get them herbs for their gut right away. I might work a little more quickly. I'll put them on a detox program to clean up their gut quickly depending on how symptomatic they are.

Graves' antibodies resolve. The symptoms go away very quickly, so they feel much better. I've had a lot of good success with Graves', and a lot of people end up not needing medication. Some of it has to do with how anxious they are. Don't forget that conventional medicine puts the fear of God in people. It's a question of how anxious they are, how sick they are, and whether together we decide that we can buy a little time, and if they're comfortable with that.

Q: In conclusion, what advice do you have for a person who has just been diagnosed with an autoimmune thyroid condition?
A: They have to find a functional medicine doctor to help them understand that they should try to find out why they have it.

It's really the question of "why?" Don't just accept that you have this for the rest of your life. Find out why. It's usually a functional medicine person, but you can also go to a naturopath and there are also some chiropractors that are trained in functional medicine too. But they need a functional medicine evaluation to understand why. Don't stop without knowing why.

Q: Thank you so much for your time and this interview. I'm sure this will be very empowering for my readers.

You can learn more about Dr. Blum at her Web site http://www.blumcenterforhealth.com/

Dr. Alexander Haskell

Dr. Haskell is a licensed Naturopathic Physician with 27 years of clinical experience. He completed his premed at San Francisco State University and graduated from the four-year medical program at The National College of Natural Medicine.

Dr. Haskell's specialty is the thyroid and endocrine system and has published two books, *Hope for Hypothyroidism* and *Hope for Hashimoto's*. Both books dedicate a special chapter to the prevention and treatment of breast disease and breast cancer.

Through applying medical research and his discoveries in his clinical practice, Dr. Haskell is able to help people with Hashimoto's to reduce their thyroid inflammation, and thus reduce their levels of thyroid antibodies.

Q: Statistics show that there are roughly 15 million people in the US with autoimmune thyroid disease. Approximately 12.5 million of these have been diagnosed with Hashimoto's and 2.5 million with Graves' disease. Can you tell us what might be causing such an epidemic?

A: That's a good question, Michelle. There are probably several factors. The primary one is the nutrient deficiency of iodide, but that usually accompanies a deficiency of iodine as well. Part of the reason for the deficiency is due to poor eating habits and not selecting foods that are rich in those trace minerals. Our soils have become depleted of a lot of nutrients and trace minerals including iodine and iodide. Additionally, people have been told by their physician or subliminally programmed to think that salt is bad. Iodized salt does not include iodine but iodide. I think those are the primary reasons why people become deficient in that trace mineral.

When that happens the thyroid cells are unable to manufacture thyroid hormones. As thyroid hormones decline, then the endocrine system, the pituitary gland, recognizes that deficiency of thyroid hormone and begins to produce larger concentrations of thyroid stimulating hormone (TSH).

TSH is a hormone that does many things in the body in different cells. One of those things is to stimulate the production of hydrogen peroxide in thyroid cells, which is an important catalyst or enzyme to promote the conversion of iodide into iodine. If there's an iodide deficiency, the thyroid cells will be unable to produce thyroid hormones, TSH will remain elevated, and hydrogen peroxide production within the thyroid cells will remain elevated, which causes irritation and inflammation. Inflammation causes thyroid cells to prematurely age, and then die-off or turn over more rapidly—to open up and release thyroid hormones along with thyroperoxidase, an enzyme, and thyroglobulin, a protein. This enzyme and protein then enter the circulation causing the activation of the immune system to produce antibodies that clean up the resulting debris.

Q: Why do you feel that women are more affected then men?
A: I think it is primarily because women's bodies have a higher demand for iodine and iodide. Besides the thyroid, the ovaries and breast tissue require iodine. During pregnancy, for example, the breasts absorb a lot more iodine in the last trimester in preparation for lactation. So a woman's demand for trace minerals is much higher than for a man, even though a man does require iodine for a healthy prostate.

Q: In your book Hope for Hashimoto's, *you talk about other factors that contribute to the autoimmune process. Can you tell me what those are?*
A: I would say that the primary one would be problems in the intestinal tract. When you look at the initial insemination of the ovum, the egg splits into three different layers and from those are formed basically every tissue in the body. The endoderm is the layer that goes on to form the intestinal tract, as well as the thyroid gland. I think there's a relationship between gut ecology and the thyroid—gut inflammation somehow affects the thyroid to some extent. The first issue seems to be a gluten intolerance, a gluten sensitivity. Food sensitivity, food allergies, Candida, and parasites in the gut really should be addressed with a person who has Hashimoto's.

Other factors include heavy metals, primarily from dental amalgams. Those amalgams actually increase their vaporization of mercury in the process of chewing food or taking hot drinks. Mercury at room temperature is a liquid. That's the reason why it's used in dentistry to make the other alloys of the amalgam more malleable so that they can be pushed and fitted into a cavity. At a certain temperature mercury changes from a liquid to a gas, and as it mixes with food, it gets into the mucosa, the mouth cavity, and the lymphatic system and drains straight down the throat. So I think mercury is another factor because it disrupts the activity of white blood cells. Often if there is a focus of the heavy metal in a certain tissue, then white blood cells are repelled by those heavy metals. I don't understand the reason why.

Another factor is chronic infections. With a low white blood cell count, the immune system becomes kind of trepidacious. It knows something is wrong and goes on alert, trying to fight infection but it can't. It becomes overwhelmed and triggered more easily by the thyroid peroxidase that's coming out of those thyroid cells that are breaking apart. There are probably other factors as well concerning the emotions and not being able to express yourself.

Q: If you don't mind, it may be more interesting to go into a case.

A: A woman with Hashimoto's called me long distance asking what she could do. I could hear in her voice that something was going on with her throat. We talked for awhile and I asked, "When did it start?" She said, "I was doing fine until a conversation with my sisters-in-law. It was very stressful but I did very well. I just tried to make it as harmonious of a conversation as possible, but from that point on for a week afterwards I was totally exhausted." I discovered that this kind of emotional pattern was going in her life—trying to adapt well to a situation but being totally exhausted from it for days and weeks afterwards.

I asked her, "How do you feel about your sisters-in-law?"

"I was really upset with them because they were taking advantage of me and my husband."

I could tell by her voice she was still very emotional about it. We talked about the psychological or emotional side of illness in general, and for her Hashimoto's specifically. She's doing really well now. We used homeopathy and she's seeking a counselor who can help her express herself more clearly and to be more in touch with her immediate feelings and how to communicate them. So I do think that our emotions are another important factor with Hashimoto's and for any illness for that matter.

Q: I'm so glad you brought that up because I did recover from Hashimoto's and the emotional aspect was directly related to my particular autoimmune process. I had a hard time expressing myself, and was always clearing my throat. I don't know how to explain that in a physiological way but I definitely had that going on. That brings me to my next question: What is your approach to treating people with autoimmune thyroid disease?

A: In some respects, every person is different. As far as the medical diagnosis is concerned everybody is the same, but you really have to personalize the approach partly based on the thyroid lab results. Those are really important to assess in a certain way, but all the other underlying factors that we have already spoken about have to be considered for each individual.

This is the crux of the problem: a woman may suffer for five or ten years and nobody can figure out what's going on. The doctor doesn't have answers until finally someone does the test for thyroid antibodies and then the conventional thinking is, "Ah, we finally found the problem!" But it is seldom the whole problem. There are other things that are related to their symptoms that have to be addressed. I try to help women become aware and encourage them to realize that if we can address all these other factors besides the Hashimoto's, they will regain their health. If we treat just Hashimoto's alone, you may see a 10 to 50 percent improvement; however, we really need to address all the reasons why they are not feeling well.

Getting back to Hashimoto's: there are pretty much two types, which is separate from the level of antibodies. I'm talking about just the thyroid now. Both types have elevated antibodies. One type has low TSH and low thyroid hormone T4 and T3. The other type with elevated antibodies has a high or elevated TSH with low thyroid hormone. There's a little bit of a difference between how they are treated. The high TSH is a lot easier to treat. The low TSH is more difficult because they probably have already passed through the period of elevated TSH. What we have to do, no matter what the level of TSH is, is to get it down to at least .5, if not a little bit lower, because the TSH is stimulating the thyroid cells to produce hydrogen peroxide. Depending on what they are already taking for thyroid medication, I've got to slowly increase the thyroid medication to bring down the TSH, and at the same time nourish their thyroid cells with what those cells require to make hormones. They must avoid iodide. The reason for that is iodide and iodine are precious to the body, and the best way the body knows of to absorb those nutrients is by stimulating certain channels called sodium iodine symports, which are pretty much in every cell, but especially ovary, breast, thyroid and prostate cells. The way these channels are stimulated to absorb iodide and iodine is by the hormone TSH. When we ingest iodide and iodine, the body senses we need to hold on to these trace minerals probably because early man may not have had iodide and iodine available all the time due to migration. So the body wants to hold on to it as a reserve. The pituitary will increase the production of TSH when it senses there's more iodide and iodine coming into the circulation, and in the case of Hashimoto's we don't want TSH to go up. We want it to stay down. Otherwise it's going to keep stimulating the thyroid cells to make hydrogen peroxide.

Q: As part of your treatment do you do testing to find out what some of the other issues might be going on for the person as well as the autoimmune thyroid condition?

A: Yes, we do a general lab test initially for most people because they haven't had recent labs done. Besides the thyroid component of that comprehensive panel, I also want to see about their immune system, which is tested by what is called a "complete blood count" that includes both the white blood cells and the red blood cells. There's also what's called a "differential," which shows the levels of different types of white blood cells. This might point in the direction of a potential viral, parasitic or bacterial problem. The red blood cell count lets us know if there is some degree of anemia contributing to a person's fatigue. Then there's also the hematocrit and hemoglobin, and what's called the MCV (mean corpuscular volume), which tests the size of the red blood cells. This points us toward nutrient deficiencies such as iron and B12, folic acid, and/or B6. And then a lipid panel is really important because many people think that cholesterol is evil and it's actually very important to have plenty of cholesterol so that the body can make important hormones like progesterone, estrogen, testosterone, cortisol, and aldosterone. All these steroid hormones require cholesterol to be made by different glands. So I want to make sure they have plenty of cholesterol—at least about 185 or 190.

Also we do what's called a "c-reactive protein" to see if there is inflammation in the blood vessels that can indicate general inflammation. We will do a liver panel that helps to understand why a person may have a normal T4 with a low Free T4. If Free T4 is low it can be due to liver problems, liver congestion or the poor breakdown of different metabolites or hormones in the body. It's typical to run a urine specimen since a woman might have frequent urination or recurring urinary tract infections, which have not been treated properly.

That's pretty much what we do besides the thyroid. We also do saliva hormone testing for male and female hormones, which helps to assess levels of estradiol, progesterone and a hormone produced by the adrenals called cortisol. Cortisol plays a very important role in the conversion of the less active thyroid hormone T4 to the more activating thyroid hormone T3.

Q: If you suspect that there is some kind of infection or something going on in the gut, do you do any kind of special testing for gastrointestinal health?

A: Sometimes we will do a test from Metametrix, which checks for the RNA and DNA of different types of parasites and yeast and things like that, but I don't usually start with that. I'll use my clinical experience and their history with what they've been through as far as medications. The testing from Metametrix is pretty expensive so I tend not to do that unless we're not getting anywhere. Most people have some degree of Candida overgrowth so we'll start them on a Candida program. Usually just clearing the Candida is a great shift in gut ecology. Often parasites will leave when bowels become more balanced or more acid.

Q: Many people who go on an anti-Candida diet have to eliminate sugars and cheese, wine, gluten and a lot of things that people are really in love with. Do you find that people have to stay on these programs, at least with respect to the gluten, for the rest of their lives, or do you find that these sensitivities resolve? The reason I ask is that I have found that many doctors tell me, "You didn't reverse anything in your body, and as soon as you go back to eating like the rest of us, your Hashimoto's will come back." And I thought, "Well, I suppose if I started to live the way that I lived before and eating gluten every day, that may be true." What are your thoughts on nutrition and how that plays a role in the autoimmune process?

A: I think that some people with Hashimoto's don't have a gluten problem, but for me it's impossible to know at the beginning. Usually people say, "Oh no! Do I have to avoid that? I don't know if I can do that." Sometimes in as little as three to four days they see an improvement just avoiding gluten. Usually when their antibodies are down and we're on the second phase of the treatment program for Hashimoto's, they're feeling pretty good at that point. I will say, "Go ahead and have some gluten once, and just watch your body's reaction. If you're feeling fine, try it again, and then we'll go from there." Sometimes people know from that experience they have to avoid the gluten because they have symptoms. They know because they've avoided it for two, three, or four months, and there's a fairly immediate reaction within the first 24 hours. Either they start sneezing or coughing at the meal, or they have a headache, or they feel really foggy—or whatever symptoms they may experience. Their reaction confirms that it's very important to avoid. With other people, they take it and they're fine. Maybe those people never had a gluten intolerance to begin with. But, I ask everyone to stop gluten during the first phase.

Q: As patients, we're told over and over again that autoimmune disease is incurable and can only be "managed." Do you have an opinion on that?

A: I think it's totally curable. In my experience, it's only a condition initiated by a nutritional deficiency, and if you understand the mechanism, you realize it's not a disease. It may be that the immune system will always be on guard. The thing is that people and doctors don't realize that every single person has these antibodies. It's not like only people with Hashimoto's have antibodies. Everybody has them because thyroid cells have a natural life span: they open up, release the thyroperoxides and the antibodies are there. Everybody has antibodies, so how can we call this a disease that is incurable when everybody has antibodies? All you have to do is bring these antibodies down to within the normal range and make sure you're providing the nutrients the body requires to make thyroid hormones and those things that help people decrease inflammation such as selenium, and essential fatty acids. I don't think that doctors in general are very intelligent on this subject.

Q: The standard of care protocol, at least in this country, with a diagnosis of Hashimoto's, is that you are put on some type of T4. A lot of Hashimoto's patients think that that's fine. Do you think there's a danger in accepting that treatment protocol, moving on with your life and just taking a pill every morning?

A: I've never treated someone with Hashimoto's with T4 and done nothing else, so I don't know. It may be that some people would be fine with that as long as the T4 is added on to the T4 their own thyroid cells are making and that's enough to bring your TSH down at least below 1.0. It's possible, but I think that giving T4 alone shows that doctors don't really understand Hashimoto's; it's just a protocol that they've been taught. They don't really understand the reason why a person should take this medication, thinking they will either be fine or that this is all they can do. I'm certain there are so many other things that can be done. If you look at the other underlying factors that should be addressed, those will not be taken care of either. I would say that probably most people with Hashimoto's who are just given thyroid medication are probably not going to feel much different unless they were very deficient in thyroid hormones. The thing about Hashimoto's is that it's a chronic condition that someone usually has had for many years, maybe a decade or even two, and most of the time low thyroid hormone accompanies Hashimoto's. Most people cannot keep up with the demands of their life with low thyroid hormones. The second gland that has to take over and support the energy requirements for those people are the adrenals, and when the adrenals get exhausted, the production of cortisol starts going down and they start having chronic infections. Cortisol is extremely important for the conversion of T4 to T3, so usually the T3 levels are also dropping. Cortisol is important for helping T3 cross the membrane of cells. Cortisol also helps to prime the nuclear receptors where T3 binds. Usually taking a thyroid medication is not going to really resolve anything. You may see an improvement in 15-30 percent of patients but that's the maximum you could expect with taking that narrow singular approach.

Q: In my experience, the women who come to me for help with their thyroid protocol were on the standard treatment. Sure, their blood tests were coming in "within normal limits," but they weren't feeling well.

A: Most docs are only testing TSH. It used to be TSH and T4. Now a lot of docs are doing TSH and free T4, which I think is also a mistake. Not many physicians are checking T3. If you are just looking at the TSH and T4, a person's hormones can look pretty good but if you don't look at the T3 and how well a person is converting T4 to T3 then you're really prescribing in the dark. A lot of the people who consult with me have low levels of both T4 and free T4, and their levels of T3 are even lower. The usual first prescription at this point is a compounded T4 and T3 because their conversion was so low that their free T3 levels are suboptimal, even lower then their free T4. After awhile when their adrenals improve—and I may have to give them some cortisol—I've noticed their conversion is much better. That compounded T4 and T3 is then switched over to just T4, whether that's Synthroid, L-thyroxin or compounded T4 alone, because their conversion is so much better. The problem is that a lot of doctors and alternative physicians think, "We'll just do compounded T4 and T3." As the person's health improves because their T4 levels improve, their T3 level starts going too high because they're on the compounded T3. A lot of docs don't get that—that this patient's body is now able to convert T4 to T3 and there's no reason to be giving T3 anymore.

Q: I have a lot of clients that say, "I don't want to stop taking my T3 because I feel so good." I know that a lot of conventional doctors have a hard time prescribing T3. They point to studies that show that it can cause bone loss and osteoporosis or osteopenia. In your estimation, is the T3 prescription something that you would only do in short term until the person starts converting the T4 to T3, or is this something that some people would stay on for life? What are your feelings on that?

A: It depends on the individual and how healthy their liver is as well as a few other factors. It used to be that physicians didn't have lab tests. I think the first lab test was in 1962 for TSH, so what were doctors doing before this? They were prescribing and watching the person's symptoms, and if they went into hyperthyroid they'd reduce the dose. I'm usually giving a dose, which I think is less than what they probably would need ideally, and there's reasons for that. I'll have them monitor their resting heart rate at night several times per week and their basal body temperature when they wake up in the morning. We're monitoring those because the heart is so sensitive to thyroid medication and we need to see if there's an increase in heart rate. We don't usually see an increase in body temperature that soon, but we have them do it anyway just to get into the habit. When we see the heart rate starting to increase—let's say they start at 60 beats per minute and get up to 70—we know we're probably on the right medication. If they don't change, we'll bump them up again until they start to have an increase in their heart rate. Once that's happened, I'll have them stay on that dose for three to four weeks and then recheck their labs to see where things are.

Q: You've developed your own glutathione solution. Can you tell us a little bit about that and how glutathione helps people with autoimmune thyroid dysfunction?

A: The body should normally make it's own glutathione from a number of other nutrients. Selenium is probably the most important nutrient the body requires to make glutathione but there are a few amino acids as well. When a person is fatigued and nutrient deficient at the beginning, I feel like the most important nutrient they could have to improve levels would be glutathione. The problem is that I don't know if there is a product on the market at this time that you can take that's actually assimilated before it's broken down in the gut. I'm becoming much more cynical about supplement companies and what they say their products do, so I feel that the most important or most direct way to get glutathione into the thyroid is either taking it sublingually so it is absorbed both in the bloodstream and in the lymphatics of the mouth and drained down through the thyroid area, or to actually mix it with a medical grade DMSO, which will be absorbed through the skin. People apply it over the thyroid and the glutathione goes directly into the thyroid area. DMSO, from what research I've read, is also an anti-inflammatory although we can't use it medically for those reasons, so I decided to combine them both together, the DMSO and the pure glutathione, and give people very clear directions on how to use it. Glutathione is a solvent. People have to use it cautiously to make sure anything that comes in contact with it isn't absorbed through the skin and into the thyroid. For example, the skin must be washed before applying. No fingernail polish can be on the nails. But I think it's a great preparation, and, thus far, it seems to have really catalyzed the improvement in antibody levels.

Q: I did purchase some from your Web site and was a little unclear on how many treatments are in one bottle?

A: Usually the bottle will last from six to eight weeks, depending on how many times people apply it. If there's some redness or irritation then people are directed to dilute it with half water and half DMSO preparation. At the minimum, applying it twice a day to the left or right side of the trachea so it doesn't drip—just a moist application—lasts about six weeks. Otherwise, if they dilute it, it's going to last a lot longer, of course.

Q: If you could sum it up in conclusion, what advice do you have for a person who has just been diagnosed with autoimmune thyroid disease?

A: The MOST important thing is to become educated: to understand your condition, know about the steps to treat it, request a personalized assessment, and be geared up and ready to go. Most of the people I talk to are desperate and want answers. They'll do basically anything to get help, and they're willing to make major changes in their lifestyles and their eating habits. If a person is informed, they're self-empowered. I think that's probably the most important thing, but that's probably not what you're looking for. You're looking for something else.

Q: No, that's exactly what I'm looking for. The first chapter of my book is on personal empowerment, because we can't rely on someone else to take care of us.

A: And that's why you and I love teaching so much.

Q: Exactly!

You can learn more about Dr. Haskell by visiting his Web site http://hopeforhashimotos.com/

CHAPTER 20

Conclusion

"Look deep into nature and then you will understand everything better."
— Albert Einstein

In my research into the many factors underlying the autoimmune process, I was genuinely surprised at the vast amount of existing information. My intuition about why we're getting sick is substantiated by thousands of scholarly articles. When you begin to review the science, it becomes clear that the many faces of stress: emotional, gastrointestinal, toxic, infectious, and so on, *ALL* tax our health and immune system in measurable ways. I realized that science knows all these stresses are bad for us, but they're hesitant to point to these factors as causal because they don't cause autoimmunity in everyone.

When I stopped doing everything that was bad for me and starting doing things that were good for me, I got better.

It turns out that we know what is bad for us – we're just not happy about it.

We humans are fairly unreasonable and headstrong. We like to bend the rules. That can be a wonderful thing when it comes to creativity and innovation, but when it comes to arguing with nature, it's a losing battle. She always wins.

What we are faced with is a choice – We can resist our biology and demand that we be able to do exactly what we want to our bodies and our planet without consequences, or accept that we don't make the rules and live in harmony with nature. I suggest the latter. The inconvenient truth is that living out of sync with nature is making us sick. We will never win the battle against nature anyway, so why not work with her? I know we'll get better results.

When I started writing this book, there were very few people writing about the connection between leaky gut, gluten, toxins and infections; and autoimmunity. Today, there are several. In fact, hundreds, if not thousands of their readers are taking the message to heart and reversing, not only autoimmune conditions, but other chronic illness as well.

You don't have to "believe" in this book for it to work. If you optimize your nutrition, reduce stress, sleep, heal your gut, improve your detoxification and clear infections, YOU WILL GET BETTER! *This is not philosophy – this is biology!*

Three years ago, I set out to write a book, and instead the book wrote me. Writing this book has forced me to look at all of the ways stress *still* manifests in my life. Even though I've stopped the autoimmune process in my body, and I'm free of autoantibodies and symptoms, I'm still vulnerable to emotional stress. I have much better coping strategies now. I'm aware of my mind-body type, and what my body and soul needs to feel balanced and centered. Although I feel much more empowered than I did 10 years ago, I still have fears and insecurities; I worry about the future – not just my own – but the future of our planet.

I've had to look at how I my feelings of shame still drive me to seek approval and pursue "perfectionism." I've had to laugh at the irony of stressing out about writing a book that connects stress with chronic illness.

Before writing *The Thyroid Cure,* I was really stuck on having a purpose. In questioning my own purpose, I began to wonder if my true purpose was to simply love myself. What if my only job was to get to know who I am? What if that self-knowledge allowed me to make more compassionate choices? What if honoring myself was the best way to honor others?

What I've learned so far along this journey is that love is an inside job. I've learned that forgiving myself is difficult, but probably the most important thing I can do. I've learned that integrity is not simply being good, or ethical, or "right"; it's being true to myself *while* acting for the greater good. I've learned that integrity means living and speaking my truth without needing others to affirm that I am right. Integrity means loving myself enough to take my health into my own hands and make healthy choices. I've learned that being in integrity means the alignment of thought, word and deed; body, mind and soul. When my mind, body and soul are in alignment, I can make conscious choices for my planet and myself. Talk about a revolution.

Please join me in this quiet revolution. You count. With every conscious choice you count.

Namaste.

Gratitude

I give thanks first to Creator for this wonderful gift of life, and for a body that knows how to heal. Thank you grandpa Norman Corey for your unconditional love, and for teaching me how to think. You are my favorite person and I miss you everyday.

I am sincerely grateful to everyone who helped me bring this book to the world. Andrew, you have been my greatest supporter and closest friend. Thank you for your patience and for believing in me, even when I didn't believe in myself.

To my clients: you entrusted me with your personal life stories; I thank each one of you and applaud your courage to heal.

To the editors and writers who contributed to this book: I extend a heart full of gratitude... To my first editor and proofer, Christian Leahy, for understanding and holding the space for my vision and helping me articulate the essence of this message. To my dear friend Jennifer Lightwood, for helping me make sense of the initial draft and organizing the chapters. To Scott Glackman, for transcribing my voice notes and editing my stories. To Jonathan Zap, for spending a week at my home in Taos, interviewing me extensively and then helping me make my personal narrative and client's stories come alive. To Dr. Gant, for being the medical editor. To Celanie Polanick, for your research and editing of the clinical sections and for your loving encouragement. To Karl "Baba" Bralich, I could not have completed this work without you. Thank you for your tireless research, and attention to detail. Your writing and editing helped shape the book. Thank you for bringing an open heart to this project, and sharing your spiritual wisdom with all of us. Thank you for loving me all the way through this process and supporting me through some of the darker moments, which were many.

Herb Bigalow, you are an amazing graphic designer and an absolute dream to work with. I can't imagine where I would be without you. Thank you from the bottom of my heart for a beautiful cover design.

Caroline De Vita, you were a total blast to work with, thank you for your sense of humor and your beautiful and funny illustrations.

I'd like to thank the team at Shelfish; Jeffrey Fuller for your creative direction, efficiency and wonderful attention to detail in the layout of this book. Thank you for appreciating my aesthetic and delivering a beautiful work of art. Thank you to Barbara Richardson for your encouragement and wonderful suggestions along the way. You both have made this process as painless as possible for a new author.

Thank you to the maverick integrative and functional doctors, C.E. Gant M.D., Susan Blum M.D. and Alexander Haskell N.D., who granted me interviews for this book. We are all blessed by your work in this world and for reminding us about the body's natural ability to heal. I also extend a heartfelt thanks to all the medical doctors, and health practitioners who work in the field everyday.

I'd like to thank Dr. Jeffrey Bland and the Institute for Functional Medicine for introducing a new paradigm to Western medicine, and advancing the ancient ways of healing through modern science.

To Dr. Gant and the Academy of Functional Medicine and Genomics: Thank you for your visionary awareness and for teaching doctors how to apply functional medicine in their practices.

Thank you to thyroid patient advocate, Mary Shomon, for sticking your neck out there for all of us and demanding a higher level of care for thyroid patients. Your research has raised consumer awareness and resulted in a better quality of life for thousands of people.

To my dear friend and mentor, Krishna Madappa; my life has been transformed by meeting you. I am so grateful for all you have shown me. You are a beacon of light in this world. OM!

To all my coaches, teachers and mentors who have helped me heal: I give my heartfelt thanks.

I am grateful to my chosen family, Beth, Eric, (baby Indira) and Gordy for your love and support. You all mean the world to me.

To my family: even though we are divided, I love you. I forgive you. I pray for healing and happiness for all of us.

Namaste! ♥

RESOURCES

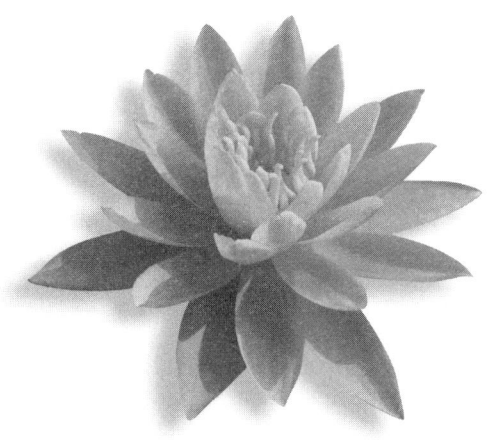

"Never memorize something that you can look up."
— Albert Einstein

Appendix I: Recommended Supplements

There are several high-quality supplements available on the market today. I have listed the ones that I take myself and recommend to my clients, family, and friends. You do not have to take these supplements to heal your condition, but I have found them to be extremely helpful. Most of these products may be purchased through your integrative/functional practitioner or online at www.thethyroidcure.com. Some may be purchased at your local health food store or vitamin shop. Remember that any nutritional supplement, plant or substance, whether used as food or medicine, externally or internally, can cause an allergic reaction in some people. Working with a qualified integrative or functional practitioner before self-prescribing supplements will save you time and money!

Multi-Vitamins
- Empowerment Formula®, by Vibrant Way®
- Damage Control Master Formula, by Primal Blueprint
- Nutrient 950® without Cu, Fe & Iodine, by Pure Encapsulations®

Essential Support
- Vitamin D3 Liquid, by Pure Encapsulations®
- Selenium (selenomethionine), by Pure Encapsulations®
- Zinc Picolinate 30, by Pure Encapsulations®
- Ester C® and flavonoids, by Pure Encapsulations®
- Alpha Lipoic Acid, by Pure Encapsulations®
- Ubiquinol QH, by Pure Encapsulations®

Essential Fatty Acids
- EPA/DHA Essentials, by Pure Encapsulations®
- Ultimate Omega®, by Nordic Naturals®
- Borage Oil, by Pure Encapsulations®

Better sleep
- Natural Calm, by Natural Vitality®
- Magnesium (citrate), by Pure Encapsulations®
- GlyMag-Z 30 stick packs, by Pure Encapsulations®

Better Mood
- Emotional Wellness, by Pure Encapsulations®
- GABA 500 mg, by Now Foods

Adrenal support
- Adreset®, by Metagenics®
- Cortisol Calm, by Pure Encapsulations®
- Daily Stress Formula, by Pure Encapsulations®
- ADR Formula®, by Pure Encapsulations® (Note: This formula contains raw adrenal cortex from cows and may be antigenic in certain individuals. Please consult with an integrative or functional practitioner before taking a bovine glandular).
- Rhodiola Rosea, by Pure Encapsulations®
- Ashwagandha, by Pure Encapsulations®

Heal Your Gut

Antifungal, Antibacterial and Antiparasitic Herbs and Supplements
- GSE – Grapefruit Seed Extract, by NutriBiotic
- Caprylic Acid, by Pure Encapsulations®
- Olive Leaf Extract, by Pure Encapsulations®
- A.C. Formula II, by Pure Encapsulations®
- Organic Neem tablets, by Banyan Botanicals

Enzymes
- Pancreatin 500 mg, by Pure Encapsulations®
- Vital-Zymes™, by ProThera®
- Digestive Enzymes Ultra, by Pure Encapsulations®
- Betaine hydrochloric acid (HCL) Pepsin, by Pure Encapsulations®

Probiotics
- Ther-Biotic®, by Klair Labs®
- Saccharomyces boulardii, by Klair Labs®
- Probiotic 50B (Soy and Dairy Free), by Pure Encapsulations®

Fiber Supplements

- Arabinogalactan Powder, by Vital Nutrients
- Now® Glucomannan Powder
- PGX® (PolyGlycopleX®)
- Organic India Whole Husk Psyllium 100% certified organic fiber.

Repair Inflammation and Leaky Gut

- GI Sustain™, by Metagenics®
- UltraInflamex 360™, by Metagenics®
- Glutagenics®, by Metagenics®
- L-Glutamine powder, by Pure Encapsulations®
- DGL Plus®, by Pure Encapsulations®

Support Liver and Immune Function

- Pure Clear, by Pure Encapsulations®
- True Whey™, by Source Naturals® (note: contains milk, dairy)

Methylation and Glutathione Support

- MethylAssist, by Pure Encapsulations®
- Sam E 200, by Pro Thera®
- NAC (N-acetyl-l-cysteine) 600 mg, by Pure Encapsulations®

Specialty Products

- Thyroid Emergency Repair Kit, www.thethyroidcure.com
- G.I. Emergency Repair Kit, www.thethyroidcure.com
- Empowerment Formula, www.thethyroidcure.com

Organic Raw and Sprouted Food Companies

Go Raw
http://www.goraw.com

Lydia's Organics
http://www.lydiasorganics.com/welcome.html

Rejuvenative Foods
http://www.rejuvenative.com

Better Than Roasted
http://www.bluemountainorganics.com/betterthanroasted/

Paleo Foods Online

Barefoot Provisions
http://barefootprovisions.com

Wild Mountain Paleo
www.wildmountainpaleo.com

Essential Oils

The Essence of Life
www.krishnamadappa.com

dōTERRA Essential Oils
www.doterra.com

Ayurveda

Banyan Botanicals
http://www.banyanbotanicals.com

Appendix II: Recommended Reading and Resources

Michelle Corey, Websites

www.thethyroidcure.com
www.vibrantway.com

Recommended Reading

Autoimmune Conditions

The Immune System Recovery Plan: A Doctor's 4-Step Program to Treat Autoimmune Disease
Susan Blum M.D.
Scribner, 2013

The Autoimmune Epidemic
Donna Jackson Nakazawa
Touchstone, Scribner, 2008

Overcoming Thyroid Disorders
David Brownstein
Medical Alternatives Press, Inc., 2002

Hope for Hashimoto's
Alexander Haskell
CreateSpace, 2011

The Autoimmune Paleo Plan: A Revolutionary Protocol To Rapidly Decrease Inflammation and Balance Your Immune System
Anne Angelone L.Ac.
CreateSpace, 2013

Hashimoto's Thyroiditis: Lifestyle Interventions for Finding and Treating the Root Cause
Izabella Wentz
Wentz, 2013

Environment

Our Stolen Future: Are We Threatening Our Fertility, Intelligence, and Survival? A Scientific Detective Story
Theo Colborn, Dianne Dumanoski, John Peter Meyers
Plume, 1997

Seeds of Deception
Jeffrey Smith
Yes! Books, 2003

Exposed: The Toxic Chemistry of Everyday Products and What's at Stake for American Power
Mark Schapiro
Chelsea Green Publishing, 2007

Not Just a Pretty Face: The Ugly Side of the Beauty Industry
Stacy Malkan
New Society Publishers, 2007

Toxic Beauty: How Cosmetics and Personal-Care Products Endanger Your Health... and What You Can Do About It
Samuel S. Epstein
BenBella Books, 2009

What's Toxic, What's Not
Gary Ginsberg
Berkley Trade, 2006

Mold Warriors
Ritchie C Shoemaker, M.D. with Patti Schmidt
Gateway Press, 2007

Psychology, and Spirituality

Minding the Body, Mending the Mind
Joan Borysenko, Ph.D.
De Capo Press 2007

I Thought It Was Just Me (but it isn't): Making the Journey from "What Will People Think?" to "I Am Enough"
Brene Brown, Ph.D.
Gotham, 2007

The Gifts of Imperfection: Let Go of Who You Think You're Supposed to Be and Embrace Who You Are
Brene Brown, Ph.D.
Hazelden, 2010

Return to Love: Reflections on the Principles of a Course in Miracles
Marianne Williamson
HarperCollins, 1992

Why People Don't Heal and How they Can
Caroline Myss
Harmony, Random House, 2010

Anatomy of the Spirit: The Seven Stages of Power and Healing
Caroline Myss
Harmony, Random House, 2010

The Power of Now: A Guide to Spiritual Enlightenment
Echardt Tolle
New World Library, 1999

Radical Self-Forgiveness: The Direct Path to True Self-Acceptance
Colin Tipping
Sounds True, 2010

Conscious Loving: The Journey to Co-Commitment
Gay Hendricks, Kathlyn Hendricks
Bantam, 1992

Loving What Is: Four Questions That Can Change Your Life
Byron Katie
Three Rivers Press, 2003

The Biology of Belief: Unleashing the Power of Consciousness, Matter, & Miracles
Bruce H. Lipton Ph.D.
Hay House, 2007

Spontaneous Evolution: Our Positive Future (and a Way to Get There from Here)
Bruce H. Lipton Ph.D.
Hay House, 2009

The Wisdom of Your Cells: How Your Beliefs Control Your Biology
Bruce H. Lipton Ph.D.
Hay House, 2009

You Can Heal Your Life
Louise L. Hay
Hay House, 1984

Women's Health and Sexuality

Women's Bodies, Women's Wisdom (Revised Edition): Creating Physical and Emotional Health and Healing
Christiane Northrup M.D.
Bantam; Rev Upd edition, 2010

The Emergence of The Sensual Woman, Awakening Our Erotic Innocence
Saida Desilets
Jade Goddess Publishing, 2006

Addiction

End Your Addiction Now: The Proven Nutritional Supplement Program That Can Set You Free
Charles Gant, M.D.; Greg Lewis, Ph.D.
Square One Publishers, 2010

Women Food and God, An Unexpected Path to Almost Anything
Geneen Roth
Scribner, 2010

Is It Love or Is It Addiction? The Book That Changed the Way We Think About Romance and Intimacy
Brenda Schaeffer
Hazelden, 2009

Paleo Lifestyle

The Primal Blueprint: Reprogram your Genes for Effortless Weight Loss, Vibrant Health, and Boundless Energy
Mark Sisson
Primal Nutrition, Inc., 2009

Primal Body, Primal Mind: Beyond the Paleo Diet for Total Health and a Longer Life
Nora T. Gedgaudas CNS CNT
Healing Arts Press, 2011

The Paleo Solution: The Original Human Diet
Robb Wolf
Victory Belt Publishing, 2010

The Paleo Diet Revised: Lose Weight and Get Healthy by Eating the Foods You Were Designed to Eat
Loren Cordain
Houghton Mifflin Harcourt, 2010

The Autoimmune Paleo Cookbook: An Allergen-Free Approach to Managing Chronic Illness
Mickey Trescott
Trescott LLC, 2014

Integrative and Functional Medicine

When the Body Says No: Exploring the Stress-Disease Connection
Gabor Mate
Wiley, 2011

The Blood Sugar Solution: The UltraHealthy Program for Losing Weight, Preventing Disease, and Feeling Great Now!
Mark Hyman
Little, Brown and Company, 2012

The UltraMind Solution: Fix Your Broken Brain by Healing Your Body First
Mark Hyman
Scribner, Simon & Schuster, 2010

Ayurveda

Ayurveda: A Life of Balance: The Complete Guide to Ayurvedic Nutrition & Body Types with Recipes
Maya Tiwari
Healing Arts Press, 1995

The Complete Book of Ayurvedic Home Remedies
Vasant Lad, B.A.M.&S., M.A.Sc.
Harmony, 1999

The Ingredients Matter: India Healing with Restorative Recipes
TheIM LLC, 2013

Nutrition

The Body Ecology Diet: Recovering Your Health and Rebuilding Your Immunity
Donna Gates
Hay House, 2011

Nourishing Traditions: The Cookbook that Challenges Politically Correct Nutrition and the Diet Dictocrats
Sally Fallon
Newtrends, 1999

The Fat Flush Plan
Anne Louise Gittleman, M.S.,C.N.S.
McGraw Hill, 2002

Prescription for Nutritional Healing: A practical A-to-Z Reference to Drug-Free Remedies Using Vitamins, Minerals, Herbs, & Food Supplements
Fourth Edition
Phyllis A. Balch, CNC
Avery, 2007

Wheat Belly: Lose the Wheat, Lose the Weight, and Find Your Path Back to Health
William Davis
Rodale Books, 2011

Grain Brain: The Surprising Truth about Wheat, Carbs, and Sugar-- Your Brain's Silent Killers
David Perlmutter
Little, Brown and Company, 2013

Clean: The Revolutionary Program to Restore the Body's Natural Ability to Heal Itself
Alejandro Junger
HarperOne, 2009

Fast Food Nation: The Dark Side of the All-American Meal
Eric Schlosser
Mariner Books; Reprint edition, 2012

Organizations and Websites

Functional Medicine

The Institute for Functional Medicine
www.functionalmedicine.org

The Academy of Functional Medicine and Genomics
www.academyoffunctionalmedicine.com

Nutrition

The Weston A. Price Foundation
http://www.westonaprice.org

Environment

The Collaborative on Health and the Environment
http://www.healthandenvironment.org

Environmental Working Group
http://www.ewg.org

Database of Environmental Health Concerns and toxic chemicals
http://toxtown.nlm.nih.gov

Scorecard pollution information site: In-depth local information on pollution sources
www.scorecard.org

Science, Spirituality and Sustainability

Institute for Science, Spirituality and Sustainability
http://www.issstaos.org

Center for Systemic and Family Constellation
http://www.familyconstellationwork.net

The Forgiveness Institute
www.internationalforgiveness.com

Adverse Childhood Experience Studies

The Adverse Childhood Experiences Study
www.acestudy.org

ACEs Too High
www.acestoohigh.com

Cool Paleo Blogs

Mark's Daily Apple
http://www.marksdailyapple.com

Robb Wolfe
www.robwolfe.com

Living Paleo
http://www.livingpaleo.com

The Paleo Mom
www.thepaleomom.com

Mindfulness Practice

The Mindful Center
http://themindfulcenter.com

Mindful Living Programs
http://www.mindfullivingprograms.com/index.php

Life & Relationship Coaching

The Hendricks Institute
http://www.hendricks.com

Diana Chapman
http://www.dianachapman.com

Grace Caitlin
http://www.gracecaitlin.com

Christine Brondyke
http://www.christinebrondyke.com

Compounding Pharmacies

The Compounding Pharmacy of Beverly Hills
www.compounding-expert.com
9629 West Olympic Boulevard
Beverly Hills, CA 90212
Phone: 310-284-8675
Toll free: 1-888-799-0212

Women's International Pharmacy
http://www.womensinternational.com
Arizona
  12012 N. 111th Avenue
  Youngtown, AZ 85363
  Ph: 623-214-7700
Wisconsin
  2 Marsh Court
  Madison, WI 53718
  Ph: 608-221-7800

Pharmaca Integrative Pharmacy
Multiple locations: http://www.pharmaca.com/stores.aspx

Functional Labs

Metametrix Clinical Laboratory
www.metametrix.com

Genova Diagnostics
www.gdx.net
For questions about insurance, billing and Medicare programs go to www.gdx.net/billing

SpectraCell Laboratories
http://www.spectracell.com

ZRT Laboratory
www.zrtlab.com

Online Labs

MyMedLab
www.mymedlab.com

Direct Labs
https://www.directlabs.com

Natural Pet Care

Only Natural Pet
http://www.onlynaturalpet.com

Dogs Naturally Magazine
www.dogsnaturallymagazine.com

Natural Living and Gardening

Mother Earth News
http://www.motherearthnews.com

Planet Natural
www.planetnatural.com

Films

Escape Fire: Fight to Rescue American Healthcare
Starring Don Berwick, Dean Ornish, Andrew Weil and Shanon Brownlee, 2013

Food, Inc
Starring Eric Schlosser, 2008

Fast Food Nation
Starring: Greg Kinnear, Wilmer Valerrama, 2006

Vitality
Starring: Dr. Pedram Shojai, 2006

The Quantum Activist
Starring: Dr. Amit Goswami, 2009

Appendix III: Finding Your ACE Score

What's Your ACE Score?

There are 10 types of childhood trauma measured in the ACE Study. Five are personal — physical abuse, verbal abuse, sexual abuse, physical neglect, and emotional neglect. Five are related to other family members: a parent who's an alcoholic, a mother who's a victim of domestic violence, a family member in jail, a family member diagnosed with a mental illness, and the disappearance of a parent through divorce, death or abandonment. Each type of trauma counts as one.

While you were growing up, during your first 18 years of life:

1. Did a parent or other adult in the household **often or very often**...
Swear at you, insult you, put you down, or humiliate you?
or
Act in a way that made you afraid that you might be physically hurt?
Yes No   If yes enter 1 _____

2. Did a parent or other adult in the household **often or very often**...
Push, grab, slap, or throw something at you?
or
Ever hit you so hard that you had marks or were injured?
Yes No   If yes enter 1 _____

3. Did an adult or person at least 5 years older than you **ever**...
Touch or fondle you or have you touch their body in a sexual way?
or
Attempt or actually have oral, anal, or vaginal intercourse with you?
Yes No   If yes enter 1 _____

4. Did you **often or very often** feel that ...
No one in your family loved you or thought you were important or special?
or
Your family didn't look out for each other, feel close to each other, or support each other?
Yes No   If yes enter 1 _____

5. Did you **often or very often** feel that ...
   You didn't have enough to eat, had to wear dirty clothes, and had no one to protect you?

   or

   Your parents were too drunk or high to take care of you or take you to the doctor if you needed it?
   Yes No   If yes enter 1 _____

6. Were your parents **ever** separated or divorced?
   Yes No   If yes enter 1 _____

7. Was your mother or stepmother: **Often or very often** pushed, grabbed, slapped, or had something thrown at her?

   or

   Sometimes, often, or very often kicked, bitten, hit with a fist, or hit with something hard?

   or

   Ever repeatedly hit at least a few minutes or threatened with a gun or knife?
   Yes No   If yes enter 1 _____

8. Did you live with anyone who was a problem drinker or alcoholic or who used street drugs?
   Yes No   If yes enter 1 _____

9. Was a household member depressed or mentally ill, or did a household member attempt suicide?
   Yes No   If yes enter 1 _____

10. Did a household member go to prison?
    Yes No   If yes enter 1 _____

    Now add up your "Yes" answers: _____ **This is your ACE Score.**

To learn more about the Ace Study go to www.acestudy.org

Endnotes

Introductory Section

1. Amino N. Autoimmunity and hypothyroidism. Baillieres Clin Endocrinol Metab. 1988 Aug;2(3):591-617. http://www.ncbi.nlm.nih.gov/pubmed/3066320
2. Lipton B, Bhaerman S. Spontaneous Evolution Our Positive Future and a Way to Get There From Here. 3rd Edition. Hay House; 2010
3. American Autoimmune Related Diseases Association. Questions and Answers. http://www.aarda.org/autoimmune-information/questions-and-answers/
4. American Association of Clinical Endocrinologists. Hashimoto's Thyroiditis. (2008) https://www.aace.com/files/hashimotos.pdf
5. "cure." Dictionary.com Unabridged. Random House, Inc. http://dictionary.reference.com/browse/cure

Part One

CHAPTER 1

1. John Hopkins Medical. Autoimmune Disease Research. http://www.hopkinsmedicine.org/fox
2. American Autoimmune Related Diseases Association. Questions and Answers. http://www.aarda.org/autoimmune-information/questions-and-answers/

CHAPTER 2

1. Kornfeld R. The "New" Standard for Care in Medicine. Huffington Post. 12/2/2011 http://www.huffingtonpost.com/dr-robert-a-kornfeld/new-standard-medical-care_b_1117409.html
2. IMS Institute for Healthcare Informatics, The Use of Medicines in the United States: Review of 2010, http://www.imshealth.com/deployedfiles/imshealth/Global/Content/IMS%20Institute/Static%20File/IHII_UseOfMed_report.pdf
3. Centers for Medicare and Medicaid Services. National Health Expenditures 2011 Highlights. http://www.cms.gov/Research-Statistics-Data-and-Systems/Statistics-Trends-and-Reports/NationalHealthExpendData/downloads/highlights.pdf,
4. Herper M. The Best Selling Drugs in America. Forbes. 4/19/2011 http://www.forbes.com/sites/matthewherper/2011/04/19/the-best-selling-drugs-in-america/2/

CHAPTER 3

1. MacIntosh A. Understanding the Differences Between Conventional, Alternative, Complementary, Integrative and Natural Medicine. Townsend Letter, July 1999, http://tldp.com/medicine.htm
2. MacIntosh A. Understanding the Differences Between Conventional, Alternative, Complementary, Integrative and Natural Medicine. Townsend Letter, July 1999, http://tldp.com/medicine.htm
3. The National Center for Complementary and Alternative Medicine, NCCAM Facts-at-a-Glance and Mission, http://nccam.nih.gov/about/ataglance
4. Avik S. A. Roy, Senior Fellow, Manhattan Institute for Policy Research, Stifling New Cures: The True Cost of Lengthy Clinical Drug Trials, Project FDA Report No. 5 April 2012 http://www.manhattan-institute.org/html/fda_05.htm#01
5. MacIntosh A. Understanding the Differences Between Conventional, Alternative, Complementary, Integrative and Natural Medicine. Townsend Letter, July 1999, http://tldp.com/medicine.htm

CHAPTER 6

1. Eggleton P. Stress protein–polypeptide complexes acting as autoimmune triggers. Clin Exp Immunol. 2003 October; 134(1): 6–8. http://www.ncbi.nlm.nih.gov/pmc/articles/PMC1808840/
2. Stojanovich L, Marisavljevich D. Stress as a trigger of autoimmune disease. Autoimmun Rev. 2008 Jan;7(3):209-13. http://www.sciencedirect.com/science/article/pii/B9780123739476000477
3. Richardson B. DNA methylation and autoimmune disease. Clin Immunol. 2003 Oct;109(1):72-9. http://www.ncbi.nlm.nih.gov/pubmed/14585278
4. Ercolini A M, Miller S D. The role of infections in autoimmune disease. Clin Exp Immunol. 2009 January; 155(1): 1–15. http://www.ncbi.nlm.nih.gov/pmc/articles/PMC2665673
5. Kivity S, Agmon-Levin N, Blank M, Shoenfeld Y. Infections and autoimmunity – friends or foes? Trends in Immunology - 1 August 2009 (Vol. 30, Issue 8, pp. 409-414) http://www.sciencedirect.com/science/article/pii/S1471490609001252
6. Velavan TP, Ojurongbe O. Regulatory T cells and parasites. J Biomed Biotechnol. 2011;201(1):520940. http://www.ncbi.nlm.nih.gov/pmc/articles/PMC3255565/
7. Biagi F, Pezzimenti D, Campanella J, Corazza GR. Gluten exposure and risk of autoimmune disorders. Gut. 2002;51(1):140–141. http://www.ncbi.nlm.nih.gov/pmc/articles/PMC1773261/
8. Negro R. Selenium and thyroid autoimmunity. Biologics. 2008 June; 2(2): 265–273. http://www.ncbi.nlm.nih.gov/pmc/articles/PMC2721352/

9. Bigazzi P E. Autoimmunity and Heavy Metals. Lupus December 1994 vol. 3 no. 6 449-453 http://lup.sagepub.com/content/3/6/449.abstract
10. Orbach H, Agmon-Levin N, Zandman-Goddard G. Vaccines and autoimmune diseases of the adult. Discov Med. 2010 Feb;9(45):90-7. http://www.ncbi.nlm.nih.gov/pubmed/20193633
11. Vial T, Descotes J. Autoimmune diseases and vaccinations. Eur J Dermatol. 2004 Mar-Apr;14(2):86-90. http://www.ncbi.nlm.nih.gov/pubmed/15196997
12. Burek C L, Monica V. Talor M V. Environmental Triggers of Autoimmune Thyroiditis. J Autoimmun. 2009 Nov–Dec; 33(3-4): 183–189. http://www.ncbi.nlm.nih.gov/pmc/articles/PMC2790188/
13. Akis M, Verhagen J, Taylor A, et al. Immune responses in healthy and allergic individuals are characterized by a fine balance between allergen specific T regulatory 1 and T helper 2 cells. J Exp Med 2004;199:1567-75
14. Rook GA, Brunet LR. Old friends for breakfast. Clin Exp Allergy 2005;35:841-2
15. Kidd P, Th1/Th2 Balance: The Hypothesis, its Limitations, and Implications for Health and Disease Alternative Medicine Review Vol. 8, Number 3 2003 (pp.223-246) http://www.altmedrev.com/publications/8/3/223.pdf
16. Rappaport S M, Smith M T. Environment and Disease Risks. Science 22 October 2010: Vol. 330 no. 6003 pp. 460-461 http://www.sciencemag.org/content/330/6003/460.summary

CHAPTER 7

1. Georgetown University Medical School. Thyroid Disease. http://medicine.georgetown.edu/divisions/endocrinology/knowledge/thyroid-disease
2. Weetman A. Review Article: Graves' Disease. N Engl J Med Online. Oct. 2000 http://isites.harvard.edu/fs/docs/icb.topic442065.files/Endocrine_Readings/Graves_Disease.pdf
3. American Association of Clinical Endocrinologists. Hashimoto's Thyroiditis. (2008) https://www.aace.com/files/hashimotos.pdf

CHAPTER 9

1. Sword R, Zimbardo P, Hurry Sickness; Is Our Quest to Do All and Be All Costing Us Our Health? Psychology Today Online Feb. 8, 2013 http://www.psychologytoday.com/blog/the-time-cure/201302/hurry-sickness
2. The American Institute of Stress (AIS) http://www.stress.org
3. Olpin N, Perceived Stress Levels and Sources of Stress Among College Students: Methods, Frequency, and Effectiveness of Managing Stress by College Students. Health Education PhD Dissertation. Southern Illinois University at Carbondale Mar. 29, 1996. http://faculty.weber.edu/molpin/dissertation.htm
4. Centers for Disease Control and Prevention. Crude and Age-Adjusted

Percentage of Civilian, Non-institutionalized Population with Diagnosed Diabetes, United States, 1980–2011 http://www.cdc.gov/diabetes/statistics/prev/national/figage.htm

5. Kadiyala R, Peter R, Okosieme OE. Thyroid dysfunction in patients with diabetes: clinical implications and screening strategies. Int J Clin Pract. 2010 Jul;64(8):1130-9 http://www.ncbi.nlm.nih.gov/pubmed/20642711

6. Hyman M. Why Your Genes Don't Determine Your Health. Huffington Post Online. 01/01/11 http://www.huffingtonpost.com/dr-mark-hyman/human-genome_b_803069.html

7. Bronwell K.D. and Warner K.E. The Perils of Ignoring History: Big Tobacco Played Dirty and Millions Died. How Similar Is Big Food? The Milbank Quarterly, Vol. 87, No. 1, 2009 (pp. 259–294) http://www.yalerudds.org/resources/upload/docs/what/industry/Foodtobacco.pdf

8. Nordlee J, Taylor S, Townsend J, Thomas L, Bush R, Identification of A Brazil-Nut Allergen In Transgenic Soybeans. N Engl J Med 1996;334:688-92 http://genetica.ufcspa.edu.br/nutric/seminarios%20monitores/IDENTIFICATION_OF_A_BRAZIL-NUT_ALLERGEN_IN_TRANSGENIC_SOYBEANS%202008.pdf

9. Aris A, Leblanc S. Maternal and fetal exposure to pesticides associated to genetically modified foods in Eastern Townships of Quebec, Canada. Reprod Toxicol. 2011;31(4):528–533. http://www.sciencedirect.com/science/article/pii/S0890623811000566

10. Lin Z, Dongxia H, Xi C, et al. Exogenous plant MIR168a specifically targets mammalian LDLRAP1: evidence of cross-kingdom regulation by microRNA Cell Research. 2011;22:107–126 http://www.nature.com/cr/journal/v22/n1/full/cr2011158a.html

11. Miyake K, Tanaka T, McNeil PL Lectin-Based Food Poisoning: A New Mechanism of Protein Toxicity. PLoS ONE (2007) 2(8): e687. http://www.plosone.org/article/info %3Adoi%2F10.1371%2Fjournal.pone.0000687

12. Cordain L., Toohey L., Smith M.J., Hickey M.S. Modulation of immune function by dietary lectins in rheumatoid arthritis. Br. J. Nutr. 2000;83:207–217 http://www.ncbi.nlm.nih.gov/pubmed/10884708

13. Jones L. Genetically modified foods. BMJ. 1999;318:581–584 http://www.ncbi.nlm.nih.gov/pmc/articles/PMC1115027/?report=reader#B14

14. Bishnoi S, Khetarpaul N, Yadav R. Effect of domestic processing and cooking methods on phytic acid and polyphenol contents of pea cultivars (Pisum sativum) Bishnoi S, Khetarpaul N, Yadav R. Effect of domestic processing and cooking methods on phytic acid and polyphenol contents of pea cultivars (Pisum sativum) Plant Foods for Human Nutrition June 1994, Volume 45, Issue 4, pp 381-388 http://link.springer.com/article/10.1007%2FBF01088088?LI=true#page-1

15. Tracy B. How did genetically altered wheat end up in Oregon field? CBS

News June 6, 2013 http://www.cbsnews.com/8301-18563_162-57588150/how-did-genetically-altered-wheat-end-up-in-oregon-field/
16. Kasarda D, Can an Increase in Celiac Disease Be Attributed to an Increase in the Gluten Content of Wheat as a Consequence of Wheat Breeding? Journal of Agricultural and Food Chemistry 2013 61 (6), 1155-1159 http://pubs.acs.org/doi/full/10.1021/jf305122s#
17. Davis W. Is gluten on the increase? Blog Online. Feb. 15, 2013 http://www.wheatbellyblog.com/2013/02/is-gluten-on-the-increase/
18. Monetini L, Cavallo MG, Manfrini S, et al. Antibodies to bovine beta-casein in diabetes and other autoimmune diseases. Horm Metab Res. 2002 Aug;34(8):455-9 http://www.ncbi.nlm.nih.gov/pubmed/12198602
19. US Dept. Of Agriculture. Genetically engineered varieties of corn, upland cotton, and soybeans, by State and for the Unites States, 2000-13. http://www.ers.usda.gov/data-products/adoption-of-genetically-engineered-crops-in-the-us.aspx#.Ua58DGTb1bs
20. Bray G, Nielsen S, Popkin B. Consumption of high-fructose corn syrup in beverages may play a role in the epidemic of obesity. Am J Clin Nutr 2004 79: 4 537-543 http://ajcn.nutrition.org/content/79/4/537.abstract
21. Dufault R, LeBlanc B, Schnoll R, et al. Mercury from chlor-alkali plants: measured concentrations in food product sugar. Environmental Health. 2009;8:2. http://www.ncbi.nlm.nih.gov/pubmed/19171026
22. Siegmund B, Leitner E, Pfannhauser W. Determination of the nicotine content of various edible nightshades (solanaceae) and their products and estimation of the associated dietary nicotine intake. J Agric Food Chem 1999;47:3113–20 http://www.ncbi.nlm.nih.gov/pubmed/10552617
23. US Dept. Of Agriculture. Genetically engineered varieties of corn, upland cotton, and soybeans, by State and for the Unites States, 2000-13. http://www.ers.usda.gov/data-products/adoption-of-genetically-engineered-crops-in-the-us.aspx#.Ua58DGTb1bs
24. Doerge D, Sheehan D. Goitrogenic and Estrogenic Activity of Soy Isoflavones. Environmental Health Perspectives. v110 June 2002. http://www.ncbi.nlm.nih.gov/pmc/articles/PMC1241182/pdf/ehp110s-000349.pdf
25. Persky VW, Turyk ME, Wang L, et al. Effect of soy protein on endogenous hormones in postmenopausal women. Am J Clin Nutr 2002;75:145-153. http://ajcn.nutrition.org/content/75/1/145.abstract
26. Asthma and Allergy Foundation of America. Peanut Allergy. Updated 2005 http://www.aafa.org/display.cfm?id=9&sub=20&cont=517
27. Kritchevsky D, Tepper SA, Klurfeld DM. Lectin may contribute to the atherogenicity of peanut oil. Lipids. 1998;33:821–3. http://www.ncbi.nlm.nih.gov/pubmed/9727614
28. Pramod SN, Venkatesh YP, Mahesh PA. Potato lectin activates basophils and

mast cells of atopic subjects by its interaction with core chitobiose of cell-bound non-specific immunoglobulin E. Clin Exp Immunol. 2007;148:391–401. http://www.ncbi.nlm.nih.gov/pmc/articles/PMC1941928/
29. Singh R, Subramanian S, Rhodes JM, Campbell BJ. Peanut lectin stimulates proliferation of colon cancer cells by interaction with glycosylated CD44v6 isoforms and consequential activation of c-Met and MAPK: functional implications for disease-associated glycosylation changes. Glycobiology.2006;16:594–601 http://glycob.oxfordjournals.org/content/16/7/594.full
30. Sategna-Guidetti C, Volta U, Ciacci C, et al. Prevalence of thyroid disorders in untreated adult celiac disease patients and effect of gluten withdrawal: an Italian multicenter study. American Journal of Gastroenterology. 2001;96(3):751–757. http://www.ncbi.nlm.nih.gov/pubmed/11280546
31. Brown A.C. Gluten Sensitivity, Problems of an Emerging Condition Separate From Celiac Disease Expert Rev Gastroenterol Hepatol. 2012;6(1):43-55. http://www.ncbi.nlm.nih.gov/pubmed/22149581
32. Tucková L, Tlaskalová-Hogenová H, Farré MA, et al. Molecular mimicry as a possible cause of autoimmune reactions in celiac disease? Antibodies to gliadin cross-react with epitopes on enterocytes. Department of Immunology and Gnotobiology, First Faculty of Medicine, Prague, Czech Republic. Clinical Immunology and Immunopathology [1995, 74(2):170-176 http://www1.lf1.cuni.cz/~kocna/docum/cs_tucko.pdf
33. Miyake K, Tanaka T, McNeil PL. Lectin-Based Food Poisoning: A New Mechanism of Protein Toxicity. PLoS ONE (2007) 2(8): e687. http://www.plosone.org/article/info%3Adoi%2F10.1371%2Fjournal.pone.0000687
34. Fasano A. Zonulin and Its Regulation of Intestinal Barrier Function: The Biological Door to Inflammation, Autoimmunity, and Cancer. Physiol Rev. Vol 91. Jan 2011. 151175 http://www.ncbi.nlm.nih.gov/pubmed/21248165
35. Fasano A. Physiological, pathological, and therapeutic implications of zonulin-mediated intestinal barrier modulation: living life on the edge of the wall. Am J Pathol. 2008;173:1243–1252.http://www.ncbi.nlm.nih.gov/pmc/articles/PMC2570116/
36. Arrieta MC, Bistritz L, Meddings JB, Alterations in intestinal permeability. Gut. 55: 1512–1520 (2006) http://www.ncbi.nlm.nih.gov/pmc/articles/PMC1856434/pdf/1512.pdf
37. Ulluwishewa D, Anderson RC, Mcnabb WC, Moughan PJ, Wells JM, Roy NC. Regulation of tight junction permeability by intestinal bacteria and dietary components. J Nutr. 2011;141:769–76 http://jn.nutrition.org/content/141/5/769.full
38. Mishra A, Liu S, Sams G. H, et al. Aberrant Overexpression of IL-15 Initiates Large Granular Lymphocyte Leukemia through Chromosomal Instability and DNA Hypermethylation. Cancer Cell, 2012; 22 (5): 645 http://www.

cell.com/cancer-cell/abstract/S1535-6108(12)00394-7
39. Baker S, Bennett P, Bland J. Textbook of functional medicine. Institute for Functional Medicine; Second edition (2005) Page 139
40. Inadera H. The immune system as a target for environmental chemicals: xenoestrogens and other compounds. Toxicol Letters 2006;164: 191–206 http://www.ncbi.nlm.nih.gov/pubmed/16697129
41. Ahmed SA, Hissong BD, Verthelyi D, Donner K, Becker K, Karpuzoglu-Sahin E. Gender and risk of autoimmune diseases: possible role of estrogenic compounds. Environ Health Perspect. 1999;107 (Suppl 5):681–686. http://www.ncbi.nlm.nih.gov/pmc/articles/PMC1566250/
42. Straub RH. 2007. The complex role of estrogens in inflammation. Endocr. Rev. 28: 521–574 http://edrv.endojournals.org/content/28/5/521.full
43. Mayes M, Epidemiologic studies of environmental agents and systemic autoimmune diseases. Environmental Health Perspectives 11/1999; 107 Suppl 5:743-8. http://www.ncbi.nlm.nih.gov/pmc/articles/PMC1566245/pdf/envhper00522-0088.pdf
44. Weidler C, Härle P, Schedel J, Schmidt M, Schölmerich J, Straub RH. Patients with rheumatoid arthritis and systemic lupus erythematosus have increased renal excretion of mitogenic estrogens in relation to endogenous antiestrogens. J Rheumatol 31:489–494 2004 http://www.jrheum.org/content/31/3/489.short
45. Vedhara K, Cox NK, Wilcock GK, et al. Chronic stress in elderly carers of dementia patients and antibody response to influenza vaccination. Lancet. 1999 Feb 20;353(9153):627–31 http://www.ncbi.nlm.nih.gov/pmc/articles/PMC166443/
46. Miller GE, Cohen S, Ritchey AK. Chronic psychological stress and the regulation of pro-inflammatory cytokines: a glucocorticoid-resistance model. Health Psychol 2002; 21: 531–541. http://www.ncbi.nlm.nih.gov/pubmed/12433005
47. Abou-Donia MB, El-Masry EM, Abdel-Rahman AA, McLendon RE, Schiffman SS. Splenda alters gut microflora and increases intestinal p-glycoprotein and cytochrome p-450 in male rats. J Toxicol Environ Health A 71:1415–1429 2008. http://www.ncbi.nlm.nih.gov/pubmed/18800291
48. Myers, RL and Myers, RL. The 100 most important chemical compounds: a reference guide. Westport, Conn: Greenwood Press. 2007.
49. Mayo Clinic: Dept of Otorhinolaryngology. Research on Chronic Sinusitis. http://www.mayoclinic.org/ent-rst/chronicsinus.html
50. Colborn T, Dumanoski D, Meyers J, Our Stolen Future: Are We Threatening Our Fertility, Intelligence, and Survival?--A Scientific Detective Story. Plume (Mar. 1997) http://www.ourstolenfuture.org
51. Department of Health and Human Services. Third National Report on Human Exposure to Environmental Chemicals. Atlanta, GA: Centers for

Disease Control and Prevention; July 2005.
52. Yurino H, Ishikawa S, Sato T, Akadegawa K, Ito T, Ueha S, et al. Endocrine disruptors (environmental estrogens) enhance autoantibody production by B1 cells. Toxicol Sci. 2004;81:139–47 http://www.ncbi.nlm.nih.gov/pubmed/15166399
53. Richter CA, Birnbaum LS, Farabollini F, Newbold RR, Rubin BS, et al. In vivo effects of bisphenol A in laboratory rodent studies. Reprod Toxicol 2007; 24: 199–224. http://www.ncbi.nlm.nih.gov/pmc/articles/PMC2151845/
54. Ye X, Bishop AM, Reidy JA, Needham LL, Calafat AM. Parabens as urinary biomarkers of exposure in humans. Environ Health Perspect. 2006a;114:1843–1846. http://www.ncbi.nlm.nih.gov/pmc/articles/PMC1764178/
55. Menegaux F, Baruchel A, Bertrand Y, et al. Household exposure to pesticides and risk of childhood acute leukaemia. Occupational and Environmental Medicine. 2006;63(2):131–134. http://www.ncbi.nlm.nih.gov/pmc/articles/PMC2078075/
56. Zhang Y, Guo GL, Han X, et al. Do polybrominated diphenyl ethers (PBDE) increase the risk of thyroid cancer? Bioscience Hypotheses. 2008;1(4):195–199 http://www.ncbi.nlm.nih.gov/pmc/articles/PMC2612591/figure/F1/
57. Zhang Y, Guo GL, Han X, et al. Do polybrominated diphenyl ethers (PBDE) increase the risk of thyroid cancer? Bioscience Hypotheses. 2008;1(4):195–199 http://www.ncbi.nlm.nih.gov/pmc/articles/PMC2612591/
58. Yi J, Cao J. Tea and fluorosis. Journal of Fluorine Chemistry 129:1976-81. (2008).
59. Whitford G. Tea contains more fluoride than once thought. Georgia Health Sciences University. Jul. 2010 http://www.eurekalert.org/pub_releases/2010-07/mcog-tcm071410.php
60. Diesendorf M. The mystery of declining tooth decay. Nature 1986 Jul 10;322:125- 9 http://www.nature.com/nature/journal/v322/n6075/pdf/322125a0.pdf
61. Braathen M, Derocher AE, Wiig O, Sormo EG, Lie E, Skaare JU, Jenssen BM. Relationships between PCBs and thyroid hormones and retinol in female and male polar bears. Environ Health Perspect. 2004,112.826–833 http://www.ncbi.nlm.nih.gov/pmc/articles/PMC1242008/
62. Schiraldi M., Monestier M. How can a chemical element elicit complex immunopathology? Lessons from mercury-induced autoimmunity. (2009) Trends Immunol. 30, 502–509. http://toxcenter.org/artikel/Quecksilber-crasht-Autoimmunitaet.pdf
63. Exley C, Begum A, Woolley MP, Bloor RN. Aluminum in tobacco and cannabis and smoking-related disease. Am. J. Med. 2006;119:276 e9–276 http://www.ncbi.nlm.nih.gov/pubmed/16490479
64. Tomljenovic L. Aluminum and Alzheimer's disease: after a century of

controversy, is there a plausible link? J Alzheimers Dis. 2011;23:567–598 http://www.ncbi.nlm.nih.gov/pubmed/21157018

65. Sterzl I, Procházková J, Hrda P, Matucha P, Bartova J, Stejskal V. Removal of dental amalgam decreases anto-TPO and anti-Tg autoantibodies in patients with autoimmune thyroiditis. Neuro Endocrinol Lett. 2006;5(27(Suppl 1):25–30 http://www.ncbi.nlm.nih.gov/pubmed/16804512

66. Geier D, Kern J, Garver C, et al. Biomarkers of environmental toxicity and susceptibility in autism, Journal of the Neurological Sciences, Volume 280, Issues 1–2, 15 May 2009, Pages 101-10 http://www.sciencedirect.com/science/article/pii/S0022510X08004310

67. Shoenfeld Y, Agmon-Levin N. 'ASIA' - autoimmune/inflammatory syndrome induced by adjuvants. J Autoimmun. 2011;11:4–8 http://www.ncbi.nlm.nih.gov/pubmed/20708902?dopt=Abstract&holding=f1000,f1000m,isrctn

68. Tomljenovic L, Shaw CA. Aluminum Vaccine Adjuvants: Are they Safe? Curr Med Chem. 2011;18:2630–2637 http://www.ncbi.nlm.nih.gov/pubmed/21568886

69. Tomljenovic L, Shaw CA. Mechanisms of aluminum adjuvant toxicity and autoimmunity in pediatric populations. Lupus February 2012 21: 223-230 http://lup.sagepub.com/content/21/2/223

70. National Network for Immunization Information. Aluminum Adjuvants in Vaccines. Nov. 2008 http://www.immunizationinfo.org/issues/vaccine-components/aluminum-adjuvants-vaccines

71. Cherry JD. Why do pertussis vaccines fail? Pediatrics 129: 968–970 (2012)

72. Centers for Disease Control and Prevention. Interim Adjusted Estimates of Seasonal Influenza Vaccine Effectiveness — United States, February 2013 http://www.cdc.gov/mmwr/preview/mmwrhtml/mm6207a2.htm?s_cid=mm6207a2_w

73. Orenstein WA, Heseltine PN, LeGagnoux SJ, Portnoy B. Rubella vaccine and susceptible hospital employees. Poor physician participation. JAMA. 1981 Feb 20;245(7):711–713 http://www.ncbi.nlm.nih.gov/pubmed/7463660

Part Two

CHAPTER 12

1. The American Academy of Clinical Endocrinologists www.aacc.org/SiteCollectionDocuments/NACB/LMPG/.../3c_thyroid.doc
2. American Association of Clinical Endocrinologists. Over 13 Million Americans with Thyroid Disease Remain Undiagnosed. January 2003 Press Release. http://www.hospitalsoup.com/public/AACEPress_release-highlighted.pdf

CHAPTER 13

1. Takasu N, Komiya I, Asawa T, Nagasawa Y, Yamada T. Test for recovery from

hypothyroidism during thyroxine therapy in Hashimoto's thyroiditis. Lancet. 1990;336(8723):1084–6 http://www.ncbi.nlm.nih.gov/pubmed/1977978
2. Takasu N, Komiya I, Asawa T, Nagasawa Y, Yamada T. Test for recovery from hypothyroidism during thyroxine therapy in Hashimoto's thyroiditis. Lancet. 1990;336(8723):1084–6 http://www.ncbi.nlm.nih.gov/pubmed/1977978

CHAPTER 14

1. Intahphuak S, Khonsung P, Panthong A. Anti-inflammatory, analgesic, and antipyretic activities of virgin coconut oil. Pharmaceutical Biology. 2010;48(2):151–157 http://www.ncbi.nlm.nih.gov/pubmed/20645831
2. Takahashi M, Inoue S, Hayama K, Ninomiya K, Abe S. Inhibition of Candida mycelia growth by a medium chain fatty acids, capric acid in vitoro and its therapeutic efficacy in murine oral candidiasis. Med Mycol J. 2012;53(4):255-61. http://www.ncbi.nlm.nih.gov/pubmed/23257726
3. Reger MA, Henderson ST, Hale C. Effects of beta-hydroxybutyrate on cognition in memory-impaired adults. Neurobiol Aging. 2004 Mar;25(3):311-4 http://www.ncbi.nlm.nih.gov/pubmed?term=Neurobiol%20Aging.%202004%20Mar;25(3):311-4
4. St-Onge MP, Jones PJ. Physiological effects of medium-chain triglycerides: potential agents in the prevention of obesity. J Nutr. 2002 Mar;132(3):329-32. http://www.ncbi.nlm.nih.gov/pubmed/11880549?dopt=Abstract
5. Bergsson G, Arnfinnsson J, Ólafur Steingrímsson, Thormar H. In Vitro Killing of Candida albicans by Fatty Acids and Monoglycerides. Antimicrob. Agents Chemother. November 2001 vol. 45 no. 11 3209-3212 http://aac.asm.org/content/45/11/3209.full
6. Boyages S. Progress in Understanding the Clinical Consequences of Endemic Iodine Deficiency. Current Opinion in Endocrinology, Diabetes and Obesity 4.5 (1997): 320-327. http://www.researchgate.net/publication/232133920_Progress_in_understanding_the_clinical_consequences_of_endemic_iodine_deficiency
7. Keck AS, Finley JW. Cruciferous Vegetables: Cancer Protective Mechanisms of Glucosinolate Hydrolysis Products and Selenium. Integr Cancer Ther March 2004 3: 5-12 http://www.ncbi.nlm.nih.gov/pubmed/15035868 -
8. Barrera LN, Cassidy A, Wang W, et al. TrxR1 and GPx2 are potently induced by isothiocyanates and selenium, and mutually cooperate to protect Caco-2 cells against free radical-mediated cell death. Biochimica et Biophysica Acta (BBA) - Molecular Cell Research. Oct 2012, Vol. 1823, No. 10: 1914-192 http://www.ncbi.nlm.nih.gov/pubmed/22820176

CHAPTER 15

1. Kaushik RM, Kaushik R, Mahajan SK, Rajesh V. Effects of mental relaxation and slow breathing in essential hypertension. Complement Ther Med. 2006;14:120–6. http://www.complementarytherapiesinmedicine.com/

article/S0965-2299(05)00148-2/fulltext
2. National Sleep Foundation. Annual Sleep in America Poll Exploring Connections with Communications Technology Use and Sleep. Published Online. March 7, 2011. http://www.sleepfoundation.org/article/press-release/annual-sleep-america-poll-exploring-connections-communications-technology-use-
3. National Sleep Foundation. How Much Sleep Do Adults Need? http://www.sleepfoundation.org/article/white-papers/how-much-sleep-do-adults-need
4. Lashley FR. A review of sleep in selected immune and autoimmune disorders. Holist Nurs Pract. 2003 Mar-Apr;17(2):65-80. http://www.anapsid.org/cnd/files/sleep-in-selected-ai.pdf
5. Yu X, Rollins D, Ruhn KA, et al. TH17 cell differentiation is regulated by the circadian clock. Science. 2013 Nov 8;342(6159):727-30. http://www.ncbi.nlm.nih.gov/pubmed/24202171
6. Waite JC, Skokos D. Th17 Response and Inflammatory Autoimmune Diseases. Int J Inflam. 2012;2012:819467 http://www.ncbi.nlm.nih.gov/pubmed/22229105
7. Nedergaard M, Xie L, Kang H, et al. Sleep Drives Metabolite Clearance from the Adult Brain. Science 18 October 2013: 342 (6156), 373-377. http://www.sciencemag.org/content/342/6156/373
8. Roehrs T, Roth T. Sleep, sleepiness, sleep disorders and alcohol use and abuse. Sleep Medicine Reviews. 2001;5(4):287–297. http://www.ncbi.nlm.nih.gov/pubmed/12530993
9. Leggio L, Ray LA, Kenna GA, Swift RM. Blood glucose level, alcohol heavy drinking, and alcohol craving during treatment for alcohol dependence: results from the Combined Pharmacotherapies and Behavioral Interventions for Alcohol Dependence (COMBINE) Study. Alcoholism: Clinical and Experimental Research. 2009b;33:1539–1544. http://www.ncbi.nlm.nih.gov/pubmed/19485973
10. Mirrakhimov A, Mirrakhimov E M. Obstructive Sleep Apnea and Autoimmune Disease: A Two-Way Process. J Clin Sleep Med. 2013 April 15; 9(4): 409. http://www.ncbi.nlm.nih.gov/pmc/articles/PMC3601322/
11. Coughlin SR, Mawdsley L, Mugarza JA, Calverley PM, Wilding JP (2004) Obstructive sleep apnoea is independently associated with an increased prevalence of metabolic syndrome. Eur Heart J 25: 735–741. http://www.ncbi.nlm.nih.gov/pubmed/15120883
12. Ip MS, Lam B, Ng MM, Lam WK, Tsang KW, Lam KS. Obstructive sleep apnea is independently associated with insulin resistance. Am J Respir Crit Care Med. 2002;13(5):670–676. http://www.ncbi.nlm.nih.gov/pubmed/11874812
13. Yu JC, Berger P 3rd. Sleep apnea and obesity. S D Med. 2011;Spec No:28-34. http://www.ncbi.nlm.nih.gov/pubmed/21717814

14. Schwartz AR, Gold AR, Schubert N, et al. Effect of weight loss on upper airway collapsibility in obstructive sleep apnea. Am Rev Respir Dis. 1991;144(3 Pt 1):494–498. http://www.ncbi.nlm.nih.gov/pubmed/1892285
15. Puhan M. A., Suarez A., Lo Cascio C., Zahn A., Heitz M., Braendli O. (2006). Didgeridoo playing as alternative treatment for obstructive sleep apnoea syndrome: randomised controlled trial. Br. Med. J. (Clin. Res. Ed.) 332, 266–270.10.1136/bmj.38705.470590.55 http://www.ncbi.nlm.nih.gov/pubmed/16377643
16. Ryan RM, Weinstein N, Bernstein J, Brown KW, Mistretta L, Gagne´ M. Vitalizing effects of being outdoors and in nature. Journal of Environmental Psychology 30 (2010) 159–168. http://www.researchgate.net/publication/228478393_Vitalizing_effects_of_being_outdoors_and_in_nature/file/32bfe513dd5917a305.pdf.
17. Howell AJ, Dopko RL, Passmore HA, Buro K. Nature connectedness: Associations with well-being and mindfulness. Personality and Individual Differences Vol. 51, Issue 2, July 2011, Pages 166–171. http://www.sciencedirect.com/science/article/pii/S0191886911001711
18. Berk LS, Tan SA, Fry WF, et al. Neuroendocrine and stress hormone changes during mirthful laughter. Am J Med Sci. 1989;298:390–6. http://www.ncbi.nlm.nih.gov/pubmed/2556917
19. Hori M, Hayashi T, Nakagawa Y, Sakamoto S, Urayama O, Murakami K. Positive emotion-specific changes in the gene expression profile of tickled rats. Mol Med Rep. 2009 Mar-Apr;2(2):157-61. http://www.spandidos-publications.com/mmr/2/2/157

CHAPTER 16

1. Prakash S, Rodes L, Coussa-Charley M, Tomaro-Duchesneau C (2011) Gut microbiota: next frontier in understanding human health and development of biotherapeutics. Biol Targ Ther 5: 71-86. http://www.ncbi.nlm.nih.gov/pmc/articles/PMC3156250/
2. Fasano A. Leaky gut and autoimmune diseases. Clin Rev Allergy Immunol. 2012;5:71–78. http://www.ncbi.nlm.nih.gov/pubmed/22109896
3. Andrès E, Noel E, Ben Abdelghani M. Vitamin B12 deficiency associated with chronic acid suppression therapy. Ann Pharmacother 2003;37:1730 http://www.ncbi.nlm.nih.gov/pubmed/14565839
4. Gardner MLG. Gastrointestinal absorption of intact proteins. Annu Rev Nutr. 1988;8:329–50. http://www.ncbi.nlm.nih.gov/pubmed/3060169
5. Kwon H-K, Lee C-G, So J-S, et al. Generation of regulatory dendritic cells and CD4+Foxp3+ T cells by probiotics administration suppresses immune disorders. Proceedings of the National Academy of Sciences of the United States of America. 2010;107(5):2159–2164. http://www.ncbi.nlm.nih.gov/pubmed/20080669

6. Ghadimi D., Folster-Holst R., de Vrese M., Winkler P., Heller K.J., Schrezenmeir J. Effects of probiotic bacteria and their genomic DNA on TH1/TH2-cytokine production by peripheral blood mononuclear cells (PBMCs) of healthy and allergic subjects. Immunobiology. 2008;213:677–692. http://www.ncbi.nlm.nih.gov/pubmed/18950596
7. Hougee S, Vriesema AJM, Wijering SC, et al. Oral treatment with probiotics reduces allergic symptoms in ovalbumin-sensitized mice: a bacterial strain comparative study. International Archives of Allergy and Immunology. 2010;151(2):107–117. http://www.ncbi.nlm.nih.gov/pubmed/19752564
8. Rossi M, Amaretti A, Raimondi S. Folate production by probiotic bacteria. Nutrients 2011;3:118-34. http://www.ncbi.nlm.nih.gov/pmc/articles/PMC3257725/
9. Dan Lukaczar, ND. The "4" R Program. Textbook of functional medicine. Institute for Functional Medicine; Second edition (2010) Page 468.
10. Souba WW, Klimberg VS, Plumley DA, Salloum RM, Flynn TC, Bland KI, Copeland EM 3rd. The role of glutamine in maintaining a healthy gut and supporting the metabolic response to injury and infection. J Surg Res. 1990 Apr;48(4):383-91. http://www.ncbi.nlm.nih.gov/pubmed/2187115
11. Rhoads JM, Argenzio RA, Chen W, Rippe RA, Westwick JK et al. (1997) L-glutamine stimulates intestinal cell proliferation and activates mitogen-activated protein kinases. Am J Physiol 272: G943-G953. http://www.ncbi.nlm.nih.gov/pubmed/9176200
12. Cho C.H. Zinc: Absorption and Role in Gastrointestinal Metabolism and Disorders Dig Dis. 1991;9(1):49-60. http://www.ncbi.nlm.nih.gov/pubmed/2009637
13. Semrad CE. Zinc, and intestinal function. Curr Gastroenterol Rep 1: 398–403, 1999. http://www.ncbi.nlm.nih.gov/pubmed/10980978
14. Wapnir R. Zinc Deficiency, Malnutrition and the Gastrointestinal Tract. J. Nutr. May 1, 2000 vol. 130 no. 5 1388S-1392S. http://jn.nutrition.org/content/130/5/1388S.full
15. Sturniolo GC, Leo DiV, Ferronato A, D'Odorico A, D'Inca R. Zinc supplementation tightens "leaky gut" in Crohn's disease. Inflamm Bowel Dis. 2001;7:94–98. http://www.ncbi.nlm.nih.gov/pubmed/11383597
16. Centanni M, Gargano L, Canettieri G, et al. Thyroxine in goiter, Helicobacter pylori infection, and chronic gastritis. N Engl J Med. 2006;354(17):1787–1795. http://www.ncbi.nlm.nih.gov/pubmed/16641395
17. Reimer C, Søndergaard B, Hilsted L, Bytzer P. Proton-Pump Inhibitor Therapy Induces Acid-Related Symptoms in Healthy Volunteers After Withdrawal of Therapy. Gastroenterology 1 July 2009 vol. 137 issue 1 Pages 80-87. http://www.gastrojournal.org/article/S0016-5085(09)00522-8/fulltext
18. Medical News Today Online. Gelatin Treats Ulcers. August 2006 http://

      www.medicalnewstoday.com/releases/50126.php
19. Hering NA, Schulzke JD. Therapeutic options to modulate barrier defects in inflammatory bowel disease. Dig Dis. 2009;27:450–454. http://www.ncbi.nlm.nih.gov/pubmed/19897959
20. Russell RI, Morgan RJ, Nelson LM. Studies on the protective effect of deglycyrrhinised liquorice against aspirin (ASA) and ASA plus bile acid-induced gastric mucosal damage, and ASA absorption in rats. Scand J Gastroenterol Suppl. 1984;92:97-100. http://www.ncbi.nlm.nih.gov/pubmed/6588541
21. Naliboff B, Mayer M, Fass R, et al. The Effect of Stress on Symptoms of Heartburn. Psychosomatic Medicine May 1, 2004 vol. 66 no. 3 426-434 http://www.psychosomaticmedicine.org/content/66/3/426.full
22. Bradley LA, Richter JE, Pulliam TJ, et al. The relationship between stress and symptoms of gastroesophageal reflux: the influence of psychological factors. Am J Gastroenterol 1993; 88:11-19. http://www.ncbi.nlm.nih.gov/pubmed/8420248
23. Naliboff B, Mayer M, Fass R, et al. The Effect of Stress on Symptoms of Heartburn. Psychosomatic Medicine May 1, 2004 vol. 66 no. 3 426-434 http://www.psychosomaticmedicine.org/content/66/3/426.full
24. Centanni M, Gargano L, Canettieri G, et al. Thyroxine in goiter, Helicobacter pylori infection, and chronic gastritis. N Engl J Med. 2006;354(17):1787–1795. http://www.ncbi.nlm.nih.gov/pubmed/16641395
25. Yancy WS Jr, Provenzale D, Westman EC. Improvement of gastroesophageal reflux disease after initiation of a low-carbohydrate diet: five brief case reports. Altern Ther Health Med. 2001 Nov-Dec;7(6):120, 116-9. http://www.ncbi.nlm.nih.gov/pubmed/11712463
26. Austin GL, Thiny MT, Westman EC, Yancy WS Jr, Shaheen NJ. A very low-carbohydrate diet improves gastroesophageal reflux and its symptoms. Dig Dis Sci. 2006 Aug;51(8):1307-12. Epub 2006 Jul 27. http://www.ncbi.nlm.nih.gov/pubmed/16871438

CHAPTER 17

1. Nomura S, Pittman CS, Chambers JB, Buck MW, Shimizu T, Reduced peripheral conversion of thyroxine to triiodothyronine in patients with hepatic cirrhosis. J Clin Invest. 1975 September; 56(3): 643–652. http://www.ncbi.nlm.nih.gov/pmc/articles/PMC301912/
2. Richardson B. DNA methylation and autoimmune disease. Clin Immunol. 2003 Oct;109(1):72-9. http://www.ncbi.nlm.nih.gov/pubmed/14585278
3. Richardson B, Scheinbart L, Strahler J, Gross L, Hanash S, Johnson M. Evidence for impaired T cell DNA methylation in systemic lupus erythematosus and rheumatoid arthritis. Arthritis Rheum. 1990 Nov;33(11):1665-73. http://www.ncbi.nlm.nih.gov/pubmed/2242063

4. Sekigawa I, Kawasaki M, Ogasawara H, et al. DNA methylation: its contribution to systemic lupus erythematosus. Clin Exp Med. 2006;6:99–106. http://www.ncbi.nlm.nih.gov/pubmed/17061057
5. Reprinted with permission from: Methylation: The Molecule That Unlocks The Body's Healing Response; A Key To: Detoxification, Cell Repair, Graceful Aging, Weight Loss, Neurotransmitter Balance, Healthy Immunity, Disease Prevention, Nerve Protection, and so much more. By Dr. Jack Tips, N.D., Ph.D., C.Hom., C.C.N. Published Online: http://www.anma.org/pdf/Methylation_by_Dr_Jack_Tips_Complete_and_Illustrated_Article.pdf
6. Lim U, Song MA. Dietary and lifestyle factors of DNA methylation. Methods Mol Biol. 2012;863:359-76 http://www.ncbi.nlm.nih.gov/pubmed/22359306
7. Tapp HS, Commane DM, Bradburn DM, et al. Nutritional factors and gender influence age-related DNA methylation in the human rectal mucosa. Aging Cell. 2013 Feb;12(1):148-55. http://www.ncbi.nlm.nih.gov/pubmed/23157586
8. Reprinted with permission from: Methylation: The Molecule That Unlocks The Body's Healing Response; A Key To: Detoxification, Cell Repair, Graceful Aging, Weight Loss, Neurotransmitter Balance, Healthy Immunity, Disease Prevention, Nerve Protection, and so much more. By Dr. Jack Tips, N.D., Ph.D., C.Hom., C.C.N. Published Online: http://www.anma.org/pdf/Methylation_by_Dr_Jack_Tips_Complete_and_Illustrated_Article.pdf
9. Perricone C, De Carolis C, Perricone R. Glutathione: a key player in autoimmunity. Autoimmun Rev. 2009 Jul;8(8):697-701. http://www.ncbi.nlm.nih.gov/pubmed/19393193
10. Habdous M, Siest G, Herbeth B, Vincent-Viry M, Visvikis S. [Glutathione S-transferases genetic polymorphisms and human diseases: overview of epidemiological studies]. [Article in French] Ann Biol Clin (Paris). 2004 Jan-Feb;62(1):15-24. http://www.ncbi.nlm.nih.gov/pubmed/15047486
11. Choi SW, Friso S. Epigenetics: A New Bridge between Nutrition and Health. Adv Nutr November 2010 Adv Nutr vol. 1: 8-16, 2010. http://advances.nutrition.org/content/1/1/8.full
12. Eckmekcioglu C, Strauss-Blasche G, Holzer F, Marktl W. Effect of sulfur baths on antioxidative defense systems, peroxide concentrations and lipid levels in patients with degenerative osteoarthritis. Forsch Komplementarmed Klass Naturheilkd. 2002;9:216–20. http://www.ncbi.nlm.nih.gov/pubmed/12232493
13. Marshall K. Therapeutic applications of whey protein. Altern Med Rev. 2004 Jun;9(2):136-56. http://www.ncbi.nlm.nih.gov/pubmed/15253675
14. Rotruck JT, Pope AL, Ganther HE, Swanson AB, Hafeman DG, Hoekstra WG. Selenium: biochemical role as a component of glutathione peroxidase.

Science. 1973 Feb 9;179 (4073):588-90. http://www.ncbi.nlm.nih.gov/pubmed/4686466
15. Johnston CS, Meyer CG, Srilakshmi JC. Vitamin C elevates red blood cell glutathione in healthy adults. Am J Clin Nutr. 1993 Jul;58(1):103-5. http://ajcn.nutrition.org/content/58/1/103.full.pdf
16. Jain SK, Micinski D. Vitamin D upregulates glutamate cysteine ligase and glutathione reductase, and GSH formation, and decreases ROS and MCP-1 and IL-8 secretion in high-glucose exposed U937 monocytes. Biochem Biophys Res Commun. 2013 Jul 19;437(1):7-11. http://www.ncbi.nlm.nih.gov/pubmed/23770363
17. Kechrid Z, Hamdi M, Naziroğlu M, Flores-Arce M. Vitamin D supplementation modulates blood and tissue zinc, liver glutathione and blood biochemical parameters in diabetic rats on a zinc-deficient diet. Biol Trace Elem Res. 2012 Sep;148(3):371-7. http://www.ncbi.nlm.nih.gov/pubmed/22410949
18. Milad K, Racz O, Ipulova A, Bajova V, Kovae G. Effect of vitamin E and selenium on blood glutathione peroxidase activity and some immunological parameters in sheep. Vet. Med. – Czech., 46, 2001 (1): 1–5 http://vri.cz/docs/vetmed/46-1-1.pdf
19. Powers SK, Ji LL, Leeuwenburgh C. Exercise training-induced alterations in skeletal muscle antioxidant capacity: a brief review. Med Sci Sports Exerc. 1999 Jul;31(7):987-97. http://www.ncbi.nlm.nih.gov/pubmed/10416560
20. Everson CA, Laatsch CD, Hogg N (2005) Antioxidant defense responses to sleep loss and sleep recovery. Am J Physiol Regul Integr Comp Physiol 288: R374-R383. http://ajpregu.physiology.org/content/288/2/R374.long
21. Valenzuela, A.; Aspillaga, M.; Vial, S.; Guerra, R. Selectivity of silymarin on the increase of the glutathione content in different tissues of the rat. *Planta Med.* **1989**, 55, 420–422. http://www.ncbi.nlm.nih.gov/pubmed/2813578
22. Zheng S, Yumei F, Chen A.De novo synthesis of glutathione is a prerequisite for curcumin to inhibit hepatic stellate cell (HSC) activation. Free Radic Biol Med. 2007 Aug 1;43(3):444-53. http://www.ncbi.nlm.nih.gov/pubmed/17602960
23. Burgunder JM, Varriale A, Lauterburg BH (1989) Effect of N-acetylcysteine on plasma cysteine and glutathione following paracetamol administration. Eur J Clin Pharmacol 36: 127–131. http://www.ncbi.nlm.nih.gov/pubmed/2721538
24. Shay KP, Moreau RF, Smith EJ, Smith AR, Hagen TM.Alpha-lipoic acid as a dietary supplement: molecular mechanisms and therapeutic potential. Biochim Biophys Acta. 2009 Oct;1790(10):1149-60. http://www.ncbi.nlm.nih.gov/pubmed/19664690
25. Vendemiale G, Altomare E, Trizio T, et al. Effects of oral S-adenosyl-L-methionine on hepatic glutathione in patients with liver disease. Scand J

Gastroenterol. 1989 May;24(4):407-15. http://www.ncbi.nlm.nih.gov/pubmed/2781235
26. Heim K. Glutathione bioavailability:_New technology confronts old questions. Published online 2013 Feb 27 http://www.pureencapsulations.com/education-research/newscaps/newscap-02-27-13
27. 2004 Global Amphibian Assessment (GAA), http://www.iucnredlist.org/initiatives/amphibians/analysis
28. Colson D G. A Safe Protocol for Amalgam Removal. J Environ Public Health. 2012; 2012: 517391. http://www.hindawi.com/journals/jeph/2012/517391/
29. Environmental Protection Agency. Mercury: Laws and Regulations: http://www.epa.gov/hg/regs.htm
30. Prochazkova J, Sterzl I, Kucerova H, Bartova J, Stejskal VD. The beneficial effect of amalgam replacement on health in patients with autoimmunity. NeuroendocrinologyLetters No.3 June Vol.25, 2004. http://www.nel.edu/pdf_/25_3/NEL250304A07_Prochazkova_.pdf

CHAPTER 18

1. Cusick MF1, Libbey JE, Fujinami RS. Molecular mimicry as a mechanism of autoimmune disease. Clin Rev Allergy Immunol. 2012 Feb;42(1):102-11. http://www.ncbi.nlm.nih.gov/pubmed/22095454
2. Oldstone MB. Molecular mimicry and immune-mediated diseases. FASEB J. 1998 Oct;12(13):1255-65. http://www.ncbi.nlm.nih.gov/pubmed/9761770
3. Fujinami RS, von Herrath MG, Christen U, Whitton JL. Molecular mimicry, bystander activation, or viral persistence: infections and autoimmune disease. Clin Microbiol Rev. 2006;19:80–94. http://www.ncbi.nlm.nih.gov/pmc/articles/PMC1360274/
4. Sfriso P, Ghirardello A, Botsios C, et al. Infections and autoimmunity: the multifaceted relationship. J Leukoc Biol. 2010 Mar;87(3):385-95. http://www.jleukbio.org/content/87/3/385.full.pdf
5. Pancewicz SA, Skrzydlewska E, Hermanowska-Szpakowicz T, Zajkowska JM, Kondrusik M. Role of reactive oxygen species (ROS) in patients with erythema migrans, an early manifestation of Lyme borreliosis. Med Sci Monit. 2001;7:1230–1235. http://www.ncbi.nlm.nih.gov/pubmed/11687735
6. Roederer M.; Raju P.A.; Staal F.J.T.; Herzenberg L.A.; Herzenberg L.A., 1991: N acetylcysteine inhibits latent hiv expression in chronically infected cells. Aids Research & Human Retroviruses. 7(6): 563-567. http://eurekamag.com/research/007/581/n-acetylcysteine-inhibits-latent-hiv-expression-chronically-infested-cells.php
7. Staal FJ, Roederer M, Israelski DM, Bubp J, Mole LA, et al. (1992) Intracellular glutathione levels in T cell subsets decrease in HIV-infected

8. Ciriolo MR, Palamara AT, Incerpi S, et al. Loss of GSH, oxidative stress, and decrease of intracellular pH as sequential steps in viral infection. J. Biol. Chem. (1997); 272 (5): 2700-2708. http://www.jbc.org/content/272/5/2700.full
9. Cai J, Chen Y, Seth S, Furukawa S, Compans RW, Jones DP. Inhibition of influenza infection by glutathione. Free Radical Biology & Medicine (2003); 34 (7): 928-936. http://www.ncbi.nlm.nih.gov/pubmed/12654482
10. Palamara AT, Perno CF, Ciriolo MR, Dini L, Balestra E, et al. (1995) Evidence for antiviral activity of glutathione: in vitro inhibition of herpes simplex virus type 1 replication. Antiviral Res 27: 237–253. http://www.ncbi.nlm.nih.gov/pubmed/8540746
11. Van Konynenburg, R.A. Glutathione Depletion—Methylation Cycle Block, A Hypothesis for the Pathogenesis of Chronic Fatigue Syndrome. Poster paper, 8th Intl. IACFS Conf. on CFS, Fibromyalgia, and Other Related Illnesses, Fort Lauderdale, FL, January 10-14, 2007. http://goo.gl/OflJeA
12. Taylor, E.W., Selenium and viral diseases: facts and hypotheses, J. Orthomolec. Med. (1997); 12 (4): 227-239. http://orthomolecular.org/library/jom/1997/pdf/1997-v12n04-p227.pdf
13. Sfriso P, Ghirardello A, Botsios C, et al. Infections and autoimmunity: the multifaceted relationship. J Leukoc Biol. 2010 Mar;87(3):385-95. http://www.jleukbio.org/content/87/3/385.full.pdf
14. Almas K, Al-Sanawi E, Al-Shahrani B. The effect of tongue scraper on mutans streptococci and lactobacilli in patients with caries and periodontal disease. Odontostomatol Trop. 2005;28:5–10. http://www.ncbi.nlm.nih.gov/pubmed/16032940
15. Quirynen M, Avontroodt P, Soers C, Zhao H, Pauwels M, van Steenberghe D. Impact of tongue cleansers on microbial load and taste. J Clin Periodontol. 2004;3:506–10. http://www.ncbi.nlm.nih.gov/pubmed/15191584
16. University At Buffalo. Researchers Show Chronic Sinusitis Is Immune Disorder; Antifungal Medicine Effective Treatment. ScienceDaily. www.sciencedaily.com/releases/2004/03/040324072619.htm (accessed March 2, 2014).
17. Kern E, Sherris D, Ponikau J, et al. Diagnosis and treatment of chronic rhinosinusitis: focus on intranasal Amphotericin B. Ther Clin Risk Manag. Jun 2007; 3(2): 319–325. http://www.ncbi.nlm.nih.gov/pmc/articles/PMC1936313/
18. Choudhary TS, Mishra R, Choudhary A. Effect of yoga intervention in chronic rhinosinusitis. International Journal of Bioassays, [S.l.], v. 1, n. 12, p. 214-216, nov. 2012. ISSN 2278-778X. http://www.academia.edu/2515039/EFFECT_OF_YOGA_INTERVENTION_IN_CHRONIC_RHINOSINUSITIS

19. Sengupta P. Health impacts of yoga and pranayama: A state-of-the-art review. Int J Prev Med. 2012;3:444–58. http://www.ncbi.nlm.nih.gov/pmc/articles/PMC3415184/
20. Ginde AA, Liu MC, Camargo CA., Jr. Demographic differences and trends of vitamin D insufficiency in the US population, 1988-2004. Arch Intern Med. 2009;169:626–32. http://www.ncbi.nlm.nih.gov/pmc/articles/PMC3447083/
21. Vos T, Flaxman AD, Naghavi M, et al. Years lived with disability (YLDs) for 1160 sequelae of 289 diseases and injuries 1990–2010: a systematic analysis for the Global Burden of Disease Study 2010. Lancet. 2012;380(9859):2163–2196. http://www.ncbi.nlm.nih.gov/pubmed/23245607
22. Fisher JF, Kavanagh K, Sobel JD, Kauffman CA, Newman CA. Candida urinary tract infections—epidemiology, pathogenesis, diagnosis, and treatment: executive summary. Clinical Infectious Diseases. 2011;52(6):S429–S432. http://cid.oxfordjournals.org/content/52/suppl_6/S437.full
23. Ledezma E, DeSousa L, Jorquera A, et al. Efficacy of ajoene, an organosulphur derived from garlic, in the short-term therapy of tinea pedis. Mycoses. 1996 Sep-Oct;39(9-10):393-5. http://www.ncbi.nlm.nih.gov/pubmed/9009665
24. Cvetnić Z, Vladimir-Knezević S. Antimicrobial activity of grapefruit seed and pulp ethanolic extract. Acta Pharm 54.3 (2004): 243-250. http://www.ncbi.nlm.nih.gov/pubmed/15610620
25. Omar SH. Oleuropein in olive and its pharmacological effects. Scientia Pharmaceutica. 2010;13:133–154. http://www.ncbi.nlm.nih.gov/pubmed/21179340
26. Sudjana AN, D'Orazio C, Ryan V, Rasool N, Ng J, Islam N, et al. Antimicrobial activity of commercial Olea europaea (olive) leaf extract. Int J Antimicrob Agents. 2009;33:461–3. http://www.ncbi.nlm.nih.gov/pubmed/19135874
27. Bao J, Zhang DW, Zhang JZH, Huang PL, Huang PL, Lee-Huang S. Computational study of bindings of olive leaf extract (OLE) to HIV-1 fusion protein gp41. FEBS Lett. 2007;581:2737–2742. http://www.ncbi.nlm.nih.gov/pubmed/17537437
28. Mahmoud DA. Hassanein NM. Youssef KA. Abou Zeid MA. Antifungal activity of different neem leaf extracts and the nimonol against some important human pathogens. Braz. J. Microbiol. vol.42 no.3 São Paulo July/Sept. 2011 http://www.scielo.br/scielo.php?script=sci_arttext&pid=S1517-83822011000300021
29. Mohanty SS, Raghavendra K, Dash AP. Influence of growth medium on antifungal activity of neem oil (Azadirachta indica) against Lagenidium giganteum and Metarhizium anisopliae. Mycoscience (Impact Factor: 1.17). 01/2008; 49(5):318-320. http://www.sciencedirect.com/science/article/pii/S1340354008702742

30. Bounous G, Gold P. The biological activity of undenatured dietary whey proteins: role of glutathione. Clin Invest Med 1991;14:296–309. http://www.ncbi.nlm.nih.gov/pubmed/1782728

CHAPTER 19

1. Babich, H, Babich, JP. Sodium lauryl sulfate and triclosan: in vitro cytotoxicity studies with gingival cells. Toxicology Letters, Volume 91, issue 3 (May 16, 1997), p. 189-196. http://www.ncbi.nlm.nih.gov/pubmed/9217239
2. Lee CH, Kim HW, Han HJ, Park CW. A Comparison Study of Nonanoic Acid and Sodium Lauryl Sulfate in Skin Irritation. Exog Dermatol 2004;3:19–25. http://www.karger.com/Article/FullText/84139
3. Mercola J. Deadly and Dangerous Shampoos, Toothpastes, and Detergents: Could 16,000 Studies Be Wrong About SLS? July 13 2013 http://articles.mercola.com/sites/articles/archive/2010/07/13/sodium-lauryl-sulfate.aspx
4. Donn J, Mendoza M, Pritchard J, PHARMAWATER I Pharmaceuticals found in drinking water, affecting wildlife and maybe humans. Associated Press. http://hosted.ap.org/specials/interactives/pharmawater_site/index.html
5. Al-Saleh I, Shinwari N, Alsabbaheen A. Phthalates residues in plastic bottled waters. J Toxicol Sci. 2011;21:469–478. http://www.ncbi.nlm.nih.gov/pubmed/21804311
6. Zock JP, Plana E, Jarvis D, Antó JM, et al. The use of household cleaning sprays and adult asthma: an international longitudinal study. Am J Respir Crit Care Med. 2007;176:735–741. http://www.ncbi.nlm.nih.gov/pmc/articles/PMC2020829/?tool=pubmed
7. AromaWeb. Aromatherapy Diffusers. http://www.aromaweb.com/articles/diffu.asp
8. Anne C. Steinemann, Lisa G. Gallagher, Amy L. Davis, Ian C. MacGregor. Chemical emissions from residential dryer vents during use of fragranced laundry products. Air Quality, Atmosphere & Health. March 2013, Volume 6, Issue 1, pp 151-156 http://link.springer.com/content/pdf/10.1007%2Fs11869-011-0156-1.pdf
9. The Honest Company. Hypoallergenic & Natural Dryer Sheets. https://www.honest.com/cleaning/honest-dryer-cloths
10. Zhu K, Hunter S, Payne-Wilks K, Roland CL, Forbes DS (2003) Use of Electric Bedding Devices and Risk of Breast Cancer in African-American Women. American Journal of Epidemiology 158: 798–806. http://www.ncbi.nlm.nih.gov/pubmed/14561670
11. IARC Classifies Radiofrequency Electromagnetic Fields As Possibly Carcinogenic to Humans. WHO/International Agency for Research on Cancer (IARC) Press Release N° 208 May 31, 2011http://www.iarc.fr/en/media-centre/pr/2011/pdfs/pr208_E.pdf
12. Mandalà M, Colletti V, Sacchetto L, Manganotti P, et al. Effect of Bluetooth

headset and mobile phone electromagnetic fields on the human auditory nerve. Laryngoscope. 2013 Apr 25.
13. Environmental Protection Agency. Home Buyer's and Seller's Guide to Radon. EPA 402/K-09/002 | January 2009 http://www.epa.gov/radon/pubs/hmbyguid.html
14. Environmental Protection Agency. A Brief Guide to Mold, Moisture, and Your Home. EPA 402-K-02-003 (Reprinted 09/2010) http://www.epa.gov/iedmold1/moldbasics.html
15. Gray MR, Thrasher JD, Crago R, et al. Mixed mold mycotoxicosis: immunological changes in humans following exposure in water-damaged buildings. Archives of Environmental Health. 2004;58(7):410–420. http://www.ncbi.nlm.nih.gov/pubmed/15143854
16. Andersson MA, Nikulin M, Koljalg U, et al. Bacteria, molds, and toxins in water-damaged building materials. Appl Environ Microbiol 1997;63:387–393. http://www.ncbi.nlm.nih.gov/pubmed/9023919
17. Kuhn DM, Ghannoum MA. Indoor Mold, Toxigenic Fungi, and Stachybotrys chartarum: Infectious Disease Perspective. Clin Microbiol Rev. 2003 January; 16(1): 144–172. http://cmr.asm.org/content/16/1/144.full
18. The California Department of Public Health. Occupational Health Hazard Alert Methylene Chloride in Paint Strippers and Bathtub Refinishing. http://www.cdph.ca.gov/programs/hesis/Documents/MethyleneChlorideAlert.pdf
19. Urbansky E.T., Brown S.K., Magnuson M.L., Kelty C.A. Perchlorate levels in samples of sodium nitrate fertilizer derived from Chilean caliche. Environmental Pollution 112 (2001) 299±302 http://www.tera.org/ART/Perchlorate/EPClO4.pdf
20. Centers for Disease Control and Prevention. National Center for Environmental Health. Perchlorate Fact Sheet October 5, 2006. http://www.cdc.gov/nceh/publications/factsheets/perchlorate.htm
21. Medline Plus, National Institutes of Health. Magnesium. Page last updated: 13 September 2013 http://www.nlm.nih.gov/medlineplus/druginfo/natural/998.html
22. Nimni ME. Han B. Cordoba F. Are we getting enough sulfur in our diet? Nutr Metab (Lond) 2007;4:24. http://www.nutritionandmetabolism.com/content/4/1/24
23. Eckmekcioglu C, Strauss-Blasche G, Holzer F, Marktl W. Effect of sulfur baths on antioxidative defense systems, peroxide concentrations and lipid levels in patients with degenerative osteoarthritis. Forsch Komplementarmed Klass Naturheilkd. 2002;9:216–20. http://www.ncbi.nlm.nih.gov/pubmed/12232493
24. 2004 Global Amphibian Assessment (GAA), http://www.iucnredlist.org/initiatives/amphibians/analysis

Part Three

1. Viljoen M, Panzer A, Roos J.L, Bodemer W. Psychoneuroimmunology: From Philosophy, Intuition and Folklore to a Recognized Science. South African Journal of Science 99 July/August 2003: 332. http://connection.ebscohost.com/c/articles/11532011/psychoneuroimmunology-from-philosophy-intuition-folklore-recognized-science
2. Viljoen M, Panzer A, Roos J.L, Bodemer W. Psychoneuroimmunology: From Philosophy, Intuition and Folklore to a Recognized Science. South African Journal of Science 99 July/August 2003: 332. http://connection.ebscohost.com/c/articles/11532011/psychoneuroimmunology-from-philosophy-intuition-folklore-recognized-science
3. Felitti V, Anda F, Nordenberg D, et al. Relationship of Childhood Abuse and Household Dysfunction to Many of the Leading Causes of Death in Adults: The Adverse Childhood Experiences (ACE) Study. American Journal of Preventive Medicine - May 1998 ;Vol. 14, Issue 4, p 245-258 http://www.acestudy.org
4. Kiecolt-Glaser J.K., McGuire L., Robles T.F., Glaser R. (2002) Emotions, morbidity, and mortality: new perspectives from psychoneuroimmunology. Annual Review Psycholgy 53, 83-107. http://www.ncbi.nlm.nih.gov/pubmed/11752480
5. Barak Y. The immune system and happiness. Autoimmun Rev. 2006;5:523–527. http://www.ncbi.nlm.nih.gov/pubmed/17027886
6. O'Connor M-F, Irwin MR, Wellisch DK. When grief heats up: pro-inflammatory cytokines predict regional brain activation. Neuroimage. 2009; 47:891-896
7. Mayo Clinic. Complicated Grief. Sept. 29, 2011. http://www.mayoclinic.com/health/complicated-grief/DS01023
8. Dickerson SS, Kemeny ME, Aziz N, Kim KH, Fahey JL. Immunological Effects of Induced Shame and Guilt. Psychosom Med. 2004 Jan-Feb;66(1):124-31. http://www.ncbi.nlm.nih.gov/pubmed/14747646
9. Lawler K. A., Younger J. W., Piferi R. L., Jobe R. L., Edmondson K. A., Jones W. H. (2005). The unique effects of forgiveness on health: an exploration of pathways. J.Behav. Med. 28, 157–167. http://www.ncbi.nlm.nih.gov/pubmed/15957571
10. Lawler K. A., Younger J. W., Piferi R. L., Jobe R. L., Edmondson K. A., Jones W. H. (2005). The unique effects of forgiveness on health: an exploration of pathways. J.Behav. Med. 28, 157–167. http://www.ncbi.nlm.nih.gov/pubmed/15957571

Index

A

Academy of Functional Medicine & Genomics, 29
Acetylation, 315
N-Acetyl-cysteine, 249, 328
Acid-blockers, 306–307
Acid reflux, 304, 306
Acrylic acid esters, 177
Acupuncture, 70
Adaptogens, 277
Addison's disease, 274
Adrenal burnout. *See* Adrenal fatigue
Adrenal exhaustion. *See* Adrenal fatigue
Adrenal fatigue, 188
    healing of, 221–222, 276–278
    role of stress in, 100, 155–157, 221–222, 273–275, 278–279
    stress-protective hormones in, 82
    symptoms of, 157–158
Adrenal glands, in insulin sensitivity, 18
Adrenal hormone deficiency, 275
Adrenal hormone tests, 278–279
Adrenaline, 100, 123–124
Adrenal Stress Assessment, 194–195, 276, 278, 290, 293
Adrenal Stress Profile, 278–279
Adrenal testing, 275–276
Adrenocorticotropic hormone (ACTH), 122
Advanced glycation end-products (AGEs), 166
Adverse Childhood Experiences (ACE) Study, 376
Advocacy, for health care, 49, 50–54
Aerobic exercise, 290
Affirmations, 237–238
Aggravating factors, of autoimmune conditions. *See* "Splinters," of autoimmune conditions
Aging
    advanced glycation end-products and, 166
    high-glycemic foods and, 167
    protein and, 247
    thyroid hormones and, 82

Air filtration devices, 356
Air fresheners, 171, 354, 355–356
Alcohol
    annual expenditures on, 63
    arsenic in, 181
    as coping mechanism, 131–132
    craving for, 5, 265
    Cymbalta use and, 18
    effect on the liver, 327
    elimination from diet, 19
    as gastrointestinal stress cause, 148
    glutathione-depleting effect of, 320
    reintroduction into diet, 265
    as sleep disturbance cause, 281, 282
Aleve (Naproxen), 151
Alfalfa, 256, 258
Alkaloids, 142, 143
Allergens, air-borne, 356
Allergies, 24. *See also* Food allergies
    as inflammation cause, 169
    pet-related, 360–361
Allopathic medicine, 65–67
Almonds, 266
Aloe, 306
Alpha-linoleic acid, 243
Alpha-lipoic acid, 23, 328–329
Alternative medicine, definition of, 68
Aluminum, 180–181
    in vaccines, 183, 184
Alzheimer's disease, 181, 244
American Academy of Pediatrics, 13
American Association of Clinical Endocrinologists (AACE), 31, 44–45, 113, 212
American Autoimmune Related Disease Association (AARDA), 31
American College of Rheumatology, 290
American Institute of Stress, 131
American Journal of Preventive Medicine, 376
Amines, 145
Amino acids, 23, 315
Amphibians, as environmental indicators, 330
Anatomy of an Illness (Cousins), 292

Anemia, 83, 300, 305
  testing for, 230
Anger, 384, 392
Anorexia, 148–150
Antacids, 151, 304
Anti-anxiety medications, 227, 293
Antibiotic-resistant organisms, 152
Antibiotics, 152
Antibodies, 94. *See also specific* antibodies
Antidepressants, 17, 18, 293
Antifungal medications, 341, 345
Antigen-presenting cells, 95
Antigens, 92
  cryptic, 335–336
Anti-inflammatory compounds, natural, 299
Anti-inflammatory drugs. *See also* Nonsteroidal anti-inflammatory drugs (NSAIDs)
  adverse effects of, 66, 151
Antinuclear antibodies (ANA), in Graves' thyrotoxicosis, 110
Antinuclear antibodies (ANA) tests, 7–8, 211, 214
Antioxidants, 223
  deficiency in, 171
  glucosinolate-derived, 248
  neutralization of free radicals by, 315
  role in glutathione production, 328
  sources of, 23, 222
Antithyroglobulin antibodies (TgAb), 113, 116
Antithyroglobulin antibodies (TgAb) test, 210, 214, 216, 217
Antithyroid drugs
  as Graves' thyrotoxicosis treatment, 111–112
Antithyroid peroxidase antibodies (anti-TPO), 110, 113, 116
Antithyroid peroxidase antibodies (anti-TPO) test, 210, 214, 215–217
Antithyroid-stimulating immunoglobulins (TSI), 110
Apple cider vinegar, 307
Armour Thyroid, 218, 219
Arsenic, 181
Artemesia (sweet wormwood), 299, 302
Artificial sweeteners, 168–169, 258
  in fiber supplements, 301

Ashwaganda, 277
Aspartame, 168, 258
Aspirin, 151
  aluminum in, 180–181
Astragalus, 346
Atenolol, (Tenormin), 111
Atenolol (Tenormin), 111
Attitude, changes in, 2
Autoimmune conditions
  allopathic approach to, 66–67
  chronic infectious stress-related, 101
  diagnostic tests for, 209–214
  as "incurable" disorders, 46
  pathophysiology of, 3
  prevalence of, 31, 44–45
  reversibility of, 32–34
  risk factors for, 4
  similarities among, 3
Autoimmune process
  as condition or disease, 99–100
  reversal/reframing of, 3, 32–34, 99–106
  stress-related impairment of, 100–101
Autoimmune thyroid conditions, 107-118.
  See also Graves' thyrotoxicosis; Hashimoto's thyroiditis
  "cure" of, 3
Autonomic nervous system, 121
Avocado oil, 245
Ayurvedic medicine, 68, 70, 235, 244, 340–341, 347, 375

B

Baba, Karl, 125, 287, 288, 396
Bacillus thuringiensis (Bt) pesticide toxin, 136–137, 141
Bacteria. *See also names of specific bacteria*
  antibiotic-resistant, 152
  beneficial intestinal, 295, 300–301, 303, 307, 344
  dental decay-causing, 340
  glutathione-depleting, 336
  harmful intestinal, 285, 299, 302, 309–310
Bacterial infections
  gastrointestinal, 152, 339, 348
  testing for, 348, 349
Baime, Michael, 288
Baking soda, 357

Barley grass, 256, 258
Batteries, 181–182
B-cells, 92, 93–94, 97–98, 101
Beans, 20, 256, 264
Benzyl alcohol, 355
Berberine, 299, 302
Beta-blockers, 111, 226, 227
Betaine hydrochloride, 303, 306–307
"Beyond Clean," 27, 368–369
Big Pharma, 48
Bile, 316, 325
Birth control pills, 161
Bisphenol-A (BPA), 174, 333
"Black mold," 359–360
Bladder infections, 342–343, 344
Blame, *versus* responsibility, 397–399
Bland, Jeffrey, 125
Bleach, 360, 363
Blood, filtration in the liver, 314
Blood draw test, 312
Blood sugar. *See also* Diabetes
    imbalances in, 131–132, 282
    regulation of, 83, 316
Blum, Susan, interview with, 423–434
Body awareness exercise, 290
Body burden, of toxins, 23, 119–121
    functional testing for, 333
Body Ecology Diet, The (Gate), 23
Body temperature, 83–84, 343–344
Body weight, 82, 236
Bone broth, 307
Bone cancer, 179
Bone marrow, immune function of, 91
Borage oil, 244, 245, 249, 301
Borrelia burgdorferi, 336, 339, 349
Borysenko, Joan, 279, 280
Brain fog, 5
Brain function, role of thyroid hormones in, 82–83
Brassica (cruciferous) vegetables, 248, 327
Bread, 166, 263–264
Breast cancer, 174, 175, 358
Breast milk, lead in, 182
Breathing techniques
    for healthful sleep, 284
    panayama, 341
    for stress management, 279–280
Breath test, for *Helicobacter pylori*, 309

Broccoli, 227–228
Bromine, 178–179, 180, 223
Brown, Brené, 385, 387–388, 391–392
Brownstein, David, 22–23
Brucella, 339, 349
Brussels sprouts, 227–228
Buddha, 190, 392
Buffett, Warren, 209
Bugleweed, 227
Bulimia, 149–150
Butter, 244, 266
Butyrate, 244
Bystander activation theory, 335

C

Cadmium, 181–182
Caffeine
    elimination from diet, 19
    as sleep disturbance cause, 281, 282
Caitlin, Grace, 14
Calcium, malabsorption of, 305
Calories, 236
Camphor, 355
Cancer. *See also specific types of* cancer
    electromagnetic fields-related, 358
    as mortality cause, 45
Candida, 7, 26, 27, 152, 343, 344
    testing for, 348
Candida-related complex, 344–345
Capric acid, 244
Caprylic acid, 299, 302
Carbohydrates
    addiction to/cravings for, 5, 131–132
    as gastrointestinal stress cause, 148
    high-glycemic, 166–167
    low-glycemic, 245–246
    reintroduction into diet, 265
Carvovirus B-19, 339
Casein, 141
CD4+ T-cells, 93
Celiac disease, 150, 153
    testing for, 312
Cell phones, 358
Centers for Disease Control and Prevention (CDC), 174, 175, 182, 360
Chambers. Ian, 12, 13, 14
Change, responsibility for, 44
Chapman, Diana, 14

Chelation therapy, 332–333
Chemical exposure, 351
  functional testing for, 333
Chief Seattle, 291
Childhood abuse and trauma, 9, 10, 376
  as source of shame, 385, 386–387, 389, 391–392, 398–399, 401–402
Chilean sodium nitrate, 363
Chinese medicine, traditional, 68, 70, 375
Chiropractors, 12, 13, 14, 278
Chlamydial infections, 338, 339
  testing for, 349
Chlorine, 178, 180, 223
  removal from drinking water, 355
Chocolate, 265
Cholesterol, 83, 158, 368
Chronic diseases
  dietary factors in, 134–135
  mismanagement of, 49
  as mortality cause, 45
  multiple causes of, 125–126
Chronic fatigue syndrome, 278, 331, 336, 347
Cinnamon leaf oil, 341
Cis-linoleic acid, 243, 244
Clayton College of Natural Health, 24
Cleaning products
  "green" (environmentally safe), 356–357
  toxins in, 27, 351, 354, 355–356
Clove oil, 341
Coconut oil, 244, 245, 301
Codependency, 14–15
Coenzyme Q10 (CoQ10), 23
Coffee drinking, 18
Cognitive stress, 129–131
Colitis, ulcerative, 3
Complementary and alternative medicine (CAM), 68–69
Condiments, 257
Condoms, 342
Conjugases, 315
Conscious Loving coaching, 28
Conservation International, 330
Conventional medicine, 65–67
Cooking oils, 244–245
Coping strategies, negative, 131–133, 400
CoQ10 (coenzyme Q10), 23
CORE test, 333

Corn
  elimination from diet, 19, 263
  gastrointestinal effects of, 264
  genetically-modified, 141–142, 264
  reintroduction into diet, 264
  sensitivity to, 141–142
Corticotropin-releasing hormone (CRH), 122
Cortisol, 82, 100, 123–124, 159
  testing for, 275–276, 278–279
Cosby, Bill, 292
Cost. See also Health insurance coverage
  of integrative/functional health care, 77, 78
  of medications, 63–64
Cousins, Norman, 292
Coxsackie viruses, 336, 339
C-reactive protein (CRP), test for, 211
Cronkite, Walter, 57
Cruciferous (brassica) vegetables, 248, 327
CT scan, of the sinuses, 348
Curcumin, 328
Cure, definition of, 33
Cushing's disease, 274
Cymbalta, 18
Cysteine, 328, 368
Cystitis, 342–343
Cytokine panels, 102
Cytokines, 97, 165, 388
Cytomel, 16, 218, 219

D

Dairy foods
  elimination from diet, 19, 254–255
  reintroduction into diet, 266
  sensitivity to, 141
Dairy substitutes, 253, 266
Dancing, 290–291
Davis, William, 140
DDT, 179
Defeat Autism Now (Yasko), 336
Deglycyrrhizinated licorice (DGL), 306, 307
Dehydroepiandrosterone. See DHEA
5'-Deiodoinase, 210, 222
De Los Santos, Visudha, 291
Dendritic cells, 95, 97
Dental fillings, silver amalgam-containing, 26, 27, 182–183, 331–332, 364
Dental hygiene, for infection control, 340–341

Dental implants, 348
Deodorants, 353
Depression, autoimmune thyroid disease misdiagnosed as, 17–19
Detoxification, 351–369
    with chelation therapy, 332–333
    factors affecting, 317
    functional/integrative practitioners' use of, 77
    functional testing for, 333–334
    of garages, 362–363
    of gardens/outdoor environment, 362–363
    glutathione in, 317
    of home environment, 353–354
    of hydrogen peroxide, 222
    in the liver, 90–91, 313, 314–315, 316, 317–321
    methylation in, 317–321
    of mold contamination, 359–360
    nutritional factors in, 321–326
    phases of, 90–91, 315
    of the workplace, 364–365
DetoxiGenomic™ Profile, 334, 350
Dextrose, as thyroid replacement medication filler, 219
DHEA (dehydroepiandrosterone), 17, 82, 158–159
    testing for, 275–276
DHEA supplements, 250
Diabetes, 3, 133, 142
Diagnosis
    components of, 45–47
    definition of, 45–46
Diagnos-Tech's, 77
Diagnostic codes, 45
Diagnostic tests, for autoimmune conditions, 77, 209–214. *See also* Functional testing
    baseline values in, 229–230
    denial of health insurance coverage for, 59
    normal *versus* optimal ranges in, 212
Dichloromethane, 363
Diet. *See also Eating for Your Good Genes! Program; Eating habits; Sensitivity Discovery Program*
    corn-based, 20
    elimination-type, 19
    low-calorie, 18
    low-carbohydrate, 310
    low-fat, 18
    low-protein, 18
    nutritionally-deficient, 133–135
    Standard American (SAD), 134–135
    vegetarian/vegan, 18, 247–248, 302–303, 320
Digestion, 83, 91
Digestive enzymes, 249, 301, 302–303
Digestive enzyme supplements, 307
Dioxin-like compounds (DLCs), 176
Dioxins, 176, 180
Disease model, of illness, 66, 67, 71
Diuretics
    alcohol as, 282
    overuse of, 149–150
DNA
    diet and, 133–134
    epigenetics and, 55, 105, 106
    of genetically-engineered food, 136–137
    methylation of, 318, 337
    repair of, 299–300
Docosahexaenoic acid (DHA), 243
Doctor(s). *See also* Functional/integrative medical practitioners
    fee-for-service, 60–61, 77
    health insurance companies' influence on, 58–59
    interviews with, 4
    of oriental medicine, 278
    successful, 51
Doctor-patient relationship, 62
    in functional/integrative health care, 76–78
    for health care advocacy, 50–54
Doctor's Data, 77
Drinking water
    antibiotics in, 152
    daily intake of, 247, 254
    filtration of, 354–355
    fluoridated, 179
    toxins in, 152, 177, 181, 354
Drinks
    elimination from diet, 257
    healing, 254
Drugs. *See* Medications
Dry skin brushing, 367
Dysbiosis, 295, 298, 305

E

Earth Friendly Products, 356
Eating disorders, 148–150
Eating for Your Good Genes! Program, 241–261, 296–297
    for adrenal health, 276
    fats in, 242, 243–245
    for liver health, 322–323
    low-glycemic carbohydrates in, 245–246
    proteins in, 246–247
    recipes, 259–260
    shopping list, 252–258
    for vegetarians, 247–248
    vitamin supplements in, 249–251
    withdrawal symptoms in, 241–242
Eating habits
    as gastrointestinal stress cause, 148
    for healthy sleep, 282
    mindful, 235–236, 299
    stressful, 299, 306, 308
Echinacea, 346
Ecover, 356
EDTA (ethylenediaminetetraacetic acid)
    baths, 27, 368–369
    powder, 27
EFT, 28
Eggplant, 142
Eggs, 19, 254
    omega-3-enriched, 242–243, 247, 262, 265
Eicosapentaenoic acid (EPA), 243
80/20 rule, 269
Electromagnetic fields (EMFs), 357–359
Elimination diets, 238, *See also Eating for Your Good Genes! Program; Sensitivity Discovery Program*
Emotional negativity, chronic, 37, 127–131, 375–407
    assessment of, 190–192, 293
    case examples of, 377–382, 399–404
    causes of, 128–129
    forms of, 382–399
    healing of, 399–407
    mind-body balance and, 399–404
    symptoms of, 130–131
Emotional state, relation to physical health, 12
Emotional stress. *See* Emotional negativity, chronic
Emotional Stress Assessment, 190–192, 293

Empowerment, 37–39, 405, 406
    Stage 1, 39, 40–41
    Stage 2, 39, 42–43
    Stage 3, 39, 44–49
    Stage 4, 39, 50–54
    Stage 5, 39, 55–56
Endocrine disrupting compounds (EDCs), 160–161, 173–176
Environmental Health Perspectives, 152
Environmental Protection Agency (EPA), 181, 359
Environmental toxins. *See* Toxins
Environmental Working Group, 175
Enzyme inhibitors, 266
    neutralization of, 267
Enzyme-linked immunosorbent assay (ELISA), 309, 349
Epichlorohydrin, 177
Epigenetics, 55, 105–106, 133–134
Epigenome, 134
Epsom salts (magnesium sulfate), 328, 367–368, 369
Epstein-Barr infections, 336, 339, 349–350
Equal®, 168
Erythrocyte sedimentation rate (ESR or SED) test, 211
Essential fatty acids (EFAs), 243–245, 301
Essential oils
    as air fresheners, 356
    for better sleep, 284
    as sinusitis treatment, 341
Esters, 177
Estradiol, testing for, 275–276
Estriol, testing for, 275–276
Estrogens, 159, 161
    elevated levels of, 161
    imbalance of, 82
    metabolites of, 161–163
Ethanol, 355
Ethers, 177
Exercise
    aerobic, 290
    effect on glutathione levels, 328
    as stress management technique, 289–291

F

Far-infrared saunas, 27, 365–367
Fasano, Alessio, 153

Fats
    breakdown of, 316
    elimination from diet, 257
    healing, 242, 243–245, 253, 301
    saturated, 167–168
Fee-for-service health care providers, 60–61, 77
Fellitti, Vincent, 376
Fermented foods, 254, 298, 300
Ferritin, 305
Fever, 241, 343
Fiber, dietary, 301
Fiber supplements, 303
Fibromyalgia, 344
    infection prevention and control in, 347
Fierstein, Harvey, 406
Fight-or-flight response, 121–124, 127, 155
    methylation in, 319
    stress hormones in, 122–124
    television-induced, 283
Fillers
    in thyroid hormone replacement preparations, 219
    in vitamin supplements, 250
Fine needle aspiration (FNA), of the thyroid gland, 117
Fish, mercury contamination in, 183
Fish oils, 298, 301. *See also* omega fatty acids
Flame-retardants, 175–176
Flea control products, 361
Flexibility exercise, 290
Flight-or-fight, 127
Flour
    bromine in, 178
    white, 166
Fluoride, 27, 179, 354
Fluorine, 179, 223
Folate/folic acid
    deficiencies, 250
    malabsorption of, 299–300, 305
    in methylation, 321, 326
Food(s)
    antibiotics in, 152
    elimination from diet. *See Eating for Your Good Genes! Program*
    goitrogenic, 248
    as inflammatory stress cause, 166–169
    reintroduction into diet. *See Sensitivity Discovery Program*

Food additives, 144–146
Food allergies, 138–139, 146
Food allergy testing, 24, 269–271
Food and Drug Administration (FDA), 47, 183
Food dyes, 145
Food hypersensitivities, 138
Food intolerance, 138–139, 269–270
Food sensitivities, 137–138, 269–270
    adrenal health and, 276
    delayed, 138–139
    hidden, 169
    symptoms of, 146
Forbes, 69
Ford, Henry, 55
Forgiveness, 28, 43, 396–397, 405
Formaldehyde, 177, 355
Foundation for Alternative and Integrative Medicine, 72–73
Fragrance-free products, 352
Fragrances, in home care products, 355–356
"Frankenfoods," 135–137
Frankl, Viktor E., 273
Free radicals, 315, 335–336
Free T3 test, 210, 216, 217
Free T4 test, 210, 216, 217
Friedlander, Joan, 31
Frogs, as environmental indicators, 330
Fruit
    elimination from diet, 256
    low-glycemic, 19, 245–246, 252
    organic, 245–246, 298
Functional/integrative medical practitioners, 61, 75–78
    for gastrointestinal disorders treatment, 310–311
    how to choose, 75–78
    for infection prevention and control, 339, 347, 348
    lists of, 75, 76, 278, 310–311
Functional medicine, 16–17, 71–73
Functional Mind-Body Approach, 314
Functional testing, 60, 74, 77
    for detoxification, 333–334
    gastrointestinal, 233–234, 297, 299, 310–312
    for heavy metals exposure, 333
    for *Helicobacter pylori* (H-Pylori), 312

for leaky gut syndrome, 312
of liver function, 329–330
for toxins, 333–334
Fungal infections. *See also Candida*
body temperature and, 343–344
gastrointestinal, 152, 154, 339, 348
locations of, 344
prevention and treatment of, 341, 345
sinusitis, 341
systemic, 338, 339
testing for, 348

G

GABA (gamma aminobutyric acid), 82–83, 284
Gallbladder function, 83
GALT (gut-associated lymphoid tissue), 87, 91, 92, 147
Gamma aminobutyric acid (GABA), 82–83, 284
Gamma-linoleic acid (GLA), 224–225, 243–244, 249
Gant, C.E., 45–46
interview with, 411–422
Garages, 362
Gardens, 362, 363
Garlic, 299, 346
Gasoline additives, 177
Gastroesophageal reflux disease (GERD), 299, 300, 304–310
proton pump inhibitor therapy for, 304–305
role of stress in, 308
self-healing program for, 305–308
Gastrointestinal infections, 152–153
parasitic, 299, 311, 339, 348
testing for, 348
Gastrointestinal stress, 101, 308
causes of, 147–154
symptoms of, 154–155
Gastrointestinal Stress Assessment, 192–194, 297
Gastrointestinal tract
anatomy of, 87–89, 147, 295, 297–298
in autoimmune disease, 89–90
functional testing of, 233–234, 297, 299, 310–312
gastroesophageal reflux disease (GERD) and, 304–310

healthy, 297
immune function of, 87–90, 295
mucus membranes of, 87
Gastrointestinal tract health, 295–312
gastroesophageal reflux disease (GERD) and, 304–310
nutritional factors in, 296, 298–300
nutritional supplements for, 300–304
Gedgaudras, Nora T., 235, 242
Gene expression, 105-106. *See also* Epigenetics; Nutrigenomics
Genetically-modified food (GMO), 135–137
Genomic testing, 329–330, 334
Genova Diagnostics, 60, 77, 272, 278–279, 333, 334, 348, 350
Ghee, 244–245, 298, 301
Gifts of Imperfection The (Brown), 388–389
Gingivitis, 339, 340, 342
testing for, 348
Gingseng, Siberian, 277–278
Gittleman, Ann Louise, 19–20, 23, 24
GLA (gamma-linoleic acid), 224–225, 243–244, 249
Glucose, 316
Glucosinolates, 248
Glucuronidation, 315
Glutamine, 315
Glutamine supplements, 301
Glutathione, 320–321, 368
how to increase levels of, 327–329, 347
infection-related depletion of, 336
methylation and, 320–321, 337
testing for, 350
Glutathione conjugation, 315
Glutathione peroxidase, 222, 248
Glutathione supplements, 329
Gluten
antibodies to, 151
elimination from diet, 231, 263–264, 298
as thyroid replacement medication filler, 219
Gluten allergy, 24
Gluten sensitivity, 23, 24, 140–141, 150–151
B-cells in, 101
in celiac disease, 150
genetic testing for, 312
as leaky gut syndrome cause, 153–154
Glycemic load, 167

Glycine, 23, 315
Glycine conjugation, 315
Glycogen, 316
Goiters, 110, 178, 248
Goitrogenic foods, 248, 327
Good Manufacturing Practices (GMP), 25, 251
Grains, elimination from diet, 19, 24, 255, 263
Granulocytes, 94–95
Grapefruit seed extract (GSE), 26, 299, 302, 340, 341, 346
Grasser, Eric, 103
Grasses, 256, 258, 263
Graves, Robert James, 107
Graves' thyrotoxicosis, 107–113
    conventional treatment for, 111–113
    diagnosis of, 108
    diagnostic tests for, 110–111
    emotional/psychological symptoms of, 109–110
    hyperthyroidism management in, 230
    physical symptoms of, 108–109
Green powders, 258
Green tea, 23, 346
Grief, 383–384
GSAS-ds questionnaire, 310
Guilt, 383
Gut-associated lymphoid tissue (GALT), 87, 91, 92, 147

H

Hahnemann, Samuel, 65
Hair loss, 84, 226, 305
Halogens, 178–179, 223
Harvard University, 51
Hashimoto, Haruko, 113
Hashimoto's thyroiditis, 113–118
    with borderline/low thyroid labs and mild symptoms, 216
    conventional treatment for, 117–118
    diagnosis of, 5–8, 113–114
    diagnostic tests for, 116–117
    emotional/psychological symptoms of, 115–116
    as "incurable" disease, 7–9
    with normal thyroid labs and no symptoms, 215–216
    personal experience of, 5–30
    physical symptoms of, 114–115
    prevalence of, 31, 114
    prognosis, 7–8
    as reversible disease, 22–30
    spontaneous remission of, 33
    symptoms of, 5
    thyroid regeneration in, 225, 226
    thyroid replacement therapy for, 215, 230
Haskell, Alexander, 85, 118, 219, 220
    interview with, 435–445
Hay, Louise, 28
Hay fever, 5, 19
Headaches, 67, 241
Healing
    length of, 55
    participants in, 15
    successful model of, 74
    unexpected sources of, 13
Health
    emotional factors in, 12
    as priority, 63–64
Health advocacy, 62
Health care, as percentage of Gross Domestic Product, 45
Health care providers. *See also* Doctor(s); Functional/integrative medical practitioners
    selection of, 75–78
    supportive, 51–52
    types of, 75–76
Healthcare quality, patient's evaluation of, 11
Health care reform, 58
Health care system, 47–49
Health insurance companies
    doctors' relationships with, 60–62
    medication coverage by, 63–64
Health insurance coverage, 57–62
    for acupuncture, 70
    for integrative and functional health care, 77
    limitations of, 57–59, 61
    for nutritional testing, 272
    out-of-pocket expenses, 61
Health Resources and Services Administration (HRSA), 183
Health savings accounts (HSAs), 61
Heartburn, 300, 304, 305, 306

Heart disease, 45, 83
Heavy metals exposure, 180–185
   chelation therapy for, 226
   detoxification of, 26
   functional testing for, 333
   T- and B-cells in, 101
Helicobacter pylori (H-Pylori), 27, 309–310, 346
   functional testing for, 312
Hematopoiesis, 91
Hendricks, Gay, 28
Hendricks, Katie, 28
HEPA technology, 356
Hepatitis B, 339, 346
Hepatitis C, 346
Herbal deficiencies, 275
Herbicides, toxicity of, 176
Herbs. *See also specific* herbs
   adaptogenic, 277
   anti-inflammatory, 298
   for gastrointestinal tract health, 302
   healing, 253
   for hyperthyroidism, 227, 228
   for liver health, 325–326
   for stress management, 277–278
Herper, Matthew, 69
Herpes, 346
Herpes simplex virus, 346
   testing for, 30
Herxheimer reaction, 326
High-fructose corn syrup, 134, 142
Hippocrates, 51, 232, 370, 375
Hippocratic Oath, 51, 59
Holistic medicine, 71–73
Home environment, detoxification of, 353–354
Home fragrances, 354, 355 356
Honey, 254
Honeybees, 176
Hope for Hashimoto's (Haskell), 118, 220
Hormonal stress, 158–164
   causes of, 160–163
   symptoms of, 163–164
Hormonal Stress Assessment, 201–203, 315
Hormone(s). *See also specific* hormones
   processing and metabolizing in the liver, 315
Hormone replacement therapy (HRT), 161

Hostility, 392–395
Household cleaning products. *See* Cleaning products
5-HTP (5-hydroxytryptophan), 284
Human growth hormone (HGH), 82, 159–160
Human papillomavirus infections, 339
Humor, 292–293
Hunter-gatherer diet, 242
"Hurry sickness," 128
Hydrogen peroxide, 118, 220
   as cleaning solution, 357
   detoxification of, 222
5-Hydroxytryptophan (5-HTP), 284
Hygiene theory, 169
Hyman, Mark, 119, 134, 233
Hyperthyroidism. *See also* Graves' thyrotoxicosis
   adrenal fatigue in, 82
   diet in, 249
   with mild symptoms, 227–228
Hypochlorhydria, 304
Hypothalamus, 79, 122
Hypothyroidism
   adrenal fatigue in, 82
   body temperature in, 343–344
   goitrogenic foods and, 248
   Hashimoto's thyroiditis-related, 3
   as heart disease risk factor, 83

I

Ibuprofen, 151
IGF-1 (insulin growth factor-1), 159–160
Immune response, 96–98
Immune system
   cells of, 91–95
   conventional medical view of, 66
   definition of, 85–86
   organs of, 95–96
   overview of, 85–98
   protective barriers in, 86–87
   role of thyroid hormones in, 82
Immunity, 86
   cell-mediated, 92–93
   humoral, 92, 93–94
Immunocal, 347
Immunoglobulins, 94
   in *Candida* infections, 344, 348

Immunosuppressive drugs, 66, 67
"Incurability," of autoimmune disorders, 44–45
Inderal (Propranolol), 111
Indiana University, Life Sciences department, 15
Infant formula, aluminum in, 181
Infections, 335–350
    case example of, 337–339
    chronic and low-grade, 169–170
    common, 339
    dental infection control and prevention, 340–341
    host environment and, 336
    nutritional supplement-based treatment of, 346–347
    testing for, 348–350
    theories of, 335–336
Infectious stress. *See* Inflammatory and infectious stress
Infectious Stress Assessment, 339, 347
Infertility, 174
Inflammation
    diagnostic tests for, 211
    food-induced, 236–237
Inflammatory and infectious stress, 165–173
    causes of, 164–171
    chronic, 165
    definition of, 97, 164
    personal assessment of, 195–198, 339
    symptoms of, 172–173
Injury, inflammation response to, 171
Insect repellents, 362
Insomnia, 5
Institute for Functional Medicine, 75, 125, 278
Insulin growth factor-1 (IGF-1), 159–160
Insulin sensitivity, 18
Integrative medicine, 71–73
Interleukins, 97, 102
Intermediary metabolites, 315
International Academy of Oral Medicine and Toxicology, 331–332
Interviews, with doctors
    about autoimmune disease treatment, 411–445
    for selection of functional medicine practitioners, 76–78
Intuition, 13
Iodide, 7, 220
Iodide supplements, 224

Iodine, 178–179, 222
    dietary sources of, 223
    high-potency, 222–223
    as inflammation cause, 223
    in multivitamins, 223
Iodine deficiency, 178–179, 221, 222–223
    artificial sweeteners and, 258
Iodine supplements, 224
Iodoral, 223, 224
ION™ Blood and Urine Test, 334
Iron, malabsorption of, 299, 300
Iron deficiency, 171, 305
Isothiocyanates, 248
I Thought It Was Just Me (but it isn't).... (Brown), 387–388

J

Johns Hopkins University, 169
Johnson-Meester score, 310
Jordan, David Starr, 207
Journaling, 40
    personalized online, 55
Journal of Biochemical and Molecular Toxicology, 17
Joy, 292
Juice "fasting," 324, 325
Juices, for liver health, 323–324
Jung, Carl, 12–13
Junger, Alejandro, 29
Junk food, 134–135, 231, 242, 263

K

Kabat-Zinn, Jon, 288
Kale, 227–228
Katie, Byron, 50
Kefir, 262, 266
Klebsiella infections, 339
    testing for, 349
Knockout Interviews with Doctors Who are Curing Cancer...(Somers), 48
Kornfeld, Robert, 58

L

Lab tests. *See* Diagnostic tests; *names of specific tests*
Lactobacillus, 340
Lactose intolerance, 141
Lao Tzu, 37

Laughter, 292–293
Laughter meditation, 292–293
Laundry detergent, 357
Lauric acid, 244
Lavender oil, 284, 356
Laxatives, overuse of, 149–150
Lead, 182
Leaky gut syndrome, 23, 24, 141, 153–154
    Candida-related, 344–345
    causes of, 153–154, 295–296, 344–345
    celiac disease and, 150
    definition of, 295
    functional testing for, 312
    healing of, 295–312
    as malnutrition cause, 223
Lectins, 139–140, 153–154, 266
Legumes, 143–144
    elimination from diet, 19, 256, 263
    gastrointestinal effects of, 264
    reintroduction into diet, 264
Lemon balm, 227–228
Lemon juice, 307
Levothroid, 117, 217
Levothyroxine
    in combination with triiodothyronine (T3), 217–218
    fillers in, 219
    as Hashimoto's thyroiditis treatment, 117, 217–222
Levoxyl, 217
    beneficial effects of, 226–227
    as Hashimoto's thyroiditis treatment, 117
Life coaching, 14
Lifestyle changes, 55–56
Light, from computers and mobile devices, 282–283
Light bulbs, mercury in, 183
Linoleic acid, 243, 244
    conjugated, 23
Lipitor, 64
Lipoic acid, 23, 328–329
Lipski, Elizabeth, 71–72
Lipton, Bruce, 28, 105
Liver
    anatomy of, 90
    detoxification process in, 90–91, 313, 314–315, 316, 317–321
    estrogen metabolism in, 161–162
    functions of, 83, 90, 314–316
    role in thyroid hormone metabolism, 81
Liver cleanses, 27
Liver restoration plan, 313–334
    functional and genomic testing in, 329–330, 333–334
    importance of, 313
    medical practitioners' role in, 330–331
    methylation in, 317–321
    nutritional factors in, 321–326
    toxins to be avoided in, 321–322
Lopressor (Metoprolol), 111
Love, 405
    of self, 43
Lower esophageal sphincter (LES), 304
Lung cancer, 359
Lupus, 8, 21, 32, 331
    anti-inflammatory drug therapy for, 67
    case example, 337–339
    discoid, 161
    infection prevention and control in, 347
    phthalates-related, 175
Lyme disease, 336, 339
    testing for, 349
Lymph nodes, 96
Lymphocytes, 92–94

M

MacIntosh, Anna, 68–69
Macrophages, 95, 97
Magnesium, 284, 367
Magnesium sulfate (Epsom salts), 328, 367–368, 369
Magnesium supplements, 327
Maharaj, Sri Nisargadatta, 397
Malabsorption
    of nutrients, 299–300
    stomach acid and, 305
Malnutrition, 133–135, 233
Marijuana smoke, aluminum in, 180–181
Marjoram oil, 284
Marley, Bob, 287
Mast cells, 95
McTaggart, Lynn, 28
Meat, organic all-natural, 19, 246, 247, 252
Medicare, 59

Medications. *See also names of specific medications*
  "antigenic," 101
  for chronic disorders, 49
  cost of, 63–64
  in drinking water, 354
  effects on the liver, 321–322
  gastrointestinal effects of, 299
Medicine
  alternative, 68
  art *versus* science in, 73
  complementary and alternative (CAM), 68–69
  functional, 71–73
  integrative/holistic, 71–73
  natural, 70
  traditional, 70
  Western/conventional/orthodox/allopathic, 65–67
Mees' lines, 181
Melasma, 5
Melatonin, 284, 358
Mercola, Joseph, 353
Mercury, 331–333
  in dental fillings, 26, 27, 182–183, 331–332, 364
  in vaccines, 183–184
Metabolic syndrome, 367
Metabolism, role of thyroid hormones in, 82
Metafolin, 326
Metametrix, 77, 278–279, 333, 334
Methimazole (Tapazole), 111
Methionine, 315
Methylation, 315, 317–321
  glutathione and, 320–321
  improvement of, 326–327
  in infections, 337
  process of, 317–318
  stress-related impairment of, 319
  testing for, 350
Methyl donors, 319, 320–321, 326
Methylene chloride, 363
Methyl tert-butyl ether (MTBE), 177
Metoprolol (Lopressor), 111
Microwaves, 358–359
Milk. *See also* Dairy foods
  sensitivity to, 141
Milk thistle (silmarin), 328

Mind-body nutrition program, 232–272
  Phase I. *See Eating for Your Good Genes! Program*
  Phase II. *See Sensitivity Discovery Program*
Mind-body types, 235
  exercises based on, 290–291
  uniqueness of, 285–286
Mindfulness, 287–289
  in eating, 235–236, 299
Minding the Body, Mending the Mind (Borysenko), 279
Mineral baths, 367–369
Mittermeier, Russell A., 330
Mold contamination, 359–360
Molecular mimicry, 335
Molecules of Emotion: The Science Between Mind-Body Medicine (Pert), 382
Monosodium glutamate, 145
Mood, effect of toxins on, 400
Mood swings, 5
MTHFR Genotyping test, 334
MTHFR trait, 321
Multiple sclerosis (MS), 3, 331
  infection prevention and control in, 347
Multivitamin supplements, 249, 277
Mycoplasma, 339
  tests for, 349
Mycotoxins, 360
Myss, Carolyn, 28

N

Naproxen (Aleve), 151
National Academy of Clinical Biochemistry (NACB), 212, 213
National Center for Complementary and Alternative Medicine (NCCAM), 69
National Institutes of Health, 31, 183
National Sleep Foundation, 285
National Toxicology Program, 175
Natural killer cells, 93, 97, 102, 346
Natural medicine, 70
Nature, reconnecting with, 291
NatureThroid, 218
Naturopathy, 70
Nedergaard, Makien, 281
Neem/neem oil, 347, 362
Negative thinking, 29
NeilMed Sinus Rinse, 341

NeuroGenomic™ Profile, 334, 350
Neurotransmitters, 82–83
New England Journal of Medicine, 136
Nexium, 64
Nightshade vegetables, 20, 142–143
    elimination from diet, 24, 256, 263
    gastrointestinal effects of, 264
Non-steroidal anti-inflammatory drugs (NSAIDS), 299
    as contraindication to betaine HCL, 307
    gastrointestinal effects of, 307
Noradrenalin/norepinephrine, 82–83, 100, 121, 123–124
Nori, 223
NSF/ANSI Standard 173, 25
NSF/GMP certification, 251
NutraSweet®, 168, 258
NutrEval® Blood and Urine Test, 333, 350
NutrEval® Plasma Test, 272
Nutribiotic, 346
Nutrigenomics, 133-134, 235, 242. *See also Eating for Your Good Genes! Program*
Nutrition
    for fungal disease prevention and control, 345
    for gastrointestinal tract health, 296, 298–300
Nutritional deficiencies, 135
    as inflammation cause, 171
    prevalence of, 250
    symptoms of, 146
Nutritional supplements
    in hyperthyroidism, 249
    for infection prevention and control, 346–347
    for promotion of sleep, 284
Nutritional testing, 250, 272, 333–334
Nutritionists, 271–272, 278
Nutrition program. *See* Mind-body nutrition program
Nuts, 144
    elimination from diet, 255–256
    enzyme inhibitor neutralization in, 267

O

Occupational Safety and Health Administration (OSHA), 364–365
O'Connor, Siobhan, 335
Odors, 353–354
Offices, 364–365
Oils
    avocado, 245
    fish, 298, 301. *See also* Omega fatty acids
    olive, 245
    partially-hydrogenated, 167–168
    vegetable, bromine in, 178
O'Keefe, Georgia, 20
Oleuropein, 346
Olive leaf extract (OLE), 302, 346
Olive oil, 245
Omega-3 fatty acid, 17, 23, 224–225, 243
    deficiency in, 171
    food sources of, 19
Omega-6 fatty acid, 243–245
Omega-9 fatty acid, 243
Omega-12 fatty acid, 243
Omega-3 fatty acid EPA/DHA supplements, 249
Oral hygiene, 340–341
Orange oil, 362
Organochlorines, 176, 179–180
Organophosphates, 176
    tests for, 333
Orthodox medicine, 65–67
Overcoming Thyroid Disorders (Brownstein), 22
Over-the-counter (OTC) medications
    effect on sleep, 282
    effect on the liver, 321–322
    elimination of, 19
Overweight, 171

P

Pain management, 67
Paint, 362
Pancreatin, 302, 303
Pantry items, 253
Parabens, 27, 175, 352
    tests for, 333
Parasitic infections, gastrointestinal, 299, 339, 348
    testing for, 311, 348
Parasympathetic nervous system, 121, 122
Passion, in health empowerment, 39, 40–41
PBDEs (polybrominated diphenyl ethers), 175–176
PCBs (polychlorinated biphenyls), 176, 180
    tests for, 333

Peanuts, 143–144
Penn Program for Mindfulness, 288
Peppers, 20, 142
Periodontal disease, 338, 339, 342
    testing for, 348
Persistent Organic Pollutants (POPs), 176
Personal assessment, of "splinters" of autoimmune conditions, 190–204
    adrenal stress, 194–195, 276, 278, 290, 293
    emotional stress, 190–192, 293
    gastrointestinal stress, 192–194, 297
    hormonal stress, 201–203, 315
    inflammatory/infectious stress, 195–198, 339, 347
    toxic stress, 198–200, 314, 329
Personal care products, 27, 352–353
Pert, Candace, 28, 382
Pesticides, 27, 136–137, 362–363
    natural alternatives to, 362
    organochlorine, 176, 179–180
    organophosphate, 176, 333
    tests for, 333
    toxicity of, 176
Petroleum-based artificial fragrances, 355
Pets, 360–361
Phagocytes, 94–95, 97–98
Pharmaceutical companies
    influence on health care system, 48
    research and development expenditures of, 69
Phenol, 355
Phenolic aids, 222
Phthalates, 174–175, 355
    tests for, 333
Phytic acid, 144, 266, 267, 298
Pilates, 23–24
Pituitary gland, 79
Pituitary tumors, 111
Placebo effect, 52
Plasma cells, 97
Plastic water bottles, 355
Polar bears, PCBs in, 180
Polybrominated diphenyl ethers (PBDEs), 175–176
Polychlorinated biphenyls (PCBs), 176, 180
Polycyclic aromatic hydrocarbons (PAHs), 177

Polycystic ovarian syndrome (PCOS), 17, 82
Polyvinyl chloride (PVC), 180
Positive thinking, 43
    in doctor-patient relationship, 51
Potatoes, 20, 142
Prakriti. *See* Mind-body types
Prayer, 12, 13
Prebiotics, 301, 306
Pregnenolone, 158–159
Premarin, 161
Prepro, 161
Prevpac, 309–310
Primal Body, Primal Mind (Gedgaudras), 235, 242
Probiotics, 249, 300, 303, 307, 345
    for liver health, 327
Processed foods, 231, 242, 263
Progesterone, 159
    imbalance in, 82
    testing for, 275–276
Prolonged Grief Disorder (PGD), 384
Propranolol (Inderal), 111
Propylthiouracil, 111
Prostaglandins, anti-inflammatory, 243, 244
Prostate cancer, 174
Proteins
    complete, 246–247
    dietary sources of, 246
    elimination from diet, 254
    as glutathioine source, 327
    organic all-natural, 19, 252, 298
    reintroduction into diet, 265
    "self" and "non-self," 335–336
ProThera Vital-Zymes™, 303
Proton pump inhibitors, 299, 300, 304–305
    as *Helicobacter pylori* treatment, 309–310
Provera, 161
Psychoneuroimmunology, 127, 375–376
Psychotherapy, 10–11
Psyllium, 301, 303
Pumpkin seeds, 266
Pure Encapsulations A.C. Formula II, 302
Pure Encapsulations Digestive Enzymes, 303
PVC (polyvinyl chloride), 180

Q

Quantum Healing Techniques, 28
Quinoa, 262, 265

R

Radioactive iodine treatment, 112
Radioactive iodine uptake test, 110–111, 117
Radio Shack, 182
Radon, 359
Rashes, 5, 20
    laboratory tests for, 239
    malar (butterfly), 337
Raynaud's disease, 161
Recipes
    for *Eating for Your Good Genes! Program*, 259–261
    for liver health, 324–326
    for *Sensitivity Discovery Program*, 268–269
Regestein, Quentin, 50
Research
    in autoimmune conditions, 31
    in complementary and alternative medicine, 69
Responsibility, 405
    versus blame, 397–399
    for change, 44
    for health, 42–43
Rest. *See also* Sleep
    role in adrenal health, 277
Resveratrol, 23
Rheumatoid arthritis, 67, 331, 347
Rheumatoid factor (RA) test, 211, 214
Rhodiola, 277
Rice
    elimination from diet, 255
    genetically-engineered, 137
    organic brown or wild, 242–243, 247, 265
Rice milk, 266
Rice protein powder, 328
Risk factor analysis, 46
Rogers, Sherry A., 295
Roman chamomile oil, 284
Root canals, infected, 338, 339, 348
Root vegetables, 252
Roth, Gabriele, 289
Rowe, Albert, 238
Rumi, 215

S

Saccharin, 169
Safe sex, 342–343
Sage, 356
Salad dressings, 257
Salicylates, 145
Saline solutions, nasal, 341
Saliva tests, for adrenal function assessment, 275–276, 278–279
SAM-e, 329
Sandalwood oil, 284
Saturated fats, 167–168
Saunas, far-infrared, 27, 365–367
Schwartzbein, Diana, 16–17, 18–19, 23
Schwartzbein Principle, The (Schwartzbein), 16–17
Schweitzer, Albert, 65
Science Magazine, 106
Scientific method, 46
Sclerderma, 161
Sea vegetables, 223
Sedentary lifestyle, 171
Seeds
    elimination from diet, 255–256
    enzyme inhibitor neutralization in, 267
    sprouted, 247, 262, 266
    used as spices, 268
Selenium, 23, 223
    in combination with isothiocyanates, 248
    in glutathione production, 328
Selenium deficiency, 222
    virus-related, 336
Selenium methionine supplements, 249
Self-awareness, 287
Self-blame, 385
Self-evaluation, of health, 53–54
Self-expression, 406
Self-pity, 10, 11
Sensitivities. *See also* Food sensitivities
    as inflammation cause, 169
Sensitivity Discovery Program, 53, 144, 145–146, 219, 237
    for adrenal health, 276
    duration of, 262–263
    80/20 rule for, 269
    family's and spouses involvement in, 240–241

for gastrointestinal health, 296–297, 298, 305–306
Journal for, 238–240
overview of, 231–232
preparation for, 238–241
timing of, 240
Serotonin, 82–83
Seuss, Dr., 285
Seventh Generation, 356
Sex hormones, 82, 159
Sexual activity, 341–343
Sexually-transmitted diseases (STDs), 342
Shame, 384–392
    as cause of chronic illness, 388
    definition of, 384
    identifying, 389–391
    origins of, 386–388
    toxic, 385–386
    transforming, 391–392
Shaw, George Bernard, 42
Siberian ginseng *(Eleutherococcus senticosus)*, 277–278
Sick, definition of, 71
Sinus Doctor, 341
Sinusitis, chronic, 5, 338, 339, 341, 348
    testing for, 348
Sjögren's syndrome, 331, 347
Skin
    detoxification of, 365–36
    functions of, 86–87
    toxin absorption in, 353
Sleep, 280–285
    effect of electromagnetic fields on, 358
    effect on glutathione levels, 328
    restorative, 280–284, 368
Sleep apnea, 285
Sleep deprivation, 280–281
Sleeping pills, 282, 293
Smoking
    effect on the liver, 327
    glutathione-depleting effect of, 320
Soda, 134, 178
Sodium fluoride, 179
Sodium iodide, 178
Sodium lauryl sulfate, 27, 352–353
Solanine, 143
Somatic integration exercises, 12
Somers, Suzanne, 48

Sore joints, laboratory tests for, 239
Soy, 143, 265
    genetically-modified, 143
SpectraCell Laboratories, 77, 334, 350
Spices
    healing, 253, 298
    seeds used as, 268
Spiritual aspect, of autoimmune healing, 404–405, 407
Spleen, 96
Splenda®, 168, 258
"Splinters," of autoimmune conditions, 125–189
    adrenal fatigue, 155–158, 188
    chronic emotional distress, 127–131, 187, 190–192
    definition of, 233
    gastrointestinal stress, 147–155, 188, 192–194
    hormonal stress, 158–164, 188, 201–203
    identification and healing of, 207–208
    inflammatory and infectious stress, 164–173, 189, 195–198
    nutritional factors, 133–147, 187
    personal assessment of, 190–204
    toxic stress, 173–186, 189
    unhealthy coping patterns, 131–133, 187
Spontaneous Evolution (Lipton), 105
Sprouted nuts and seeds, 247, 262, 266
Standard American Diet (SAD), 134–135
Standards of care, 58, 59, 60–61
Staphylococcus aureus, 339
    MRSA, 346
Steroids, 299
Stimulants. *See also* Alcohol; Caffeine
    as sleep disturbance cause, 281
Stomach acid, 299–300, 301, 327
    reducing levels of, 304–305
Stool analysis, 310–311, 348
Strengthening exercise, 290
Streptococcus, 339
Streptococcus mutans, 340
Stress
    autoimmune process in, 100–101
    chronic, 119–124, 165
    as Graves' thyrotoxicosis risk factor, 108
    as Hashimoto's thyroiditis risk factor, 18, 23

liver in, 327
methylation in, 319
physiology of, 121–124
prevalence of, 131
purposeless, 130–131
reverse T3 in, 221
T4 conversion in, 221
tolerance for, 119–120
Stress hormones, 82, 100
    effects of, 156
    in fight-or-flight response, 122–124
Stress management techniques, 27–28, 273–294
    breathing techniques, 279–280
    exercise, 289–291
    in Graves' thyrotoxicosis, 228
    herbal formulas, 277–278
    medical treatment, 293
    mind-body factors in, 285–286
    mindfulness, 287–289
    reconnecting with nature, 291
    sleep, 280–285
Stressors, 30
Stroke, as mortality cause, 45
Sucralose, 168, 258
Sugar
    craving for, 265
    elimination from diet, 263
    as gastrointestinal stress cause, 148
    as inflammation cause, 166
    refined, 134
    reintroduction into diet, 265
    as sleep disturbance cause, 281
Sulfation, 315
Sulfites, 144
Sulfur, 327–328, 367, 368
Sulfur-containing foods, 327
Sunblock, 353
Sunflower seeds, 266
"Superbugs," 152
"Sustain" (food supplement powder), 26–27
Sweeteners. *See also* Artificial sweeteners; Sugar
    elimination from diet, 256–257
    healing, 253
Sweet 'N Low', 169
Sweet potatoes, 249
Sweet wormwood (artemesia), 299, 302
Swollen joints, 5

Sympathetic nervous system, 121
Symptoms
    allopathic approach to, 66–67
    as basis for medical diagnosis, 45–46
    medication-related, 46–47
Synthroid, 16, 217
    adverse effects of, 226
    fillers in, 219
    as Hashimoto's thyroiditis treatment, 117

T

T3. *See* Triiodothyronine
T4. *See* Thyroxine
Taking control, 15–21
Tapazole (Methimazole), 111
Taurine, 315
T-cells, 95–96
    in chronic infectious stress, 101
    stress-related impairment of, 100
T-cells/CD4+ cells, 93, 98
Tea, fluoride in, 179
Tea tree oil, 345
Teeth, fluorosis of, 179
Teflon®, 179
Television, 283
Tenormin (Atenolol), 111
Testosterone, 159
    imbalance in, 82
    testing for, 275–276
T-helper cells, 93, 97
Thimerosal, 183–184
Thiocyanates, 248
Thrush, oral, 345
Th1/Th2 response, 92, 94, 346
Th1 *versus* Th2 dominance hypothesis, 102–105
Thyme oil, 341
Thymus, 95–96
Thyroid antibody tests, 210–211
    antithyroglobulin antibodies (TgAb) test, 210, 214, 216, 217
    antithyroid peroxidase antibodies (anti-TPO) test, 210, 214, 215–217
    baseline, 230
Thyroid Cure
    overview of, 370–372
    Web site of, 55, 75, 76

Thyroid disorders. *See also* Graves'
     thyrotoxicosis; Hashimoto's
     thyroiditis
  prevalence of, 44–45
Thyroidectomy, 112
Thyroid gland
  healthy functioning of, 79–81
  overactive. *See* Hyperthyroidism
  regeneration of, 226
  underactive. *See* Hypothyroidism
Thyroid hormone(s)
  functions of, 81–84
  optimal levels of, 81–84
  production and metabolism of, 79–81
Thyroid hormone replacement medications,
     217–220
  choice of, 217–218, 217–219
  dosage, 219
  duration of use, 225–226
Thyroiditis, 110
  autoimmune. *See* Hashimoto's thyroiditis
  chronic lymphocytic. *See* Hashimoto's
     thyroiditis
Thyroid panels, 116–117
Thyroid peroxidase (TPO). *See also*
     Antithyroid peroxidase antibodies
     (anti-TPO), 79
  blockage of, 248
Thyroid receptor antibodies (TRAb)/thyroid
     stimulating immunoglobulin test
     (TSI), 214
Thyroid-releasing hormone (TRH),
     production and metabolism of, 79
Thyroid-releasing hormone (TRH) test, of
     thyroid regeneration, 225, 226
Thyroid-stimulating hormone (TSH), 7
  elevated levels of, 220
  in Graves' thyrotoxicosis, 110
  in Hashimoto's thyroiditis, 116, 117, 118,
     220
  lowering of, 223–225
  optimal range of, 216
Thyroid-stimulating hormone (TSH) test,
     209–210
  in Hashimoto's thyroiditis, 215–217
  normal *versus* optimal ranges in, 212–213
Thyroid-stimulating immunoglobulin (TSI)
     test, 210

Thyroid tests, 209–210
  guidelines for, 212–213
l-Thyroxin, 217
Thyroxine replacement therapy, for
     Hashimoto's thyroiditis, 117–118
Thyroxine (T4)
  conversion into T3, 315, 316
  in Graves' thyrotoxicosis, 107, 110
  in Hashimoto's thyroiditis, 116, 117
  production and metabolism of, 79–80, 81,
     178, 209, 210
  in stress, 124
  synthetic. *See* l-Thyroxin; Levothyroxine
Tibetan medicine, 70
Tick-borne disease. *See* Lyme disease
Tick control products, 361
Time, lack of, 128
Titanium oxide, 353
T-lymphocytes, 92–93
Tobacco smoke, 180–181
Tolle, Eckhart, 28, 29
Toluene, 363
Tomatoes, 20, 142
Tongue scraping, 340–341
Toothbrushes, 340, 347
Tooth decay, 340
Toothpaste, 27, 179, 340, 353
Total stress load, 119
Toxic stress, 173–186
  causes of, 173–185
  symptoms of, 185–186
Toxic Stress Assessment, 198–200, 314, 329
Toxins, 170–171
  as autoimmune condition cause, 101
  body burden of, 23, 119–121, 333
  effect on the liver, 327
  functional testing for, 333–334
  indoor, 353–354
  list of, 363
  in personal care products, 352–353
  removal and neutralization in the liver,
     314–315
  tolerance to, 119
Trans fats, 134, 167–168
Trauma, as Graves' thyrotoxicosis risk factor, 108
Triggers, of autoimmune conditions. *See*
     Splinters, of autoimmune conditions
Triiodothyronine (T3)

in combination with levothyroxine, 217–218
in Graves' thyrotoxicosis, 107
in Hashimoto's thyroiditis, 116
production and metabolism of, 79–80, 81, 209, 221
reverse, 124, 221
in stress, 124
Triiodothyronine (T3) replacement therapy
immediate release formulations of, 218
time-released formulations of, 218
Triiodothyronine (T3)/thyroxine (T4) replacement therapy
compounded formulations of, 230
sustained-release formulations of, 218
Trisodium nitrilotriacetate (NTA), 363
T3/T4 thyroid medications, 17, 18–19, 24
Tuberculosis, 339, 349
Tumor necrosis factor alpha, 102
Tylenol (acetaminophen), 321–322

U

United States Army, 70
Unithroid, 217
University of California, Osher Center for Integrative Medicine, 71
University of Cincinnati, 287
University of Maryland School of Medicine, 153
University of Michigan, 174
University of Rochester Medical Center, Center for Translational Neuromedicine, 281
Urinary tract infections, 342–343, 344
Use of Medicines in the United States: Review of 2011 (IMS Health), 63–64

V

Vaccines
action mechanism of, 184–185
aluminum in, 183, 184
"antigenic," 101
mercury in, 183–184
without aluminum, 184
Valerian root, 227
Valium, 10, 11
Van Konynenburg, Richard A., 336
Vegetable oils, bromine in, 178

Vegetables. *See also* Brassica (cruciferous) vegetables; Nightshade vegetables; *names of specific* vegetables
as folate source, 326
good, 298
non-starchy, 245–246
organic, 245–246, 252
Vegetarian/vegan diets, 247–248
glutathione deficiency in, 320
plant-based digestive enzyme supplements in, 302–303
Vetiver oil, 284
Vibrant Way, Inc., 24–25, 29, 250
Victim role, 39, 42–43
Vinegar, 357
apple cider, 307
Viral infections, 339. *See also specific* viruses
testing for, 349–350
Vitamin(s)
malabsorption of, 305
need for, 249–251
Vitamin B complex vitamins, 23
food sources of, 326
malabsorption of, 299–300, 305
Vitamin B complex vitamin supplements, 277, 326
Vitamin B deficiencies, 250
Vitamin B12 deficiency, 300
Vitamin C, 224–225, 328
Vitamin D, 328, 343
Vitamin D3, 224–225, 249
Vitamin D deficiency, 171
Vitamin E, 328
Vitamin supplements, 250–251
Volatile organic compounds (VOCs), 176–177, 351, 355, 357
Volatile solvents, tests for, 333

W

Waitley, Denis, 44
Walking, 23–4
Walnuts, 266
Water "fasting," 324
Water filters, 354–355
Weight gain, 82
Wellness, real cost of, 57–118
Western medicine, 65–67

Wheat, 20, 140
    genetically-modified, 140
Wheat Belly (Davis), 140
Wheatgrass, 256, 258
Wherever You Go, There You Are (Kabat-Zinn), 288
Whey, 141
Whey protein
    powder, 23, 328
    undenatured, 347
Williamson, Marianne, 5, 28, 99
Winfrey, Oprah, 40
Withdrawal symptoms, 241–242
Women's Empowerment Formula, 226, 227, 250–251
Women's Empowerment Program, 24
Workplace, hazardous conditions in, 364–365
World Health Organization, 45, 176–177
World Health Organization/International Agency for Research on Cancer (IARC), 358
Worrying, 287

X

Xenoestogens, 160–161
Xylene, 363

Y

Yale University, 134
Yams, 249
Yasko, Amy, 336
Yeast. *See also Candida*
    beneficial, 300
    harmful, 299
    intestinal, 295, 297, 299
    vaginal, 345
Yeast extract, 145
Yoga, 341
Yogurt, 262, 266

Z

Zeolite, 368–369
Zinc, malabsorption of, 305
Zinc deficiency, 301–302
Zinc oxide, 353
Zinc supplements, 249, 306, 307, 327
Zonulin, 153–154
ZRT Laboratory, 278

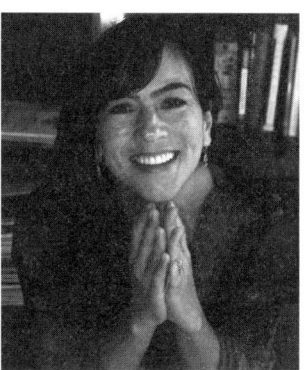

Michelle is a Certified Nutrition and Wellness Consultant, health care advocate, researcher and author. Michelle studied holistic nutrition at Clayton College of Natural Health, and Functional Medical protocols at the Academy of Functional Medicine and Genomics.

After completely reversing her autoimmune condition, Michelle founded Vibrant Way Inc., which began by creating an all-natural high-potency nutrient complex called the Empowerment Formula. Today Vibrant Way has expanded its mission to support healing and vibrant health through Vibrant Way Press.

Michelle is currently an advisor to the Academy of Functional Medicine and Genomics, and teaches doctors how to integrate Functional Medical protocols into their practices.

Michelle loves her friends and animal relatives, adventures in the wild, tending her garden, spirituality, philosophy, and expressing herself through art and dance. She is always thirsty for deeper knowledge of science and the mysteries of life.

She lives in Taos New Mexico with her magical dog Yoki, the Papillion.

Notes

Notes

Notes

Notes

Notes